Informed Consent

INFORMED CONSENT

Legal Theory and Clinical Practice

Second Edition

Jessica W. Berg, J.D.
Case Western Reserve University
Schools of Law and Medicine

Paul S. Appelbaum, M.D.
University of Massachusetts
School of Medicine

Charles W. Lidz, Ph.D.
University of Massachusetts
School of Medicine

Lisa S. Parker, Ph.D.
University of Pittsburgh
Center for Bioethics and Health Law

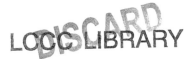
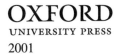
OXFORD
UNIVERSITY PRESS
2001

OXFORD
UNIVERSITY PRESS

Oxford   New York
Athens   Auckland   Bangkok   Bogotá   Buenos Aires   Calcutta
Cape Town   Chennai   Dar es Salaam   Delhi   Florence   Hong Kong   Istanbul
Karachi   Kuala Lumpur   Madrid   Melbourne   Mexico City   Mumbai
Nairobi   Paris   São Paulo   Shanghai   Singapore   Taipei   Tokyo   Toronto   Warsaw

and associated companies in
Berlin   Ibadan

Library of Congress Cataloging-in-Publication Data
Informed consent: legal theory and clinical practice/
Jessica W. Berg . . . [et al].—2nd ed.
p. cm.
Prev. ed. cataloged under: Appelbaum, Paul S.
Includes bibliographical references and index.
ISBN 0-19-512677-7
1. Informed consent (Medical law)—United States.
2. Medical ethics—United States.
3. Physician and patient—United States.
I. Appelbaum, Paul S. Informed consent.   II. Berg, Jessica W.
KF3827.15 A96   2001
344.73′0412—dc21   00-53069

9 8 7 6 5 4 3 2 1

Printed in the United States of America
on acid-free paper

J. W. B.
To John, my husband

P. S. A.
To Dede, my wife

C. W. L.
To the memory of my parents,
Ruth and Ted Lidz

L. S. P.
To my favorite lawyer, Robert Parker,
and favorite doctor, Richard Sogg

Preface

Few issues affecting the therapeutic professions are as much discussed and as little understood as informed consent. Most physicians, and other healthcare professionals who are affected by the legal requirements for informed consent, recognize that there is some legal obligation to talk with patients and obtain their agreement to proposed treatment. But often the clinicians' knowledge of the details is a mixture of myth and misunderstanding. Many healthcare professionals are not aware of the ethical principles underlying the idea of informed consent. Their actual legal obligations are often quite different from what they believe. Most important, few caregivers realize that the requirements of informed consent can be met in a manner that improves, rather than impedes, quality patient care.

This book, written with the needs of practicing clinicians in mind, aims at providing a comprehensive introduction to the theory and practice of informed consent. We trace the evolution of the doctrine of informed consent from its roots in ethical theory to its embodiment in contemporary American law. As important as it is for clinicians to recognize the basis of informed consent in deeply held notions of individual autonomy—that is, the idea that each of us, when we are patients, has the right to participate meaningfully in making decisions about our care—it is not enough. They must also have practical ways of integrating informed consent into everyday clinical care. Thus, we provide a model in which informed consent can be embedded in the doctor–patient relationship, simultaneously empowering patients and strengthening the therapeutic dyad.

Part of the robustness of this model stems from the variety of perspectives that have been blended in its formulation. We are, respectively, an attorney, a physician, a sociologist, and an ethicist, each with many years of experience dealing with these issues. Given the diverse interests that are reflected in the shape of informed consent law today, including the protection of patients' autonomy and the preservation of their health, an interdisciplinary approach is particularly useful. Although we wrote this book with the practitioner in mind, we believe that it will serve equally well students, researchers, and attorneys who want to learn more about the development of informed consent law and the problems faced when ethical and legal theories confront the realities of clinical practice.

When the first edition appeared, in 1987, the need for a comprehensive introduction for the clinician to the principles and practice of informed consent seemed clear. The response to that volume was extremely gratifying. In the years since, although the law of informed consent has changed relatively little, the context in which medical care is rendered and clinical research takes place has shifted dramatically. Thus, in addition to updating the law and research data on informed consent, this second edition contains a thoroughly revised section on consent to research, as well as new chapters on managed care and informed consent, and on the limits of informed consent in the medical setting.

Part I provides an overview of the development of the idea of informed consent and an introduction to the ethical values on which the idea rests. In Part II, the evolution and current status of the law are described; legal requirements for practitioners are detailed, with particular attention given to areas of legal ambiguity that are problematic for practitioners in formulating their approaches; and the legal theory of informed consent is critiqued.

Part III considers the problems that health professionals face when applying informed consent theory in the clinical setting and proposes a model for simplifying that task and making it clinically meaningful. Part IV delineates the unique problems created by the requirements for informed consent in the research setting, especially clinical investigations. Part V addresses the limits of the doctrine and the long-term need to improve practitioners' performance in meeting the ethical and legal mandates, and suggests a course of action.

The team responsible for this revised edition is different from the original set of authors. Alan Meisel, one of the original authors, was not involved in the revisions, but we want to acknowledge the continuing influence of his contributions on this second edition. In addition, Jessica Berg and Lisa Parker have joined our group; Paul Appelbaum and Charles Lidz have been involved from the beginning.

Our hope, as with the first edition of this work, is that this book will illuminate the significance of informed consent in clinical practice and provide a model for practitioners to follow. To the extent that we are able to do this, we will have succeeded in our task.

Acknowledgments

The first edition of this book grew out of the collaboration of Paul Appelbaum, Chuck Lidz, and Alan Meisel, whose empirical and theoretical work on informed consent culminated in the predecessor to this volume. Although he elected not to be a part of the team for this second edition, Alan Meisel's contributions continue to be reflected throughout much of the book, and we are grateful for them and for his friendship.

We acknowledge as well the enduring influence on this book of Loren Roth, who brought the authors of the first edition together in the Law and Psychiatry Program at the Western Psychiatric Institute and Clinic of the University of Pittsburgh. He was a pioneer in the study of informed consent, and his insights remain as fresh today as when they were formulated.

Other colleagues who shaped our views of informed consent include Thomas Grisso, Robert Arnold, and Cory Larkin.

Support for the empirical studies that we have conducted over the years, on which much of our understanding of informed consent is based, came from the following: the National Institute of Mental Health, the Foundations Fund for Research in Psychiatry, the President's Commission for the Study of Ethical Problems in Medicine and Biomedical and Behavioral Research, and the Research Network on Mental Health and the Law of the John D. and Catherine T. MacArthur Foundation.

We would also like to acknowledge the invaluable research assistance of many students at each of our respective institutions.

Contents

Part IV Consent to Research

Part V Advancing Informed Consent

Part I

An Introduction to Informed Consent

1

Informed Consent: Framing the Questions

What is informed consent? The answer may seem self-evident only to those who have yet to explore the many meanings of the term. Informed consent refers to legal rules that prescribe behaviors for physicians and other healthcare professionals[1] in their interactions with patients and provide for penalties, under given circumstances, if physicians deviate from those expectations; to an ethical doctrine, rooted in our society's cherished value of autonomy, that promotes patients' right of self-determination regarding medical treatment; and to an interpersonal process whereby these parties interact with each other to select an appropriate course of medical care.

Informed consent is each of these things, yet none of them alone. As a theory based on ethical principles, given effect by legal rulings and implemented by clinicians, it has been haunted by its complex lineage. When legal principles and ethical values conflict, which should take precedence? When clinical interests appear to be served by neither legal nor ethical concerns, which interests should be compromised and to what degree? The vast literature on informed consent, found in journals and books of medicine, law, bioethics, philosophy, and public policy, has been stimulated by the need to create a workable doctrine that can accommodate values that to many observers are in an irremediable state of conflict.

---

[1] In this book we use the shorthand "physician" and "patient" and trust that the reader understands that informed consent applies to all healthcare profesionals who treat patients or other types of clients.

The conflicts in theory and the need to resolve them in practice are the subjects of this book. Theory is the focus of the first half of the volume; practice is the topic of the second. Seeking to understand the fascinating theoretical problems requires us to grapple with some of the most difficult ethical and policy issues facing our society today. But let us state at the outset our belief that the clinician on the front lines need not be paralyzed by differences of opinion among legal and ethical theorists. Through the vaguely translucent wall of expertise behind which the discussion about the proper shape of the informed consent doctrine has taken place, a reasonable approach to informed consent in the clinician–patient relationship can be discerned. Our most important and challenging task in this book is to make that approach evident.

Since the goal of this volume is to help the clinician deal reasonably with legal and ethical mandates for informed consent, we begin our analysis in the clinical setting. From a consideration of informed consent in practice emerge the questions we address in the rest of this book. It is important to note at the outset that this book is based on American law,[2] American [or generally Western (1)] ethical debates, and the clinical encounters that commonly occur within the American healthcare system. The doctrine of informed consent is most fully developed within American law, and the ethical concept of autonomy is given a great deal of prominence here. Although there has been much interest in the American model, and many attempts to adapt it in other settings, we must acknowledge the significant differences between the situation in the United States and the healthcare systems in other countries—including those countries with universal health coverage systems and those third-world countries lacking substantial healthcare resources. There are not only vast differences in clinical realities, but also differences among cultural, ethical, and legal systems (2). As a result, we limit our comments to the American situation, but ask international readers to consider whether, and in what ways, our analyses and suggestions may fit their circumstances.

The Clinical Setting

John Williamson[3] is a twenty-three-year-old man who was seen in an outpatient surgical clinic of a major health center and diagnosed as suffering from an acute flare-up of chronic pancreatitis. Mr. Williamson's chief complaint was the intense abdominal pain that accompanies pancreatitis. Dr. Johnson, the chief surgical resident, had seen him a number of times before for similar problems. Dr. John-

---

[2]There is a great deal of similarity between English and American law, since the latter system developed out of the former. This includes the law of informed consent (2).

[3]All names have been altered in this history of an actual case.

son and Dr. Ricah, the senior resident, examined him and asked whether the narcotic pain relievers they had previously prescribed were doing him any good.

PATIENT: No . . . I am just getting used to them. Maybe a couple of belts (i.e., drinks) would help me out.

CHIEF RESIDENT: No, I can guarantee that that will not help. I've looked at your tests but I still want to look at your X-rays. What I think is that you will do better if we take out part of your pancreas; as long as you understand that this is a serious operation in that, while you probably won't die from it, there is a small chance that you might, although not much. But there are serious side effects from it, like you will probably have some diabetes and have trouble digesting your food. Then I think that we should go ahead and have you talk with your wife about coming in and make plans for you to come in.

SENIOR RESIDENT: I think that you ought to understand that this is not going to be a cure-all. This is not going to do away with all of your problems. You are still going to have a lot of problems from that pancreas of yours.

PATIENT: I know that.

A researcher studying informed consent, who made daily rounds with the surgical team, witnessed this conversation and later that morning interviewed Mr. Williamson.

RESEARCHER: Can you tell me what your problem is?

PATIENT: It is the pancreas.

RESEARCHER: Have any idea why?

PATIENT: No, I don't know. The doctor knows really what I'll have to do. . . . I've been having this problem about two years now. It's getting unbearable. Before, I could live with it, but now I'll take a chance on anything. . . .

RESEARCHER: Can you tell me what they are going to do in this operation?

PATIENT: They are going to take my pancreas out.

RESEARCHER: The whole pancreas?

PATIENT: Um-hm . . . It is going bad anyway. I'd rather have it out of me than if it really might ruin me on the inside. . . .

RESEARCHER: Think it will make the pain better?

PATIENT: Well, at least we won't take any chances.

Mr. Williamson was brought into the hospital one week later, after he complained that he was unable to wait the scheduled month before the operation because of the pain. Dr. Johnson described the case on rounds as being one in which he had treated the patient with painkillers for an extensive period of time. He described Mr. Williamson as an ex-alcoholic whose pancreatic deterioration was the result of alcoholism. Dr. Johnson said that he would not make a final decision about going through with the operation until he saw whether or not the X-rays showed that the lesion was limited to an operable area of the pancreas. In his view, the main advantage of the operation was that it would allow Mr. Williamson to be withdrawn from the pain medication. He also said he hoped the patient was telling the truth when he said he had quit drinking, or he would just have the same problem again.

The next day Dr. Johnson revealed to the surgical team on rounds that he planned to do a distal pancreatectomy. "That should benefit him if he has really quit drinking. . . . He has said that he wants it out. The results are not good with distal pancreatectomies but it is probably worth a try. . . . He knows we are doing it to get him off medication." The next morning Dr. Ricah told Mr. Williamson that the X-ray had come back and that they planned to do the operation the next week.

While waiting in the hospital for the tests to be completed and for the scheduled surgery, Mr. Williamson generally was told a little bit about what was happening each day. Four days before the scheduled operation, Dr. Johnson told him, "I'd say that there is a 50 percent chance that there will be no pain after the operation and an 80 to 90 percent chance that it will help you. The object is to relieve some of your pain, and as far as that is concerned the only other thing that we're concerned with is that you've got to be sure you don't drink, because that's not helping at all. So we are going ahead Wednesday, O.K.?" Mr. Williamson agreed.

The next day Mr. Williamson asked about his sugar test. The surgeon responded, "Your sugar seems to be normal. I think if we only have to take out half or two-thirds of the pancreas that you should not become diabetic. You may have to watch your diet a little bit, but that is all." In another interview that afternoon it became clear that Mr. Williamson now understood that only part of the pancreas would be removed, but his description seemed to imply that it was being removed to prevent the spread of an infection.

Two days before the operation, during rounds, the following discussion occurred:

PATIENT: How long will the operation take?

SENIOR RESIDENT: Four or five hours. It's a pretty long one. I want you to know that we may have to take out your spleen as well as your pancreas.

PATIENT: Why is that?

SENIOR RESIDENT: Oh, it's an organ that takes care of things like the breakdown of old blood cells and a few things like that. It seems to have something to do with fighting infections, so for people who have it taken out, we usually make a special effort to vaccinate them again. We will try to save it, but the blood vessels that feed it run right along the back of the pancreas and it is much better to take it out than to get all of the bleeding that is sometimes required to save the blood vessels . . . Another problem we could have is adhesions.

PATIENT: What's that?

SENIOR RESIDENT: Well, because you have had this many operations, things get sticky in there, and we may have trouble with things getting stuck together.

PATIENT: What about the diabetes thing?

SENIOR RESIDENT: The chances are that you will not have to take any medicine but you may have to watch your diet a bit.

Although Dr. Johnson was convinced that this operation was a good idea, his senior resident was not, and they argued about it more than once. Dr. Ricah felt the patient was expecting too much from the treatment and it was not going to provide him with the relief he expected. Dr. Johnson contended, "There are risks, but I've explained them to him and I'll explain them to him again tomorrow. I think we can help this kid."

The afternoon before the operation Dr. Johnson did the informed consent disclosure required of him by hospital rules.

CHIEF RESIDENT: We've talked about everything, I think. We're going to take out that area of the pancreas that is abnormal, and we will probably also have to take out your spleen as well. The problems of the operation are the possibility of bleeding during the operation. Sometimes there is a possibility of infection from the operation. We will cover you with antibiotics, of course, both before and after the operation. When you come out of the operation you'll have a drain in your nose and in your stomach for a few days. It isn't an easy operation but I am fairly confident that we can help you.

Later that evening one of the evening shift nurses went into Mr. Williamson's room to get a consent form signed.

NURSE: John, I have to get your consent, but you did talk to Dr. Johnson about it today, didn't you?

PATIENT: (nods)

NURSE: First, let me tell you what will happen tomorrow. As soon as we're through here, I am going to start an IV on you and then you're going to get a PhisoHex shower; you know that, don't you?

PATIENT: (nods)

NURSE: (Describes morning shower, blood pressure monitoring, Valium administration, and starting general anesthesia. Reports that the operation will take four or five hours and tells the patient that he will then come back up to the ward and describes some of the postoperative care. About ten minutes of description.) Well, all I have left is for you to sign this [consent form]. Read it over first. If you have any questions, just ask. (She leaves the room briefly while he reads a general consent form for surgical procedures containing information specific to his situation.)

PATIENT: Sign right here, right? (signing)

NURSE: Do you have any questions?

PATIENT: Not really. (after a moment) I do have one question. Does my spleen have anything to do with my having children?

NURSE: (surprised) No, no, nothing to do with that.

Mr. Williamson had his operation the next morning.

Mr. Williamson's case is in some ways typical of and in some ways quite different from most doctor–patient interactions. The ambiguities in communication and the unspoken motives of all participants are, current research suggests, common to the medical setting. On the other hand, despite important omissions and Mr. Williamson's less-than-perfect understanding of the reasons for and possible consequences of the procedure he was to undergo, quite a bit of information was passed to Mr. Williamson by his physicians. Existing empirical research, as we shall see, indicates that this is not universally the case.

For our purposes, any conclusions we might draw from the interaction between these physicians and their somewhat bewildered patient are of much less importance than the questions raised.

1. The discussions Drs. Johnson and Ricah had with their patient, culminating in his encounter with the nurse who brought him a consent form for his signature, are a part of the preoperative routine (some might say ritual) in all medical centers. Asked why they were doing what they did, most of the participants would probably have replied, "I am trying to live up to my responsibilities under the law of informed consent." What is the law of informed consent and how did it evolve into its current form?

2. Had Dr. Johnson been asked whether he would have behaved differently in the absence of a legal requirement for him to discuss certain issues with his patient, he might well have hesitated before responding, "I'm not sure because I've just taken for granted that this is something that we have to do. But now that I think about it, I'd feel uncomfortable operating on someone without telling him something about the operation. It's his body, after all. And besides, he'll be more cooperative if he knows what's going on." This response suggests that the conveyance of information from doctor to patient has roots that go deeper than the legal rules that usually dominate most discussions of consent. Basic notions of right and wrong and good and bad seem to be involved. What are the ethical underpinnings of informed consent in the doctor–patient relationship?

3. Although Drs. Johnson and Ricah may have felt both legal and ethical imperatives to provide Mr. Williamson with certain information concerning his medical care, they were clearly selective. Mr. Williamson was told some of the major risks of surgery, for example, but never that his physicians viewed the operation largely as a maneuver to wean him from the use of painkillers or that they had substantial doubts that the procedure would measurably reduce his pain. There was no discussion at all of possible alternatives to the distal pancreatectomy Dr. Johnson decided to perform. What information does the law require physicians to disclose to their patients when it defines what constitutes an informed consent?

4. To the extent that the physicians disclosed information to Mr. Williamson, the focus was strictly on the medical aspects of the procedure he was about to undergo. Do they have an obligation to reveal other kinds of information as well? For example, if Dr. Johnson's hospital is compensated partially on the basis of how well it holds down the costs of patient care, should Mr. Williamson be told that? What if part of Dr. Johnson's motivation in suggesting surgery is to reduce the likelihood of future readmissions to manage the patient's pain, thus diminishing the amount of money the hospital—which has accepted a capitated contract to provide all of Mr. Williamson's medical care—will have to spend on his treatment? Is that the sort of information that a reasonable person would want to know before consenting to surgery?

5. Mr. Williamson, who had barely completed high school, had obvious difficulty understanding some of the information his physicians disclosed to him. In part, this problem may have resulted from the lack of detail he was offered. The discussion of diabetes as a possible consequence of the surgery, for example, was conducted without any effort to explain to Mr. Williamson just what it might mean to cope with a surgically induced diabetic state. But some of Mr. Williamson's confusion stemmed from his own intellectual limitations. Was he able to understand enough of what he was told to make a meaningful decision about surgery? How can one determine who is able to make their own decisions—in legal terms, who is competent to decide for themselves—and who is not? When someone is found not to be competent, what alternative decisionmaking mechanisms are available?

6. Lurking in the back of the minds of the physicians in this case was the knowledge that some patients sue their doctors on the grounds that informed consent was not obtained. On what basis can such suits be brought, and according to what rules are they handled by the legal system?

7. The procedure performed on Mr. Williamson is an accepted part of the surgical repertoire, not an innovation that Dr. Johnson decided to test. Furthermore, Dr. Johnson's sole motivation for performing the surgery was to help Mr. Williamson, rather than in a formal way to gather data that might be of assistance to other patients in the future. What if the opposite had been the case? That is, what if Dr. Johnson had been introducing a new surgical procedure and intended to use information about Mr. Williamson's operation as part of a larger body of data to assess the new procedure's utility? Would the ethical or legal rules governing consent change? Should consent be obtained differently in such circumstances?

The questions stated so far address primarily the theoretical aspects of informed consent from an ethical and legal perspective. Mr. Williamson's case also raises a number of practical questions concerning informed consent in the clinical setting.

8. As we have seen, questions exist about how effective the efforts to communicate with this patient really were, and how much he was able to comprehend, regardless of the communication methods used. What do we know about various methods of disclosure? How much do patients understand as a result of using one method over another? How competent are most patients? Finally, how are decisions about medical care really made?

9. Careful review of the transcripts of Mr. Williamson's discussions with his caregivers suggests some puzzling and troubling issues. For example, Mr. Williamson was given a good deal of information about his treatment over a period of several days. However, he appears to have committed himself to proceed with the surgery well before all the information about it was made available, even before its full extent and major complications were made known to him. (He was unaware, for example, that a splenectomy would be part of the procedure until quite late in the process.) What suggestions can we make to Drs. Johnson and Ricah as to how they might better have dealt with Mr. Williamson to ensure a more informed decision?

10. One of the more curious aspects of the interactions was the late appearance on the scene of a nurse bearing a consent form for Mr. Williamson to sign. What purpose do these consent forms have, and are there ways of using them that integrate them more meaningfully into the rest of the informed consent process?

11. Mr. Williamson consented to have the procedure performed even though he evidently had some serious concerns about the possible results. He signed the consent form, after all, while still entertaining the possibility that the removal of his spleen might have an adverse impact on his ability to father children. What if he had refused to undergo the procedure? Do we have any understanding of why patients refuse treatment, what role the provision of information to them plays in their refusal, and how physicians might best respond to refusals?

12. A great deal of ink has been spilled in efforts to determine how Mr. Williamson and his doctors should interact before his consent to surgery is considered legitimate. How would critics of the present process have altered the discussions? Are legal approaches the best way to go about modifying the behavior of both sides?

These general issues, of immense significance for the delivery and receipt of medical care today, and many more related questions, form the substance of the chapters that follow.

Terminology

Informed consent is a term that has been elaborated in the context of ethics, law, and medicine. As a consequence, the term may denote quite different things to specialists in different disciplines, even at the most general level and among persons to whom informed consent is not a novelty. For example, the phrase *theory of informed consent* may signify one thing to the ethicist and quite a different thing to a person trained in law. Even within a given discipline there may be disparities of understanding as to the meaning of particular terms. The phrase *law of informed consent* may mean one thing to the legal scholar and something else to the trial attorney. As a result, it is necessary to describe here some terms and concepts that appear in discussions of informed consent and to indicate how we will employ them.

The Idea of Informed Consent

At the most general theoretical level is what we call, borrowing from Jay Katz, "the idea of informed consent" (4, p. xvi). This idea is the core notion that decisions about the medical care a person will receive, if any, are to be made in a collaborative manner between patient and physician. The concept also implies that the physician must be prepared to engage in—indeed to initiate—a discussion with the patient about the available therapeutic options and to provide relevant information on them. The influential report on informed consent of the President's Commission for the Study of Ethical Problems in Medicine was premised on the idea of informed consent, and the report's recommendations strongly reflect the associated concepts (5).

The idea of informed consent has its origins in ethics, in law, and in contemporary medicine's own understanding about the nature of the doctor–patient relationship and the advantages that accrue when patients are knowledgeable about their treatment. The ethical justification of informed consent stems from its promotion of autonomy and well-being (as individuals themselves define well-being). There are two, sometimes competing, grounds upon which policies are ethically evaluated: (*1*) based upon rights and duties, and (*2*) based upon the consequences of actions. These two types of theories, deontological and consequential, both have been applied in the development of the idea of informed consent (see Chapter 2).

Law has also played an important role in nourishing the idea of informed consent. In fact, it is probably from law that the term informed consent originated. Legally protected interests—primarily bodily integrity and individual autonomy—have contributed to the idea of informed consent. The right of bodily integrity is largely a common-law one, embodied in the protections conferred by both the civil and criminal law of assault and battery. There are also important constitutional underpinnings to this right. Individual autonomy, or the right to choose or decide, has similar common-law and constitutional antecedents.

The Legal Doctrine

The idea of informed consent is made operational by means of the *legal doctrine of informed consent*. The doctrine, which prevails in all American jurisdictions, requires that informed consent be obtained before a physician is legally entitled to administer treatment to a patient. This requirement is actually composed of two separate but related legal duties imposed on physicians: the duty first to disclose information to patients, and the duty subsequently to obtain their consent before administering treatment. (The legal doctrine of informed consent is discussed in Chapters 3 through 6.)

The extent to which the idea of informed consent is actually embodied in legal requirements has been a matter of great concern to scholarly commentators. In practice the idea of informed consent and its ethical and legal underpinnings has been seriously diluted in the duties the law actually imposes on physicians. A similar dilution has been seen in the "rules for recovery" (see *The Rules for Recovery*) that govern lawsuits brought by patients who allege that they were treated without informed consent, by which they usually mean that they believe the treatment was inadequately explained to them before they received it.

The *legal requirements for informed consent* generally specify what kind of information doctors must disclose to patients and sometimes how consent should be obtained. An example of these legal requirements is the generally accepted rule that physicians must inform patients of the nature, purpose, risks, and benefits of any treatment they propose to perform, as well as any alternative forms of treatment that may exist for the patients' conditions. Similarly, the exceptions that exist for either making such disclosure or obtaining consent, or both, are also examples of what we mean by the legal requirements for informed consent. The legal requirements and levels of specificity vary substantially from state to state and sometimes even from case to case within a given state. It is certainly safe to say that there is no single set of legal requirements for informed consent.

The Rules for Recovery

The legal requirements for obtaining informed consent define the legal obligations of physicians to their patients. The enforcement of these obligations requires further discussion. There are any number of potential means for implementing the idea of informed consent. One might be through requirements promulgated by hospitals, with penalties such as curtailment or loss of staff privileges for the physician who fails to comply. Similarly, in some jurisdictions, such failure may be grounds for state disciplinary proceedings.

By far the most familiar, however, and probably the most common means of redress for a patient who claims there was inadequate explanation and consent prior to treatment, is a lawsuit seeking damages (i.e., a monetary recovery) from the physician. Most such lawsuits are resolved either through settlement procedures or by a trial. Of those that go to trial, a small proportion are appealed. The appellate court reviews the outcome of a trial, determines whether it should be affirmed or reversed, and—most important for present purposes—writes an opinion explaining the reasons for its decision. Most of the legal requirements for informed consent are derived from the collected opinions of appellate courts. From these appellate decisions the legal *doctrine* of informed consent has been developed by scholars, as an embodiment of the *idea* of informed consent. In addition, some states have codified parts of the legal doctrine in legislation, creating statutory law on informed consent.

Because the legal opinions are written in response to particular claims by injured patients requesting compensation for their injuries, the cases (and statutes) establish a variety of rules to guide the litigation process in such lawsuits. We refer to these as the *rules for recovery,* that is, recovery by the patient of damages. Some of these rules involve the standard of care, the standard of causation, the requirement for expert testimony, and the materialized risk requirement. These are largely technical issues, most of which should have only indirect (though not necessarily insubstantial) influence on the manner in which physicians seek to comply with their duties to inform patients and obtain their consent. They deal, in effect, not with the right to informed consent, but with the remedy for the violation of that right. (These rules are discussed in Chapter 6.)

References

1. Koch, H-G., Reiter-Theil, S., and Helmchen, H. (eds) (1996) *Informed Consent in Psychiatry: European Perspectives of Ethics Law and Clinical Practice.* Baden-Baden: Nomos Verlagsgesellschaft.
2. Levine, R.J. (1991) Informed consent: some challenges to the universal validity of the Western model. *Law Med Health Care*, 19(3-4): 207–213.
3. Miller, F. (1992) Denial of health care and informed consent in English and American law. *Am J Law Med*, 18: 37–71.
4. Katz, J. (1984) *The Silent World of Doctor and Patient.* New York: Free Press.
5. President's Commission for the Study of Ethical Problems in Medicine and Biomedical and Behavioral Research (1982) *Making Health Care Decisions: The Ethical and Legal Implications of Informed Consent in the Patient-Practitioner Relationship.* Volume 1, Report. Washington, D.C.: U.S. Government Printing Office.

2

The Concept and Ethical Justification of Informed Consent

The values underlying informed consent—autonomy and concern for individual well-being—are deeply embedded in American culture, in our religious traditions, and in Western moral philosophy. It is not surprising that informed consent is a cornerstone doctrine of contemporary medical ethics and health law in the United States. There is widespread agreement about the importance of the concept, goals, and practice of informed consent. Even when there are differences of opinion about the best way to implement informed consent in clinical practice, or when there is debate about the core meaning of the concept, the attention paid to these controversies only reinforces recognition of the importance of informed consent in contemporary health care and medical research.

The concept of informed consent has multiple meanings and draws its ethical justification from several sources. Some consider informed consent to be synonymous with the ideal of shared decision making between physician and patient, or at least to embody this ideal (1). Others emphasize that informed consent is a particular sort of decision made by a particular sort of decision maker (2). Still others focus on informed consent as a norm-governed social practice that is embedded in social institutions, specifically law and medicine. This chapter discusses these different but often overlapping conceptions of informed consent.

From a patient's perspective, informed consent appears to be a right, while from the physician's viewpoint, it is a duty or obligation. In fact, informed consent imposes responsibilities on both patient and physician. The relationship between ethical rights and duties, as well as the possibility of conflict between them, form another topic of this chapter.

In this chapter we also discuss the ethical values and goals that underlie informed consent. Informed consent is grounded in some of the ethical values most prized in American society and Western ethical thought, especially autonomy— *auto* from the Greek word for self, and *nomos* from the Greek for rule—literally "self-rule." It is interesting to observe how the fundamental goals of informed consent usually coincide, but sometimes conflict, both in theory and as manifest in particular cases. The strain that can arise when its goals come into conflict reflects deep ethical tensions with which philosophers have struggled since ancient times.

Informed consent became a cornerstone doctrine of contemporary American bioethics in the 1960s and 1970s as the field attempted to help doctors, patients, and the public make sense of the possibilities and problems presented by new technological opportunities and the need to allocate these opportunities fairly. At the dawn of this new century, informed consent remains a central doctrine whose goals and underlying values influence other policies and practices in bioethics and medicine. Today, however, our understanding of informed consent and the challenges of implementing it in the clinical setting is richer because of developments in bioethics that began in the 1990s. Then, bioethicists began to examine some of the biases and blind spots the field displayed during its first three decades and to reassess the field's reliance on autonomy and its hope that informed consent could address most ethical problems in medicine (3). In its final section, this chapter examines some of these developments. It explores how autonomy can be reconceptualized and the process of informed consent modified to address these criticisms and thus make informed consent better serve the interests of patients and research subjects.

What Is Informed Consent?

There are at least three distinct senses of informed consent. In their comprehensive analysis, *A History and Theory of Informed Consent*, Ruth Faden and Tom Beauchamp distinguish between two senses of informed consent—the policy-oriented conception and the philosophical conception. A third sense—shared decision making—was promoted by the President's Commission for the Study of Ethical Problems in Medicine.

The policy-oriented conception of informed consent refers to "legally or institutionally *effective* . . . authorization from a patient or subject. Such authorization is 'effective' because it has been obtained through procedures that satisfy the rules and requirements defining a specific institutional practice in health care or in research" (2, p. 280). If those rules did not exist, the actions would not have the same meaning. It is only because of existing laws and institutional policies that a patient's saying, "Okay, I agree to have the surgery" has the effect of authorizing his doctor to cut him open and remove his tumor.

An astute observer witnessing this norm-governed process of informed consent take place in medical and research settings could derive at least some of the legal rules and requirements that govern the practice from this observation. When, in the balance of this book, we discuss these rules and requirements, we are concerned with informed consent in this sense, as a social practice governed by these social norms (i.e., rules, laws, and implicit values). These rules and requirements have evolved for particular reasons—historical, practical, and normative (i.e., because of ethical and cultural values). We believe that these rules and requirements generally seek to create conditions in which informed consent most closely approximates the philosophically fundamental sense of informed consent that Faden and Beauchamp identify: informed consent as autonomous authorization.

In this sense, informed consent is "an autonomous action undertaken by a subject or a patient that authorizes a professional either to involve the subject in research or to initiate a medical plan for the patient (or both)" (2, p. 278). "In authorizing, one both assumes responsibility for what one has authorized and transfers to another one's authority to implement it. . . . [O]ne must understand that one is assuming responsibility and warranting another to proceed" (2, p. 280). Outside of medicine, people authorize others to do things on their behalf all the time. When a homeowner hires house painters, for example, she authorizes them to scrape off the old brown paint, prime any bare wood, and paint the house the shade of gray she has selected. She retains responsibility for what she has authorized. If it turns out that the selected color, "Cloudy Day," is more sky blue than the subtle gray that she had envisioned, the responsibility is still hers. Her painters are responsible for providing a paint job that meets industry standards, but not for her choice of paint color or choice of them to do the job. Assuming that hers is an *autonomous* authorization—that, for example, she was not unduly pressured by her fiancé—she is responsible for her decision. If instead her fiancé applied overwhelming pressure on her to choose the subsequently garish "Cloudy Day," then her authorization to apply that paint is not autonomous. (She might then hold her fiancé responsible.) In most decisions of daily life, such overwhelming pressure is absent, and thus most authorizations of others to act on our behalf are autonomous authorizations. Indeed, when the process of informed consent is pursued (see Chapter 8), autonomous authorization in medicine resembles such decisions in other aspects of life.

As will become clear in subsequent chapters, informed consent as autonomous authorization is distinct from the legal and institutional rules and requirements the fulfillment of which constitutes the social practice of informed consent. Informed consent as autonomous authorization is an ideal toward which these requirements are aimed. The account of informed consent as autonomous authorization is silent, for example, on the question of how the patient or subject achieves the substantial understanding necessary to authorize the treatment or research plan. The homeowner could discuss possible paint colors with the painters, she could solicit opinions from her neighbors, or she could simply feel inspired when she discovers the "Cloudy Day" paint chip at her local store. No matter how she reached her decision, in hiring the painters to paint her house "Cloudy Day," she authorizes them to act on her behalf. In practice, the process of informed consent often demands a degree of shared decision making between physician and patient or researcher and potential subject. People often know less about medical interventions than, for example, about house painting or the effect of sunlight on a color that looks great in the store. Therefore, patients and subjects often rely upon physicians or researchers to inform them adequately, so that they can then autonomously authorize a course of action. Perhaps for this reason, psychiatrist Jay Katz and the President's Commission tend to equate informed consent with shared decision making, the third sense in which the term is used (1,4). However, informed consent is only one aspect of shared decision making in medicine. Moreover, in the sense of autonomous authorization, informed consent could actually occur without shared decision making.

These three senses of informed consent—as a specific rule-governed practice, as autonomous authorization, and as shared decision making—are obviously interrelated. For example, the rules and requirements that constitute informed consent in the institutionalized, policy-oriented sense that Faden and Beauchamp identify are designed to promote shared decision making and to enable autonomous authorization. However, it is important to recognize the distinctions among these conceptions of informed consent. Acknowledging them permits us to see that sometimes strict adherence to the rules governing informed consent may actually undermine the dialogue involved in the process of shared decision making, or may fail to enable a particular patient autonomously to authorize a treatment plan. Alternatively, placing too much emphasis on *sharing* the decision may undermine the decisional authority of some patients, for example, if they overvalue maintaining a good relationship and comfortable interaction with their physicians at the expense of expressing their own views. These patients may eventually be disappointed when they find that they, not their physicians, bear responsibility for what they authorized their doctors to do. Like the hypothetical homeowner who would like to be able to blame her painters for her own paint color choice, patients may want to blame their physicians for choices they later regret. Recognizing that in authorizing another to act on one's behalf, one still retains responsibility for what is authorized may help avoid misplacing blame. In order to be responsible for what they authorize, however, patients must be well informed and act autonomously.

Goals of Informed Consent

The primary goals of informed consent are the protection of patient or subject welfare and the promotion of autonomy [see, for example, (5), especially p. 142]. Although these goals can conflict both in theory and in practice, with a deeper understanding of each it is generally possible to reconcile them. Much of the apparent conflict centers on how welfare or well-being is defined and by whom. The welfare-protection/autonomy-promotion conflict involves a broader conflict between medical paternalism and patient autonomy, which has a long history.

Historian Martin Pernick discerns a tradition of physicians' being truthful with their patients and encouraging their participation in medical decision making "based on medical theories that taught that knowledge and autonomy had demonstrably beneficial effects on most patients' health" (6, p. 3). In this view, informing patients and soliciting their agreement to a treatment plan—elements of shared decision making, but not informed consent in a more rigorous policy-oriented sense—seek to ensure patients' compliance and thereby promote patients' health. Recent empirical studies indeed support this long-held belief that supplying information to patients can reduce anxiety and depression about health states (7–9), increase adherence (10–15), enhance patient satisfaction (16), and facilitate monitoring of symptoms (17, 18).

Nevertheless, this traditional information-giving, agreement-seeking process has a different goal from that of true informed consent. In the tradition Pernick identifies, medicine's goal of achieving health, admittedly a goal most often shared by patients, provides the justification for involving them in decision making. If in a particular case, or in general, such involvement were believed to be contrary to patient health, the warrant for informing patients and soliciting their agreement to a treatment plan would evaporate. (Indeed, such a belief is thought to justify the "therapeutic privilege" of withholding information, discussed in Chapter 4.) In this view, physicians are the ultimate decision makers; they possess decisional authority that they share with patients only insofar as they believe it is in the best health-related interests of patients to participate in decision making. As we discuss in Chapter 8, usually there are health-related benefits of involving patients in their healthcare plans, including the process of informed consent. However, this traditional justification for such involvement is paternalistic because it involves substituting the parentlike decision of the physician for the patient's own judgment, for what the physician presumes to be the patient's own good. This paternalism may involve overriding the patient's autonomous decision, or preventing the patient from acquiring information or otherwise having the opportunity to make such a decision.[1]

In contrast, contemporary informed consent serves as a counter to medical paternalism. It allows patients to exercise their autonomy and to protect their well-being as they themselves define it. In this way, both at the level of theory and in particular cases, the demands of informed consent may conflict with what medical paternalism, or the physician's desire to do good for her patient, would prescribe.

Katz recognized this conflict. In *The Silent World of Doctor and Patient*, he writes that "the history of the physician-patient relationship from ancient times to the present . . . bears testimony to physicians' inattention to their patients' right and need to make their own decisions" (1, p. 28). He believes that physicians have not only utterly failed to discuss medical matters with their patients, but they have failed "to invite patients' participation in sharing the burden of making joint decisions" (1, pp. 3–4). Katz, an advocate of the shared decisionmaking concept of informed consent, explicates this "burden" in terms akin to patients' being led to recognize and exercise their decisional authority, their right of autonomous authorization:

> I . . . postulate a duty to reflection that cannot easily be waived. Asserting such a duty sounds strange. We are accustomed to recognizing a right to choice as an aspect of the right to self-determination, but a duty to reflection as a component part of the concept of autonomy is quite another matter. Yet . . . respect for the right to self-determination requires respect for human beings' proclivities to exercise this right in both rational and irrational ways. Doctors are obligated to facilitate patients' opportunities for reflection to prevent ill-considered rational and irrational influences on choice. Patients, in turn, are obligated to participate in the process of thinking about choices. (1)

Assumption of responsibility for a treatment plan and authorization of another (the physician) to implement it is the right and burden that patients have in the contemporary context of informed consent (although, as we will see in Chapter 4, they need not carry the full weight of autonomous decision making under which Katz would have them labor). Informed consent, as Katz recognizes, is not a matter of informing patients when doing so will conveniently promote a treatment plan; it requires informing patients with the recognition that they may disagree with a recommended treatment plan and retain the authority to do so.

But why? Why should informed consent (or any justifiable doctrine) have as its goals the promotion of values that may occasionally be contrary to the goals of medicine and the recommendations of well-intentioned and knowledgeable

[1]There are several excellent and differently nuanced accounts of paternalism (see, e.g., 19–21).

physicians? How can such contrary goals be justified? If the twentieth century indeed witnessed a shift in the justification of informing and involving patients in decision making from a "beneficence model" to an "autonomy model," how is this shift itself justified?[2]

Autonomy and Well-Being

Part of the explanation for the shift from beneficent paternalism toward autonomy lies in historical events of the twentieth century, primarily related to research, that called into question the trustworthiness of the medical profession. The atrocities revealed in the Nuremberg trial of Nazi doctors, as well as highly publicized cases of human subjects abused in the United States, sparked suspicion of the general benevolence of physicians and researchers. In this context, informed consent was seen as a protection from abuse by untrustworthy professionals. Even if the medical and research establishment could not be trusted to conduct prospective review of the likely harms and benefits and to offer individuals only research and treatment opportunities that had acceptable risk–benefit ratios, individuals could safeguard their own interests if they were adequately informed and if their autonomous authorization was required before research or treatment could proceed. Individuals were thus called upon to exercise their autonomous decisional authority to safeguard their welfare.

Other historical developments coincided to shift medical decision making even further toward a patient autonomy model. Technological advances in medicine created treatment options that allowed physicians to keep patients alive even when they had few chances of recovery and very poor quality of life. Patients who did not want to be dependent on ventilators or dialysis presented the possibility that medicine's capabilities could clash with patients' deeply held values. What individual patients asserted against medical paternalism was, in essence, that health was not the only value of importance to them. Patients whose vision of a good life included a death unencumbered by technology found that their vision of their own well-being clashed with the "do everything" mandate of acute care medicine. Many physicians were themselves increasingly uncomfortable with the path charted by their perceived professional mandate to promote health and preserve life at all costs. It was growing less clear that doing "what is best for the

---

[2]Faden and Beauchamp use these terms to describe the shift from a view of informed consent as part of a physician's obligation, conceived primarily as an obligation to provide medical benefit, to a view whereby "the physician's responsibilities of disclosure and consent-seeking are established primarily (perhaps exclusively) by the principle of respect for autonomy" (2, p. 59). Another important conceptual shift focuses on the understanding of autonomy, from mere freedom from uninvited interference with one's body, to an opportunity to express one's values and preferences. Finally, as Chapter 3 describes, legal doctrine surrounding informed consent has witnessed a shift from simple voluntary consent to *informed* consent.

patient," the paternalistic mandate, entailed aggressive medical intervention. Asking what the patient wanted provided a way out of this dilemma.

The era of the late 1960s and early 1970s, however, also involved considerable changes in the larger social environment. The growing activism of African Americans and women and their assertion of individual rights challenged established social consensus on multiple fronts. The Vietnam War undercut the credibility of many different authorities. In short, the social climate was ripe for groups and individuals to assert their preferences even when those preferences conflicted with the recommendations of the (medical) establishment. In this climate, it was easy to view patients as another oppressed class who needed more freedom from their oppressive physicians. Individuality and autonomy, in the sense of freedom from interference, and even in the stronger sense of self-actualization or authenticity, gained ascendancy.

Although the time was ripe for a change, it is important to ask why controls on medical power came in the form of support for patient autonomy. Many nations would have focused on restricting physician authority directly, rather than on supporting patients' choices. However, American culture has always been supportive of individual choice. The dominant political ideology at the time the United States became a nation reflects this American ethos; enlightenment philosophy focused on the rationality of the individual, the power of reason to produce good, and the individual's right to make choices. This political philosophy reinforced emphasis on the sanctity of the individual conscience, which was central to beliefs of the Puritans and other radical Protestant groups who came to the New World from Europe. Finally, individualistic values were reinforced by the "frontier mentality" of self-reliance that emerged with the settlement of the new continent, that remains highly prized in American culture today, and that further reinforces individualistic values.

Thus, during the late 1960s and 1970s, the patients' rights movement, along with the women's and civil rights movements, joined in a long tradition of asserting the inalienable and inherent value of individual persons, and individuals' rights of self-determination. Contemporary American bioethics emerged as an interdisciplinary field of inquiry during this era of social conflict and deep ethical tension in the United States. Although the origins of the legal doctrine of informed consent predate this turbulent time (see Chapter 3), the values underlying informed consent resonated with the values asserted during this era. The right to determine what happened to one's own body became an important instrument in individuals' attempts to counter medical paternalism and the prevailing social consensus (22).

Although these historical developments help to explain the emergence of the contemporary sense of informed consent and its reliance on and valorization of autonomy, by themselves they do relatively little to justify it. For that justification, we must look to ethical theory. We must come to understand how respect for autonomy grounds a robust theory of informed consent and how ethics helps to analyze conflicts between autonomy and beneficence, between individual and community, and between individual interest and the social good.

Ethical Justification of Informed Consent

Autonomy plays its most prominent role in the ethical theory of nineteenth-century philosopher Immanuel Kant. For Kant what is unique about persons is that they self-legislate. Persons can exercise their wills, their self-ruling capacities, their autonomy. It is this feature of persons that makes them inherently valuable, unlike things in the world that are valuable only insofar as they serve people's ends. In order to act ethically, Kant argues, persons must act with respect for other persons as intrinsically valuable, self-legislating beings. Thus, to deceive a research subject into enrolling in a clinical trial, or to conceive a child for the sole purpose of procuring her stem cells to treat one's beloved, would be ethically unacceptable because in so doing, the research subject and the child would be treated solely as means to another's ends. Deception deprives the prospective subject of the information necessary to decide for himself, and thus treats him as a means to the researcher's ends, rather than respecting him as a "self-legislating" person with ends of his own. Conceiving a child for the sole purpose of using her tissue fails to treat her as an inherently valuable person; she is instead treated as valuable only insofar as she has tissue valuable to another person.

What is significant and distinctive about Kant's theory is the role played by autonomy. Autonomy, together with rules of logic, laws of nature, and facts about the world in which we live, provides the test for moral action. It is not something extrinsic to ourselves that provides the mark and measure of ethical acceptability. It is something intrinsic to us, our autonomy. It is not the consequences of our actions, nor an externally given set of laws, that determines the ethics of our action. It is recognition of our intrinsic, irreducible, inalienable value as autonomous persons, our dignity beyond price, that provides the supreme moral measure. It is the demand that we act as self-legislators, indeed as would-be self-legislators for all self-legislating people, that is the test of ethical action.

As a guide to action, Kantian ethics is notoriously difficult to interpret and apply. However, it presents an ethical ideal that suffuses many other moral philosophies and provides a criterion against which competing ethical theories may be judged. This ideal is the inherent value or dignity of persons, a quality that is explained in terms of their unique ability to be self-legislating or autonomous.

Utilitarianism, an equally prominent ethical theory, takes an action's utility to be the measure of its ethical acceptability. An action's utility is its usefulness or its ability to produce some good. The ethically best option is the one that produces the most overall utility. A common conception of utilitarianism considers the best course of action to be the one that produces the greatest good or the greatest happiness for the greatest number. Several practical and conceptual problems plague all but the most sophisticated utilitarian theories (and some would argue even they are ultimately unsatisfactory; see, for example, [23]). First, it is difficult to predict the consequences of one's actions, and for purposes of analysis, it is difficult to specify how far along the "ripple effect" of an action one is supposed to assess the possible or actual consequences. Second, it is practically impossible to assess adequately other people's preferences for or reactions to an action. Moreover, interpersonal comparisons of pains, pleasures, or utilities that utilitarianism demands are impossible.

Joe does something that makes Mark writhe in pain, but makes Jane and Jim exclaim with pleasure. Even a neutral observer would be hard-pressed to determine whether Mark's pain was exceeded by the pleasure of Jane and Jim, or not. A "gut response" might be that no matter how much pleasure Joe's action produced, he had no right to cause Mark pain. Shrinking from causing pain seems an appropriate moral intuition. However, when we realize that Joe is a nurse drawing blood from his young patient, Mark, so that his condition may be accurately diagnosed, and that his worried parents are actually exclaiming with pleasure and relief that some action is finally being taken to diagnose Mark's mysterious condition, we recognize the pitfalls in relying on gut feelings or even our somewhat more reflective intuitions, as well as the problem with incompletely described acts.

Nevertheless, this example and the initial natural response to it suggest a flaw typically identified in pure utilitarian analyses. On the basis of consequences or the balance between pleasure and pain alone, it is difficult and perhaps impossible to assign rights to respect individual dignity and to protect individuals from both harm and the "tyranny of the majority." What if, for example, a vast majority of people could significantly benefit from imposing a modest amount of suffering on a very small minority? For example, in light of the potential positive consequences, what is wrong with a well-intentioned scientist forcing a small number of people to test a new AIDS vaccine for the benefit of future generations? Recognizing this potential misuse of his own theory, John Stuart Mill, author of *Utilitarianism*, supplied respect for autonomy as the requisite corrective. In *On Liberty*, he wrote:

> The only freedom which deserves the name is that of pursuing our own good in our own way, so long as we do not attempt to deprive others of theirs or impede their efforts to obtain it. Each is the proper guardian of his own health, whether bodily or mental and spiritual. Mankind are greater gainers by suffering each other to live as seems good to themselves than by compelling each to live as seems good to the rest.

Though this doctrine is anything but new and, to some persons, may have the air of a truism, there is no doctrine that stands more directly opposed to the general tendency of existing opinion and practice (24). Mill supplies autonomy, conceived as a sphere of personal freedom, as the limiting factor on what may be required for the sake of the greater good. He also suggests the relationship between this autonomy and individual well-being.

Autonomy is the freedom from external constraints (Mill) and the capacity for self-determination (Kant) that permits individuals to pursue their own good in their own way. When they have adequate information and opportunity (i.e., freedom), individuals tend to promote their own well-being.[3] Of course, people are not entirely egoistic. They will act for the sake of others' interests, as well. The stranger who donates bone marrow may act because she has an interest in being altruistic. In other words, doing good for others (and perhaps also being recognized as doing good for others) is one of her values. The brother who donates a kidney to his sister may act both out of altruism and because he has a personal interest in her well-being.

In most cases, including most healthcare contexts, respect for an individual's autonomy coincides with promotion of her well-being. So long as an individual decides in light of adequate information, and chooses freely, she will act to promote her *subjective* well-being, her well-being as she herself defines it. Her definition, however, may not coincide with her *objectively determined* well-being, her best interest as an ostensibly objective observer may define it. The person who above all else values her independent mobility, for example, may refuse a recommended surgery that might prolong her life but might also leave her unable to walk. Her exercise of her autonomy promotes her values and thus her subjective well-being, even though another may view her autonomous decision as contrary to her (objectively determined) well-being.

Constraints on Autonomy

In clinical medicine, the great weight placed on health and longevity is perhaps the greatest external threat to autonomy, that is, to the capacity for and sphere of

---

[3]Whether individuals' acting autonomously always promotes the greatest social good is, however, doubtful. Therefore, some would argue that individuals should be encouraged, and in some cases forced, to take into account the broader social effects of their individual decisions and actions. Consider highly prized and legally protected reproductive autonomy. American women are permitted to terminate their pregnancies for any or no reason (at least within particular temporally defined constraints). If having children of one sex was generally preferred in society, and if many pregnant women decided to use prenatal genetic testing to determine the sex of their babies-to-be and to terminate pregnancies with fetuses of the undesired sex, an imbalance between the sexes could result and have socially undesirable consequences. For this reason, in a striking departure from its usual nondirective ethos, the genetic counseling profession frowns upon genetic testing for sex selection purposes (25); moreover, genetic testing for sex selection is prohibited or regulated in some jurisdictions (e.g., 26).

individual decision making. Allegedly justified by concern for a patient's health, a physician or a patient's family might coerce or unduly pressure a patient to make a healthcare decision or might submit the patient to treatment without his autonomous authorization. (In contrast, justifiable exceptions to the requirement for informed consent are discussed in Chapter 4.)

Since all actions, including healthcare decisions, are to some degree pressured by outside circumstances or influenced by others, the difficult question is how much influence must be present for a decision to be considered not to have been made autonomously? Outside influences that so overwhelm the will that the decision maker cannot decide or act otherwise so severely compromise the capacity for autonomy that such decisions and actions are clearly non-autonomous. Decisions that are made at leisure, after much deliberation, in accordance with one's own values, and without others' (undue) influence should clearly count as autonomous. There is, however, a vast gray area in between. The ethical mandate for society and its institutions is to promote, as much as possible, the conditions that enable individuals to make substantially autonomous decisions. This means avoiding as much as possible pressures of time, dictatorial presentations of information and options, and suggestions that choice of the "wrong" option will be dealt with punitively, perhaps by a withdrawal of care.

Another set of constraints on autonomy are largely *internal*. People who feel they are too ignorant or too weak to make choices, or who cannot find the emotional strength to do so, are not capable of acting autonomously. As a result, they may become overly susceptible to external influences that would otherwise not be considered undue. They may, for example, be overawed by the prestige of medical professionals or defer to an authority figure in their family. Some people may suffer from phobias or other internal constraints that overwhelm their wills so they cannot freely choose an option they would otherwise desire. A patient who has been sexually abused, for example, might feel incapable of having a physical exam despite intellectually recognizing the health-related benefits it may afford. Ignorance, on the other hand, is generally considered to be a remediable impediment to autonomous decision making. Although a person cannot autonomously choose an option she does not understand, usually patients can be provided with information relevant to their treatment decisions, in terms that they can comprehend, so they can decide whether to authorize implementation of a treatment plan.

Thus, both substantial understanding and the absence of substantially controlling influences are constituent aspects of autonomous decision making. The autonomous authorization that is informed consent also involves intent. The patient or research subject must intend to authorize the course of action consented to, or alternatively, intend to refuse such authorization. It is in the intending that the patient or subject assumes responsibility for the decision made.

Informed consent as autonomous authorization, then, is justified both by respect for patient autonomy and as a means of protecting patients' subjective well-being. Concern for individual autonomy and well-being are, in turn, justified by ethical theories like those grounded in the intrinsic value of self-legislating persons or the pursuit of individual happiness constrained by respect for others' right to the same pursuit, Kantianism and Utilitarianism, respectively. Thus, informed consent in its more philosophical sense, as well as the policy-oriented rule-governed sense, is justified not only out of respect for patient autonomy but also because of positive consequences anticipated in its pursuit. These include: protection of patients and subjects, avoidance of fraud and duress, encouragement of self-scrutiny by medical professionals, promotion of rational decisions, and involvement of the public in health care (27). These anticipated benefits constitute what are sometimes termed the "prophylactic" and the "therapeutic" arguments for autonomy and informed consent (28, pp. 18–22); they stress the prevention of abuse and the promotion of health-related benefit. Improving the doctor–patient relationship, demystifying medicine, demythologizing physicians, and reducing miscommunication and other risk factors for malpractice suits are also associated with the informed consent process (1,29–32).

Challenges to the Theory of Informed Consent

Despite these deeply rooted ethical justifications and the frequent positive consequences of informed consent, the process of informed consent faces many practical challenges in its implementation, which are addressed in the chapters that follow. However, there are also some challenges to informed consent at the theoretical level, challenges lodged at its ethical justification. These challenges center around two basic observations. First, not all patients want to assume the burdens of decision making. Second, informed consent and its underlying values of individualism and autonomy are not the only relevant ethical concerns in medical decision making. Addressing each of these challenges results in reconceptualizing autonomy and formulating a stronger theory of informed consent that more fully serves patients' interests and promotes their autonomous wishes and their well-being as they define it.

Diversity of Decision-Making Preferences

One set of theoretical concerns about informed consent stems from empirical data about what patients really want in the context of medical decision making, in their doctor–patient relationships, and in clinical research settings. If, for example, a substantial number of patients do not want to make decisions regarding their care, then it seems that it might be wrong to place upon them the burden of doing so. After all, one of the goals of informed consent is to allow patients to pursue their own conceptions of the good, to safeguard their own subjective welfare. If exercising the measure of direct control over their medical care afforded by informed consent does not coincide with their values, then demanding that patients retain decisional authority is not in their interests, at least not as they define them. Indeed, if medicine and society more generally are really committed to the right of self-determination, and if that right is to have any meaning at all, then it would seem that patients should have the right to choose not to decide themselves, but to delegate that responsibility (5).

Here we examine the implications, for informed consent doctrine, of empirical evidence that not all patients welcome the decisional authority vested in them by informed consent doctrine. Instead of suggesting that patient decision making be thrown out and medical paternalism restored, like throwing out the proverbial baby with the bath water, this examination suggests ways that the informed consent process may be improved to meet the needs of patients and fulfill the goals of promoting their autonomy and well-being. Most important, it is our premise that the theory of informed consent may be justifiably amended to meet the needs of patients and to accommodate their realities, not to increase the convenience of physicians, researchers, or healthcare institutions.

In *The Practice of Autonomy*, Carl Schneider surveys empirical studies about what patients want with respect to autonomy, informed consent, and medical decision making (28, pp. 36–46). Reviewing studies of populations ranging from the generally well public to the seriously ill, as well as personal accounts of illness that patients have shared in their memoirs, Schneider concludes that

> while patients largely wish to be informed about their medical circumstances, a substantial number of them do not want to make their own medical decisions, or perhaps even to participate in those decisions in any very significant way. The studies do not explain fully just which kinds of patients want to make their own decisions. They do reveal, however, two telling patterns. First, the elderly are less likely than the young to want to make medical decisions. Second, the graver the patient's illness, the less likely the patient is to want to make medical decisions. (28, p. 41; see also 33, 34)

Three points are of great importance: first, while a substantial number of patients may not want to make such decisions, a substantial number do. Second, even patients who do not want to make medical decisions nevertheless want to be well informed. Third, attempts to characterize patient preferences in terms of patient age or seriousness of condition are based on epidemiological data; they are generalities that may or may not apply to the individual patient.

In addition, there may also be important differences in individuals' decision-making preferences with respect to research, in contrast to treatment contexts. With respect to enrolling in a research study that does not have his individual benefit as its primary goal, a patient may be quite reluctant to entrust decisional authority to someone else, especially to the physician-researcher; however, in an individualized therapeutic context, the same patient may be most comfortable relying on his doctor to employ medical expertise and benevolent intentions to decide on his behalf.

Schneider considers various reasons that patients may prefer to entrust medical decision making to others, including their physicians (28). These reasons center either on the psychological and physical experience of being ill or on the complexity of the decisions that must be made.

First, being sick can sap patients of the usual emotional, intellectual, and physical resources that they call upon to make decisions. Getting well can be hard, sometimes all-consuming work. Moreover, some people avoid facing the harsh realities of their illnesses as a way of coping with their conditions or as a prerequisite for enjoying the balance of their lives to the fullest. For others the experience of illness calls for being cared for, or even demands being dependent. Oliver Sacks writes, "though as a sick patient one was reduced to moral infancy, this was not moral degradation, but a biological and spiritual need of the hurt creature. . . . [T]his might be felt as 'infantilizing' and degrading or as a sweet and sorely-needed nourishing" (35, pp. 165–166).

The second set of concerns focuses on the complexity of medical decisions. As various commentators note, the assumption that a lack of medical knowledge is a generally remediable impediment to autonomous decision making may be challenged by the sheer complexity of the information that patients must understand to make an informed decision (28). People have well-documented difficulties understanding probabilities (36,37). And many contemporary medical decisions involve making trade-offs, choosing the least undesirable of several onerous options, weighing probabilities, and understanding complex systems (including not only physiological systems, but social systems within which only some treatments are fully or partially reimbursed by insurance plans).

For these reasons, Schneider concludes "patients might not crave the decisional authority the autonomy paradigm [and the doctrine of informed consent] envisions for them" (28, p. 74). He comments:

> Some people may behave as autonomists [advocates of autonomy] imagine, but an imposing number of them act quite differently. Their desire for information is more equivocal than the model assumes; their taste for rational analysis is less pronounced; their personal beliefs are not as well developed, relevant, or strong; and their desire for control is more partial, ambivalent, and complex. Especially, many people do not hunger to make their own medical decisions. (28, pp. 229–230)

But Schneider stresses that the data and discussion he presents should not be taken as an argument for the restoration of medical paternalism or for the abandonment of autonomy as a legitimate goal of bioethics. Instead, he argues that in bioethics we need to accommodate people who aggressively want to make their own medical decisions, people who think they do but really do not, people who think they do not but really do, and people who aggressively do not. (28, p. 230)

We wholeheartedly concur. Far from suggesting wholesale abandonment of informed consent, the studies Schneider examines point to ways of improving the process by tailoring it to meet the needs of individual patients and to address the complexity of decisions required.

Thus, while the conditions of illness may indeed conflict with maximal autonomy, illness is compatible with the exercise of at least the rudiments of self-determination. Indeed, for some people, the experience of illness may itself inform and hone their values, bring them more in touch with what they really care about, and provide a unique opportunity for self-actualization. For some patients severely disabled by their illnesses, the realm of medical decision making may remain one domain in which they can remain effective, even if their normal activities are disrupted or largely curtailed.

The myriad ways that different patients may view informed consent—ranging from empowering to burdensome—suggest that patients should be asked about their decisionmaking preferences. Some patients may enjoy the sense of sharing in decision making but be reluctant to make the final decision. Some may like being kept informed but want to leave the direction of their care to someone else, for example, their family or doctor (e.g., 38). Those who prefer to share their decisional authority may be encouraged to do so. Chosen family members or other trusted advisors may be invited to participate in discussions with physicians, to become informed of treatment options along with the patient (or, in some cases, in accord with a patient's express preference, instead of the patient). Finally, as discussed in Chapter 4, waiver of the right of informed consent may be an option for patients who find the burden of decision making unbearable.

Some worries about the ability of patients to become sufficiently informed to make the decisions required of them may be addressed by developing innovative methods to educate patients about their conditions and possible medical interventions. Evidence about how much patients and research subjects actually understand and retain from the disclosure stage of the informed consent process indicates that informed consent best occurs against a backdrop of interventions designed to educate patients (and research subjects) over an extended period of time and with a variety of media (some of these are discussed in Chapters 8 and 9).

Just as important as improving the disclosure of information is addressing the psychological barriers to understanding. This, in turn, may require reconsideration of precisely what patients must understand to make adequately autonomous medical decisions. Some patients may feel abandoned at the crucial decisionmaking moment by the professional they have trusted and thus resist being forced to make a decision on their own. Others may feel frustrated at being asked to make what seems to be a technical decision for which they are less well equipped than their doctors. In fact, the doctrine of informed consent does not require that patients make what are primarily technical decisions, nor that they make decisions without advice from their physicians.

One model of informed consent as shared decision making imagines physicians supplying the diagnosis and treatment options and patients supplying the values and making a decision (39). For many patients this will be a desirable model, although they may need assistance in relating treatment options to their preferences and values. They may need guidance to trace out the implications of their desires in order to see how one option or another is favored by their preferences. As Schneider observes, it is possible "that doctors will already have done much of the work of integrating preferences into the decision by the time they present choices to their patients" (28, p. 107). So long as the preferences that are integrated are those of the individual patient, and not those of the physician or others, this preference-influenced presentation of options may be helpful and enhance, rather than hinder, autonomous decision making. To benefit from the expertise and experience of their physicians, however, it is crucial for patients to share their expertise to educate their physicians about the experience of their conditions and about what is important to them.

A primary benefit of recent scholarship like Schneider's and the data he examines is to illustrate the diversity of patient preferences with respect to medical decision making. As noted, appropriate responses to these diverse desires at the practical level, in the clinic, are addressed more fully in later chapters. The next section explores a further implication of the diversity of patients' preferences with respect to decision making.

Informed Consent: Right or Obligation

In *The Practice of Autonomy*, Schneider worries that bioethical argument surrounding informed consent has itself fallen prey to a sort of tyranny of the majority. He observes that bioethics has fallaciously reasoned that because a *majority* of people are thought to want to make healthcare decisions, *all* people want that decisional authority. Moreover, he argues, bioethics has been overly enamored with autonomy and independence. Some theorists have come to view the exercise of autonomy not as an entitlement, but as an obligation. While Dan Brock articulates "the moral doctrine of informed consent" as a doctrine that "*entitles, but does not require*, a patient to take an active role in decision making regarding treatment," others adopt what Schneider calls a "mandatory" model of autonomy (40, p. 33).

These advocates of autonomy "believe patients not only may, but should, or even must, make 'autonomous' decisions" (28, p. 17). Mandating that patients decide autonomously about their care is thought to combat their magical thinking about their illnesses, their myth making about their doctors, and their "false consciousness" whereby they are duped by the cultural and economic power of medicine into mistakenly believing that they want to delegate decisionmaking authority (1,28). Haavi Morreim, for example, states that "in matters of health, and of health care, it is time to expect competent patients to assume substantially greater responsibility. In the first place, they should generally make their own decisions. Not only is the patient entitled to decide these issues that affect his life so fundamentally; he has a presumptive obligation to do so" (41, p. 139). But why? It would seem that the diversity of patient preferences requires that the question of whether informed consent is a right or an obligation of patients and subjects should be resolved in favor of patients' rights.

Like Schneider, we argue against the "mandatory autonomy" view. We believe that informed consent is a right of patients (and subjects) and that as part of that right, patients may seek advice from and even share decision making with those whom they trust. The duty to disclose, to answer patient questions, and to ensure so far as possible that the patient may make a voluntary decision—these are concomitant duties of physicians (and researchers). Nevertheless, it is instructive to examine moral arguments in support of imposing an obligation to decide autonomously. The content of these arguments helps to explain the importance of ensuring that patients and subjects have the right of informed consent. In fact, properly understood, these arguments undermine attempts to mandate autonomy.

Thinking back to Kant's conception of people as self-legislating agents, we can see the roots of the moral argument for mandating autonomous decision making. In the Kantian tradition, people have a duty to exercise their power of self-legislating choice to shape their own destinies. Self-reflection and either active choice or acceptance-upon-reflection are the essence of authenticity. By making choices that reflect one's deeply held values, one can craft a life of authenticity that expresses one's uniqueness. Kant specifically claims that people have a moral duty to develop their talents, but the particular path of development is left to each to determine on her own.

Liberation and self-actualization, themes that characterized the 1960s in America, are actually mutually reinforcing moral goals and prescriptions. As free or autonomous individuals we must act. If we did not choose to act, and choose the particular course of action, our freedom would be not only meaningless but not even evident. Drawing on this ethical tradition, the sanctity of the individual conscience to which the Puritans were so dedicated, and the individualism of the frontier, the American cultural tradition of "rugged individualism" takes as its icons explorers, pioneers, and entrepreneurs, those non-conformist, action-oriented individuals who strike off on their own. Even the most conformity-demanding of all American groups, the army, urges recruits to join by appealing to authenticity: "Be all that you can be." In the latter part of the twentieth century, the drive for individualism returned to the inner frontier of the psyche from which, in its religious grounding, it originally sprang. Self-understanding and self-assertion became modern day "virtues," inculcated by the thriving self-help industry.

Drawing on these moral and cultural traditions, mandatory autonomists argue that one should not burden others with medical decisions and that one owes it to oneself to guide one's own care, as a matter of both self-protection and self-expression. Autonomous people can, and thus should, make autonomous decisions. However, just as one can sometimes pursue one's own, authentically chosen life plan by conforming to the dictates of others (e.g., by joining the army or a religious order), one can also be an autonomous moral agent without choosing autonomously all the time in every instance. A person can act autonomously and responsibly without micromanaging every decision about his car's repair, or even the details of his employment contract. In leaving the details to his mechanic or his lawyer, he does not shirk his moral responsibility, although he may indeed be acting at his own peril should they not decide as he would prefer. Although Talcott Parsons may be correct that those occupying the sick role have a responsibility to seek to get well, it is not clear that they shirk their duty if they entrust decisions about their treatment to someone else (42). Indeed, for the substantial number of people who apparently would prefer not to make their own healthcare decisions, not to delegate those decisions would seem inauthentic.

Reconceptualizing Autonomy

Trying to square the apparent actual preferences of these reluctant decision makers with the autonomy orientation of bioethics, especially a mandate of autonomy, is not merely a practical problem, but a theoretical challenge. Schneider vividly concludes: "I neither want nor expect autonomy to lose its status in the centerpiece of bioethics. But that centerpiece should be a whole bouquet of concepts, and not just the single flower of autonomy, however beguiling it may be" (28, p. 33). Some commentators have also suggested that autonomy itself is not the monolithic concept it is sometimes imagined to be; as a flower, instead of being simply an American Beauty, autonomy would be more of a varietal that comes in several hues.

Communitarian and feminist theorists have criticized as unrealistic and morally undesirable the image of an isolated, perfectly rational, prudential decision maker who privately weighs all the information disclosed, in light of her personal values and individual interests. Susan Sherwin, for example, points out that autonomy is traditionally regarded as the "instrument of agency for individuals who are perceived as separate, independent, and fully rational" (43, p. 137). Far from being an appropriate ideal of informed consent, this image is a caricature of actual informed consent and of the people it is designed to protect. No one should be expected or encouraged to make a purely self-interested decision in isolation. Patients should (and do) consult those who will be affected by their decisions and who help to inform their values (44–49). Interests are not purely individual (50). As a recent and abundant body of literature suggests, there is considerable controversy (e.g., at the level of institutional policy) and myriad opinions (at the personal level) about the role intimates should play in patients' decision making and about the relevance of familial interests in those decisions. In contrast to strict adherents to individualism, some of these more communitarian writers open the door to inquiring about the relevance for medical decision making of other interests, for example, broader social interests or interests of a patient's chosen community, like a church congregation. The consensus seems to be that if the patient (or research subject) herself considers these interests important, then she may, or even should, give them some weight. On the other hand, it would be wrong for her physician (or a researcher) to insist that she take others' interests into account.

Communitarian and feminist writers who insist that people do not make decisions in isolation force advocates of autonomy to recognize that individuals participate in webs of social relationships and bring to their decision making complicated sets of commitments, including commitments to particular others, to communities, and to ideals. Honoring those commitments and maintaining those relationships may sometimes conflict with the pursuit of medical treatment and health, and thus with narrowly defined self-interest. These theorists advocate a notion of autonomy that is cognizant of individuals' relatedness and of the social context of both decision making and the formulation of personal values. Their arguments help to make sense of how people actually make decisions that reflect their values. They also help to explain a particularly well studied class of decisions that appear to violate the demands of informed consent as autonomous authorization: decisions to donate organs to emotionally related others (51). Living related donors tend to make their decisions to donate immediately, prior to disclosure of the risks and benefits of donation. Moreover, many speak of feeling morally compelled to donate or of having no choice in the matter (52). Understanding autonomy in terms of authentic decision making, and recognizing the role of others in an individual's life plan, make sense of these donors' decisions as autonomous authorizations.

Recent attention to the concept of autonomy reflects the importance of self-determination in contemporary medicine and bioethics, as well as the vitality of autonomy in American culture more generally. It also reveals that autonomy is a more complex ideal than previously recognized and that, in some ways, respecting autonomy may be more complicated in practice than previously thought. On the other hand, reconceptualizing autonomy—to take account of how people are interrelated and how individuals' interests are rarely purely self-interested and often reflect social values—may actually bring theory in line with practice.

Bioethicists who have been critical of the field's apparent preoccupation with autonomy, particularly an individualistic conception of autonomy, and with autonomy's ascendancy over other ethical principles and concerns, are nevertheless generally supportive of the advances against medical paternalism that the implementation of informed consent represents. They believe that autonomy-oriented analyses often do not go far enough in addressing ethical concerns. They believe that while an emphasis on autonomy and informed consent has opened doors for patients to make their own values effective, it has not opened doors equally for all patients and has also closed some paths of ethical inquiry that would benefit some patients more (53). Sherwin, for example, comments that

> the concept of autonomy, rather than working to empower the oppressed and exploited among us, in practice often serves to protect the privileges of the most powerful. . . . [G]reater equality is a precondition for any meaningful exercise of autonomy by seriously disadvantaged members of society. Therefore, theories that place priority on autonomy—at least as the concept is commonly interpreted—must be understood as primarily protecting the autonomy of those who are already well-situated, while sacrificing the necessary prerequisites for autonomy for others. (54, p. 53)

Although many would find this criticism of bioethics' autonomy orientation too extreme, it is instructively ironic to note that in the 1960s, the assertion of individualism and autonomy was coupled with demands for social justice and pleas to assume social responsibility. In medicine, as in much of American society, the ethics of the individual and of the community came uncoupled. In bioethics, issues are often analyzed either in terms of autonomy or in terms of justice, and generally are considered in separate chapters of prominent texts. Thus, questions considered in terms of the demands of informed consent, with its grounding in autonomy, are somewhat isolated from background considerations of, for example, the justice of social arrangements of medicine and research within which the questions arise (3). With respect to ethics in research, there is an attempt to move analysis beyond questions of consent to issues of justice (55).

Feminist commentators have worried that so long as bioethics considered a valid informed consent to be the last word in ethical analysis, people would be asked and allowed to continue to act in ways that may be contrary to their long-term self-interest and not in accordance with the values that they would truly hold upon self-reflection. They stress, however, that the problem is not informed consent per se, but the lack of attention to considerations of equality, prevailing social norms, and unjust social conditions.

These critiques indicate that while autonomy may be losing its hegemonic hold on bioethical analysis, it is not declining in importance (56). Instead, other values and considerations are moving to the forefront of ethical attention along with autonomy. In 1988 when Edmund Pellegrino and David Thomasma published *For the Patient's Good: The Restoration of Beneficence in Health Care*, they wrote of the "boldness" of their attempt to reconcile the traditional conflict between patient autonomy and medical paternalism by viewing autonomy and attention to the patient's self-defined good as preconditions of medical beneficence (57). Today it is still somewhat heretical, even risky, to recount these challenges to informed consent in a book that seeks to convince clinicians, researchers, and the public they serve that informed consent is a practically and morally valuable social practice. Susan Wolf notes that there are "renewed challenges now to the very notion of patients' rights," (56) and Schneider takes pains not to recommend throwing out the whole bioethical enterprise of informed consent because thorny issues surrounding autonomy have taken the bloom off its initial promise (28). We do not mean to join in challenges to patients' rights. We believe that the process of informed consent is still the most promising path to patients' receiving care that is for their own good, as they themselves define it.

However, we are skeptical of a "one size fits all" process and are critical of "one shot" attempts to obtain informed consent or refusal (the event model of informed consent—see Chapter 8). We advocate increased patient and research subject education beyond the requirements of informed consent. We are also concerned both about attempts to force patients to make "autonomous" decisions when they do not want to assume that responsibility and about blithe acceptance of waivers of informed consent. Finally, perhaps more than some recent commentators, we highlight the different practical and moral pitfalls that may attend the informed consent process in research settings, as opposed to clinical care. Whereas it might be ethically acceptable for patients to delegate medical decisions in a clinical context still designed for their benefit, it seems both personally risky and unduly burdensome to others for competent persons to delegate such decisions regarding participation in research, which is by definition designed to benefit third parties, members of a future generation of patients.

With this background in the ethical underpinnings of informed consent, we turn now to consider the legal roots of the doctrine.

References

1. Katz, J. (1984) *The Silent World of Doctor and Patient.* New York: Free Press.
2. Faden, R.R. and Beauchamp, T.L. (1986) *A History and Theory of Informed Consent.* New York: Oxford University Press.
3. Wolf, S.M. (1996) Introduction: gender and feminism in bioethics. In Wolf, S.M. (ed) *Feminism and Bioethics: Beyond Reproduction.* New York: Oxford University Press.
4. President's Commission for the Study of Ethical Problems in Medicine and Biomedical and Behavioral Research (1982) *Making Health Care Decisions.* Volume 1. Washington, D.C.: U.S. Government Printing Office.

5. Beauchamp, T.L. and Childress, J.F. (1994) *Principles of Biomedical Ethics,* 4th ed. New York: Oxford University Press.
6. Pernick, M.S. (1982) The patient's role in medical decisionmaking: a social history of informed consent in medical therapy. In President's Commission for the Study of Ethical Problems in Medicine and Biomedical and Behavioral Research, *Making Health Care Decisions.* Volume 3. Washington, D.C.: U.S. Government Printing Office.
7. Gerle, B., Lundin, G., and Sandblom, P. (1960) The patient with inoperable cancer from the psychiatric and social standpoint. *Cancer,* 13:1206–1217.
8. Koocher, G.P. (1986) Psychosocial issues during the acute treatment of pediatric cancer. *Cancer,* 58:468–472.
9. Slavin, L.A., O'Malley, M.D., Koocher, G.P., and Foster, D.J. (1982) Communication of the cancer diagnosis to pediatric patients: impact on long-term adjustment. *Am J Psychiatry,* 139:179–183.
10. Davis, M. (1969) Variations in patients' compliance with doctors' advice: an empirical analysis of patterns of communication. *Am J Public Health,* 58:274–288.
11. Davis, M. (1971) Variation in patients' compliance with doctors' orders: medical practice and doctor-patient interaction. *Psychiatry Med,* 2:31–54.
12. Fox, R.C. (1974) *Experiment Perilous: Physicians and Patients Facing the Unknown.* Philadelphia: University of Pennsylvania Press.
13. Francis, V., Korsch, B.M., and Morris, M.J. (1969) Gaps in doctor-patient communications: patients' response to medical advice. *N Engl J Med,* 280:535–540.
14. Schneider, J.W. and Conrad, P. (1983) *Having Epilepsy: The Experience and Control of Illness.* Philadelphia: Temple University Press.
15. Stone, G.C. (1979) Patient compliance and the role of the expert. *J Soc Issues,* 35:34–59.
16. Roter, D.L. and Hall, J.A. (1989) Studies of doctor-patient interaction. *Ann Rev Public Health,* 10:163–180.
17. Greenfield, S., Kaplan, S., and Ware, J.E. (1985) Expanding patient involvement in care: effects on patient outcomes. *Ann Intern Med,* 102:520–528.
18. Kaplan, R.M. (1991) Health-related quality of life in patient decision making. *J Soc Issues,* 47:69–90.
19. Sartorius, R. (1983) *Paternalism.* Minneapolis: University of Minnesota Press.
20. Dworkin, G. (1988) *The Theory and Practice of Autonomy.* Cambridge: Cambridge University Press.
21. Cohen, M., Nagel, T., and Scanlon, T. (1981) *Medicine and Moral Philosophy.* Princeton: Princeton University Press.
22. Ross, J.W., Bayley, C., Michel, V., and Pugh, D. (1986) *Handbook for Hospital Ethics Committees.* Chicago: American Hospital Publishing.
23. Smart, J.C.C. and Williams, B. (1973) *Utilitarianism For and Against.* Cambridge: Cambridge University Press.
24. Mill, J.S. (1978) *On Liberty.* Indianapolis: Hackett Publishing Co. (originally published 1859).
25. National Society of Genetic Counselors (1992) Code of Ethics. URL: *http://www.nsgc.org/ethicsCode.html,* accessed October 11, 2000.
26. 18 Pa.C.S. § 3204 (1999).
27. Katz, J. and Capron, A. (1975) *Catastrophic Diseases: Who Decides What?* New York: Russell Sage Foundation.

28. Schneider, C.E. (1998) *The Practice of Autonomy: Patients, Doctors, and Medical Decisions*. New York: Oxford University Press.
29. Beckman, H.B., Markakis, K.M., Suchman, A.L., and Frankel, R.M. (1994) The doctor-patient relationship and malpractice. *Arch Intern Med*, 154:1365–1370.
30. Hickson, G.B., Clayton, E.W., Githens, P.B., and Sloan, F.A. (1992) Factors that prompted families to file medical malpractice claims following perinatal injuries. *JAMA*, 267:1359–1363.
31. Hickson, G.B., Clayton, E.W., Entman, S.S., Miller, C.S., Githens, P.B., Whetten-Goldstein, K., and Sloan, F.A. (1994) Obstetricians' prior malpractice experience and patients' satisfaction with care. *JAMA*, 272:1583–1587.
32. Levinson, W., Roter, D.L., Mullooly, J.P., Dull, V.T., and Frankel, R.M. (1997) Physician-patient communication: the relationship with malpractice claims among primary care physicians and surgeons. *JAMA*, 277:553–559.
33. Nease, R.F. and Brooks, W.B. (1995) Patient desire for information and decision making in health care decisions: the autonomy preference index and the health opinion survey. *J Gen Intern Med*, 10:593–600.
34. Ende, J., Kazis, L., Ash, A., and Moskowitz, M.A. (1989) Measuring patients' desire for autonomy: decision making and information-seeking preferences among medical patients. *J Gen Intern Med*, 4:23–30.
35. Sacks, O. (1984) *A Leg to Stand On*. New York: Summit Books.
36. Janis, I.L. (1984) The patient as decision maker. In Gentry, W.D. (ed) *Handbook of Behavioral Medicine*. New York: Guilford Press.
37. Shiloh, S. (1996) Decision-making in the context of genetic risk. In Marteau, T. and Richards, M. (eds) *The Troubled Helix: Social and Psychological Implications of the New Genetics*. Cambridge: Cambridge University Press.
38. Strull, W.M., Lo, B., and Charles, G. (1984) Do patients want to participate in medical decision making? *JAMA*, 252:2990–2994.
39. Brock, D.W. (1991) The ideal of shared decision making between physicians and patients. *Kennedy Inst Ethics J*, 1:28–47.
40. Brock, D.W. (1993) *Life and Death: Philosophical Essays in Biomedical Ethics*. Cambridge: Cambridge University Press.
41. Morreim, E.H. (1995) *Balancing Act: The New Medical Ethics of Medicine's New Economics*. Washington, D.C.: Georgetown University Press.
42. Parsons, T. (1951) *The Social System*. Glencoe: Free Press.
43. Sherwin, S. (1992) *No Longer Patient: Feminist Ethics and Health Care*. Philadelphia: Temple University Press.
44. Bluestein, J. (1993) The family in medical decision making. *Hastings Cent Rep*, 23(3):6–13.
45. Doukas, D.J. (1991) Autonomy and beneficence in the family: describing the family covenant. *J Clin Ethics*, 2:145–148.
46. Hardwig, J. (1990) What about the family? *Hastings Cent Rep*, 20(2):5–10.
47. Mappes, T.A. and Zembaty, J.S. (1994) Patient choices, family interests, and physician obligations. *Kennedy Inst Ethics J*, 4:27–46.
48. Nelson, J.L. (1992) Taking families seriously. *Hastings Cent Rep*, 22(4):6–12.
49. Strong, C. (1993) Patients should not always come first in treatment decisions. *J Clin Ethics*, 4:63–65.
50. Loewy, E.H. (1991) Families, communities, and making medical decisions. *J Clin Ethics* 2:150–153.

51. Majeske, R.A., Parker, L.S., and Frader, J. (1996) An ethical framework for consideration of decisions regarding live organ donation. In Spielman, B. (ed) *Organ and Tissue Donation: Ethical, Legal, and Policy Issues.* Carbondale: Southern Illinois University Press.
52. Simmons, R.G., Marine, S.K., and Simmons, R.L. (1987) *The Gift of Life: The Effect of Organ Transplantation on Individual, Family, and Societal Dynamics.* New Brunswick: Transaction Book.
53. Roberts, D.E. (1996) Reconstructing the patient: starting with women of color. In Wolf, S.M. (ed) *Feminism and Bioethics: Beyond Reproduction.* New York: Oxford University Press.
54. Sherwin, S. (1996) Feminism and bioethics. In Wolf, S.M. (ed) *Feminism and Bioethics: Beyond Reproduction.* New York: Oxford University Press.
55. Kahn, J.P., Mastroianni, A.C., and Sugarman, J. (1998) *Beyond Consent: Seeking Justice in Research.* New York: Oxford University Press.
56. Wolf, S. (1994) Shifting paradigms in bioethics and health law: the rise of a new pragmatism. *Am J Law Med,* 20:395–415.
57. Pellegrino, E.D. and Thomasma, D.C. (1988) *For the Patient's Good: The Restoration of Beneficence in Health Care.* New York: Oxford University Press.

Part II

The Legal Theory of Informed
Consent

3

The Legal Requirements for Disclosure and Consent: History and Current Status

The translation of ethical principles into concrete requirements for physicians' behavior has been largely a function of the courts (usually state, occasionally federal) as they consider patients' allegations that their physicians improperly obtained their consent to treatment. To a lesser extent, state legislatures have been involved in making law in this area. The combined efforts of courts and legislatures have resulted in the creation of two legal requirements: the historical requirement that physicians obtain patients' consent before proceeding with treatment, and the more recent requirement that physicians disclose such information to patients as will enable them to participate knowledgeably in making decisions about treatment. (Chapters 4 and 5 describe the exceptional circumstances in which some or all of the basic legal requirements do not apply.)

The Historical Context

Despite some uncertainty about the origins of legal actions for lack of consent to medical treatment, in theory, non-consensual medical treatment has always been remediable at common law (i.e., judge-made as opposed to statutory law). The law's concern for the bodily integrity of the individual can be traced to the writ of trespass for assault and battery and to the criminal law's proscription of homicide, battery, and mayhem (1). A similar, though less intense, concern for psychic integrity has existed for almost as long and has received increasing support in this century as evidenced by the cases recognizing causes of action in tort law for intentional and, more recently, negligent infliction of emotional distress (2, §§ 12, 54). Similarly, the development of the constitutional and tort law of privacy reflects the continued vitality of society's concern for the individual's right to be let alone, both by agents of the state and by private parties (2, §117; 3).

Early medical practice codes did not speak of consent—it was more likely that a physician would conceal his actions from the patient than seek his or her consent to treatment. However, patient consent is not completely a modern legal creation. Historically, the notion that physicians must inform patients about what will be done to them has its origins in eighteenth-century English law (4). In the 1767 case of *Slater v. Baker and Stapleton,* the court held that because the professional custom among surgeons was to obtain consent from their patients before beginning treatment, it was only fair to impose liability on a physician who failed to meet this standard of care (5).

> [I]t appears from the evidence of the surgeons that it was improper to disunite the [partially healed fracture] without consent; this is the usage and law of surgeons: then it was ignorance and unskillfulness in that very particular, to do contrary to the rule of the profession, what no surgeon ought to have done. (5)

Not only was it customary for the surgeon to obtain the patient's consent, the court observed, but "indeed it is reasonable that a patient should be told what is about to be done to him that he may take courage and put himself in such a situation as to enable him to undergo the operation" (5). Thus, one rationale for the custom was that physicians needed patients' cooperation if surgery were to be performed without the use of an anesthetic, as was then necessary. The court's observation regarding the role of communication shows a pragmatic or consequentialist justification for informed consent, rather than one focused on information disclosure as a good in itself or on a patient's right to control what happens to his body. In line with this justification, there is a good deal of evidence to suggest that physicians historically saw the requirements for consent as minimal, requiring that little or no information be disclosed before permission to proceed was obtained. Even some distortion of the facts was tolerated in the name of encouraging patients' compliance and cooperation.

The paucity of cases prior to the beginning of the twentieth century that question the legal authority of physicians to render treatment speaks equally to the previously restricted societal role of the medical profession and to the similarly restricted role of litigation as a means of resolving disputes. However, even when such cases began to arise, courts were willing to find that a patient had not provided valid consent to treatment only in the most egregious circumstances. A simple interchange between patient and physician long passed for valid consent.

In substance the physician said to the patient, "You need to do thus-and-so to get better," and the patient responded with some phrase or action indicating the intention to go along with the doctor's recommendations or not. The response may have been very broad: "O.K. Doc, whatever you say"; slightly less inclusive: "Go ahead and do thus-and-so"; somewhat more limiting: "Go ahead and do *thus*, but I don't want you to do any *so*" (6–9); or even totally restrictive: "If that's what I need, then I'd rather be sick, and don't do anything at all" (10–12).

Each of these responses (even the express prohibition!) has been considered authorization to treat by physicians at various times. The courts have generally agreed that the patient has, by speaking some phrase, authorized the physician to proceed and thereby provided the physician with a defense to an action for battery. We refer to this as a "simple consent" requirement.

It was not until the beginning of the twentieth century that litigation over the requirement of consent to medical treatment began in earnest. Slowly the realization grew that an authorization consistent with the principle of autonomy might be more complicated than it originally seemed (13). For example, the doctor might not have merely said, "You need thus-and-so to get better," but in an attempt to put an anxious patient at ease added, "Oh, it's not a serious operation at all." The patient might then have agreed to undergo the procedure, much assured that it was a simple operation, and been distraught at the conclusion of the operation when undesirable results were discovered (14–17).

As a result, a more complicated set of rules began to develop beyond the original simple proposition that a physician might not treat a patient without the patient's authorization. Not only was the physician required to obtain the patient's consent to treatment, but if the physician affirmatively misrepresented the nature of the procedure and its probable consequences, the misrepresentation might be held to invalidate the patient's consent, leaving the physician open to a claim for unauthorized treatment (12,14–16,18,19). The courts uniformly held that fraudulent, deceptive, or misleading disclosure vitiated the consent that the patient subsequently gave (14–17).

This early rule—that ordinarily no information need be provided, but if the physician did provide information, it must be truthful—contained the seed of the requirement of an affirmative duty of disclosure. Although several cases before the middle of the twentieth century intimated that this duty existed, they were greatly scattered both temporally and geographically, and even in retrospect do not constitute any coherent pattern (15,20,21).

The Transition from Simple to Informed Consent

In the 1914 case of *Schloendorff v. Society of New York Hospital*, Justice Cardozo noted that "every human being of adult years and sound mind has a right to determine what shall be done with his body" (22). The case emphasized the concept of *voluntary* consent, that is, that the patient must freely give permission for a specific procedure to occur. This was an obvious next step from the simple consent requirements identified previously, since an involuntary (or non-voluntary) consent is really no consent at all. During the next few decades there was some litigation regarding consent. But it was not until the 1950s that a clear transition from the older simple consent rule to the first contemporary *informed* consent cases began to develop.

In 1955, the Supreme Court of North Carolina stated that the failure to explain the risks involved in surgery "may be considered a mistake on the part of the surgeon" (17). Two years later, in *Salgo v. Leland Stanford Junior University Board of Trustees*, a California court—relying in part on the North Carolina precedent—specifically held that physicians had an affirmative duty of disclosure. The following year, the Supreme Court of Minnesota reinforced this duty. It held a physician liable for failing to inform a patient before surgery of alternative forms of treatment that would not have entailed the undesirable consequence of the procedure actually performed (23). Thus began the modern evolution of informed consent, which not only requires *free* consent but also requires that patients be fully *informed* by practitioners about risks and benefits and other aspects of treatment (24).

While some courts at this time were imposing this affirmative duty of disclosure upon physicians, others were reiterating the older view that physicians had no such duty (25,26). One New York court actually imposed liability upon a physician for mental anguish caused by information he disclosed to the patient about her condition and its proper treatment (27). Even the *Salgo* court failed to offer a detailed and explicit statement of what kinds of information the affirmative duty of disclosure entailed; a jury verdict for the plaintiff was reversed on appeal, on the ground that the trial court's instruction on the duty to inform went further than required.

The Doctrine Defined

Salgo is probably the most significant case in the mid-1950s, primarily because it coined the term "informed consent." The case involved a patient who underwent translumbar aortography— a now outmoded technique of puncturing the aorta through the back, in order to inject a radio-opaque dye— and suffered paralysis of the legs, a rare but not unheard-of complication. The patient alleged, among other complaints, that insufficient information had been given to him beforehand about the procedure (24). The court ruled that "a physician violates his duty to his patient and subjects himself to liability if he withholds any facts which are necessary to form the basis of an intelligent consent by the patient to the proposed treatment" (24, p. 181). At the same time, in elaborating on this principle, the court stated that the jury should be instructed that "the physician has . . . discretion [to withhold alarming information from the patient] consistent, of course, with the full disclosure of facts necessary to an informed consent" (24, p. 181). Thus *Salgo* also focused on the physician's discretion to *withhold* facts that may alarm the patient, the so-called therapeutic exception, which will be discussed later. Even as the courts were developing informed consent requirements, they were hesitant to mandate full disclosure by physicians.

The result, as Jay Katz has cogently observed, is that the case contributed substantially to the confusion that already existed and continues to exist about the requirement of the informed consent doctrine. This is because *Salgo* attempts to reconcile two inherently contradictory terms: "Only in dreams or fairy tales," Katz wrote, "can 'discretion' to withhold crucial information so easily and magically be reconciled with 'full disclosure'"(28). Nevertheless, *Salgo* did provide a certain stability to the notion of a duty to disclose by using the term informed consent, a handy (if facile) means of describing the evolving legal requirement. But despite its use of the new term, *Salgo* did not advance the developing law a great deal.

It took another three years for the courts to begin systematically to sketch the contours of the doctrine. Two cases decided in different jurisdictions within two days of each other in 1960 clearly indicated that there was to be no turning back from the imposition of an affirmative duty of disclosure. Judicial movement beyond the simple consent requirement was in evidence during the 1950s, but the decisions in *Natanson v. Kline* (29) and *Mitchell v. Robinson* (30) clearly established that the simple ways of the past would no longer suffice.

In *Natanson*, a woman had suffered substantial burns to the thorax from radiation therapy performed after a mastectomy. In *Mitchell*, the plaintiff received insulin shock and electroshock therapy for the treatment of schizophrenia, causing the fracture of several vertebrae. In both cases the patients' consents to treatment had been obtained. However, they asserted that their physicians had been under an affirmative duty to them to disclose information about the risks of treatment, that this duty had not been fulfilled, and that the breach constituted negligence. Both courts agreed. The *Mitchell* court phrased the duty as requiring the physician "to inform [the patient] generally of the possible serious collateral hazards" (30, p. 19). The *Natanson* court went further, and described the doctor's duty as requiring

> a reasonable disclosure . . . of the nature and probable consequences of the suggested or recommended . . . treatment, and . . . a reasonable disclosure of the dangers within his knowledge which were incident to, or possible in, the treatment he proposed to administer. (29, p. 1106)

Mitchell and *Natanson* both held that the central information that needed to be disclosed was the possible bad results of a particular procedure. The possible bad results, which courts have described in several ways—as side effects, collateral hazards, dangers, perils—are today generally referred to as the *risks* of the procedure. It is self-evident that if persons are to make informed, autonomous choices, they must be told not only that the procedures are intended to diagnose or treat the condition from which they suffer but also that the procedures may fail to do so, or that patients may be worse off after the procedures. Disclosure of risks does not guarantee that patients will utilize the information or that their decisions will be reasonable. Yet without this information, most patients are unable to make the kind of informed decisions that are central to the ethical notion of informed choice.

Although *Mitchell* mandated only the disclosure of risk information, *Natanson* went further, to require disclosure of the nature of the ailment, the nature of the proposed treatment, the probability of success, and possible alternative treatments. These requirements, with slight modifications of terminology, are now the bedrock elements of the disclosure requirement imposed by courts and statutes on physicians.

Standards of Disclosure

Professional Standards

In the formative years of the legal doctrine of informed consent, the 1950s and 1960s, the courts held that the degree of disclosure made to patients was primarily a question of medical judgment. Consequently, "[t]he duty of the physician to disclose . . . is limited to those disclosures which a reasonable medical practitioner would make under the same or similar circumstances" (29, p. 1106). This standard closely parallels the one used in medical negligence or malpractice cases generally: physicians are held to the standard of what is customary and usual in the profession, not only in the exercise of skill but also in the disclosure of information to patients (31,32). The courts of numerous jurisdictions adopted this rule, and few seriously questioned it for more than a decade (33).

The advantages of this professional or customary standard include the legal system's familiarity with it, and the maintenance of the medical profession's freedom (as a whole, not necessarily the freedom of individual physicians) to shape the contours of appropriate disclosure. If one believes, perhaps as a result of dealing with many patients over the years, that doctors generally know how much a patient should be told about a medical procedure (because they know what factors are objectively important and also what issues seem to be of greatest concern to patients), then the professional standard may be acceptable and even desirable. In addition, the professional standard places no extra burden on physicians to conform to an externally imposed standard, since they presumably already know about and observe professional norms.

However, three problems with the use of a professional standard quickly become apparent. First, as Judge Robinson remarked in the landmark case of *Canterbury v. Spence*, it is not at all certain for many medical procedures that there is "any discernable custom reflecting a professional concensus [*sic*] on communication of option and risk information to patients" regarding recommended treatment (32). In other words, in cases where there is no professional custom of disclosing, the legal right to obtain information is undermined by professional practice.

Second, even where professional standards exist, they may be set too low to satisfy the needs of patients who wish to participate in medical decision making in accord with the idea of informed consent. For example, the custom of physicians may be to inform patients of only the minor risks of a particular procedure, so as not to frighten off patients from receiving treatment. Although the motivation may be to help patients based on what physicians view as their patients' best interests, this degree of restriction on disclosure utterly vitiates the purposes of informed consent. In addition, even a standard of fairly complete disclosure of information that *physicians* believe to be important does not offer recourse to a patient whose injury resulted from a procedure consented to without benefit of information that most *patients* would want to know. Physicians and patients may find different information important to treatment decisions. Moreover, disclosing information does not appear to depend on medical skill, thus further calling into question a professional practice standard for disclosure.

Third, in cases where professional standards are used, the plaintiff must obtain an expert witness, in this instance a physician familiar with the relevant subject matter, to establish the standard of care (34). (See Chapter 6 for a more complete discussion.) For a variety of reasons, getting expert witness testimony has proved to be as onerous a requirement in informed consent litigation as it has been in other kinds of malpractice cases (33). A plaintiff's primary difficulty in obtaining an expert witness is the unwillingness of physicians to testify against other physicians (35). This obstacle is often reduced if the plaintiff is permitted to seek out a physician who practices in another city, county, or state. However, in the 1960s and early 1970s, many courts held firm to an old rule known as the locality rule: to establish the standard of care in a malpractice case, one had to use an expert witness familiar with the standard of practice in the defendant-doctor's own locality. The rationale was that it was manifestly unfair to hold physicians to standards of practice that their geographic isolation and limited resources might not permit them to attain.

Because of improved means of transportation and communication and a growing belief within the profession that standards should not be disparate, the rationale for the locality rule has eroded, and its use has declined (36). Nevertheless, a number of courts still adhere to it, some informed consent legislation also employs it (37–40), and it occasionally continues to be applied in informed consent cases (41,42).

Patient-Oriented Standards

Within a matter of months in 1971 and 1972, a number of courts challenged the slightly more than ten-year-old rule regarding the professional standard of disclosure (32,43–45). Because there may be no custom in the medical profession to disclose information to patients, because disclosure of information does not bring the physician's special medical knowledge and skills peculiarly into play (32), and because of the difficulty in obtaining expert witnesses, these courts rejected the professional standard of disclosure. In its place they required that physicians disclose as much information as a *patient* would want to know. This new formulation of the standard of care was variously referred to as the lay, legal, or patient-oriented standard—lay, because the adequacy of disclosure was applied by laypersons (jurors) unaided by expert witnesses; legal, because it was imposed by courts rather than by medical custom; and patient-oriented because its aim was that patients be provided with information that would enable them to make informed choices.

The question of which patient to use as the benchmark arose immediately as an important issue. A fair statement of the rule that emerged is that the physician is required to disclose all information about a proposed treatment that a reasonable person in the patient's circumstances would find material to a decision either to undergo or forgo treatment (32). The scope of the duty to disclose was determined by what is called the patient's right to decide, not by the custom or practice of either the particular physician or the larger medical profession. The patient-oriented standard of disclosure was rapidly adopted by the courts. Between 1970, when it was formulated by Waltz and Scheuneman (46), and 1978 about half of the courts considering the issue moved in this direction. Since then, however, there has been a gradual reverse trend, prompted mostly by legislatures that overturned judicial applications of the patient-oriented standard. At this time roughly half the states use a professional standard of disclosure, and half use a patient standard.

The adoption of patient-oriented standards was motivated in part by the lack of professional standards of disclosure and by plaintiffs' difficulties obtaining expert witnesses. However, the fundamental motivation was the underlying rationale of the informed consent doctrine: to permit patients to exercise choice concerning the risks to which they are willing to subject themselves. Thus, the *Canterbury* court, in the leading opinion among these cases, concluded that "[r]espect for the patient's right of self-determination on particular therapy demands a standard set by law for physicians rather than one which physicians may or may not impose upon themselves" (32, p. 784). To permit physicians to determine what information is to be disclosed by reference either to their own personal standards or to standards of the medical profession is to undercut the right of patients to have information available that they might find relevant to the decisions they must make.

This last point is particularly important because it reflects a recognition that the informed consent requirement goes beyond the older, simple consent requirement in the interests that it protects. The purpose of the simple consent requirement—protecting patients from unwanted interferences with their bodily integrity—was important, but limited in comparison with the other purpose of informed consent, which is to permit patients to make informed choices about their health care.

The patient-oriented standard imposes upon physicians more substantial obligations than the professional standard. Assuming that it actually is the custom of the profession to make disclosure to patients, physicians have reasonably ready ways of knowing what the professional standard is and of complying with it. Medical education and supervised clinical training, formal continuing education, and informal discourse among colleagues all help to inform physicians as to what it is customary to tell patients about treatment. For the same reasons that the content of the standard is easily accessible to physicians, it is relatively simple to establish in a trial, assuming that other physicians are willing to serve as expert witnesses.

By comparison, the content of the patient-oriented standard is more difficult for physicians to ascertain. The professional standard is factual and therefore empirically determinable; the patient-oriented standard is hypothetical. It requires physicians to disclose the information that a reasonably prudent person would find material to making a decision. The reasonably prudent person of tort law is a hypothetical construct used by the fact finders—usually jurors, in informed consent cases—to develop and apply what they perceive to be community standards of reasonable conduct. After a particular kind of problem is litigated, more concrete standards may begin to evolve, with the speed of their evolution depending on the frequency of litigation. But within very broad limits, the jury is free to write on a clean slate. Previous jury verdicts are not binding precedent. In every case, the jury is required to determine what would have been reasonable disclosure, taking into account all the facts and circumstances of the particular case.

The very difficulty of knowing and applying the patient-oriented standard could turn out to be its virtue, though possibly not from the physicians' perspective. To determine what a reasonable patient would find material to making a decision, physicians are compelled to engage in discussion with patients. In so doing, they act to implement one of the fundamental goals of the idea of informed consent: to involve patients in decision making about their own care. This, of course, is an idealized version of how informed consent operates under the patient-oriented standard. Empirical evidence in support of the existence of this ideal is lacking. In fact, there is some evidence to the contrary showing that physicians do not engage in discussions with patients and are just as likely unilaterally to decide what to disclose under a patient-oriented standard as under a professional standard (47).

It has been argued that even the patient-oriented standard as formulated in *Canterbury* is not entirely adequate to making the legal requirements true to the idea of informed consent. To the extent that informed consent is intended to permit patients to make medical decisions based on their *own* personal beliefs, values, and goals, even the patient-oriented standard, as applied by the overwhelming proportion of courts, undermines this objective. This standard requires physicians to tell patients what a reasonable person would find material to making a decision—hence its designation as an objective standard. It therefore compels a particular patient whose values differ from the norm to be satisfied with the nature and amount of information dictated by that norm. A patient who works as a watch repairer, for example, may be very interested to know that a medication occasionally causes a fine tremor, whereas to most patients, hence to the hypothetical reasonable patient, such information would be of little importance. If a particular patient needs information that most patients would not find useful or necessary, there may be no legal entitlement to that information unless the patient specifically asks for it or the physician knows or should have reason to know of the patient's particularized needs.

A very small number of courts and legislatures have recognized this deficiency in the objective patient-oriented standard and applied as a remedy a *subjective* patient-oriented standard (48, p. 62). Under this standard, a physician is obligated to disclose the information that the *particular* patient would find material to making a decision about treatment (49). Thus, the standard is subjective and personal to each patient. To determine what the patient needs to know to make a decision, the physician is compelled, even more than under the objective patient-oriented standard, to engage in a conversation with the patient about treatment.

Although it maximizes the underlying basis for informed consent by focusing completely on the information that a particular individual needs or wants to know in order to make a decision, the subjective standard has not been well received. First, it is even more difficult for physicians to ascertain their responsibilities under a subjective than an objective standard. Thus, there is some concern that this is too high a standard to impose upon physicians and would be extremely difficult to implement. Second, the standard is difficult to evaluate in court. The best witness to testify about what the individual patient would have wanted to know is the patient herself. This opens the possibility of hindsight abuse. In fact, only two states (Oklahoma and West Virginia) appear to have adopted such a subjective standard, tailoring the disclosure requirement to the specific patient (50).

In an effort to remedy these deficiencies and still address the concerns of applying a reasonable person standard in the general tort law context, Martha Minnow has suggested a modified reasonable person standard that would take into account group identity rather than individual specifics (51). Thus, one might apply a reasonable woman standard or reasonable gay man standard in contrast to the now applied "reasonable white-middle-class-Protestant-able-bodied man" standard (51, p. 100). No court or state has yet adopted such a standard nor explored the enormous practical and theoretical difficulties in application (e.g., how do you decide whether and with which group to identify someone). Nonetheless, some authors have argued that such a standard should be applied in the context of informed consent for medical treatment (52,53, see also 54).

Mixed Standards

The distinction between professional and patient-oriented standards is useful for conceptual purposes, but in practice the boundary between these two standards is often blurred. First, the professional standard really embodies two different standards, one a pure approach looking to professional self-regulation, and the other a mixed model. The first leaves the issue of disclosure entirely in medical hands. In *Bly v. Rhoads*, for example, the Virginia Supreme Court required the plaintiffs to show "that prevailing medical practice requires disclosure of certain information" and did not limit professional practices in any way by creating an affirmative duty to disclose particular information (34). Alternatively, some courts use a "mixed" model, establishing boundaries within which medical opinion may be determinative.

The decision in *Natanson v. Kline*, for example, is frequently cited as the paradigmatic example of the adoption of a professional standard for disclosure (29). The term professional standard as applied to this case, however, is something of a misnomer. The *Natanson* court attempted to keep the newly defined duty to obtain informed consent within the bounds of traditional negligence law by referring to the behavior of a "reasonable medical practitioner," but the opinion went further than this phrase suggests. Apparently recognizing the unlikeliness of the medical profession disclosing much information to patients at the time, the court itself defined the framework within which medical discretion might operate (55). The court not only described the areas that the physician's disclosure was required to cover—the nature of the illness and proposed treatment, the probability of success and of "unfortunate results and unforeseen consequences," and the alternative treatments available—but also required that the disclosure be "sufficient to insure an informed consent," and that it be made "in language as simple as necessary." These statements represented a potentially significant limitation on the medical profession's capacity to set its own standards. If the usual medical practice were to explain operations to patients in highly technical terms, or to limit disclosure severely, this practice would presumably not provide an adequate defense to a charge of negligence under *Natanson*.

The approach of the *Natanson* court might better be called a "modified professional standard" (56). The court seemed to say: "So long as you physicians operate within the parameters of behavior that we consider reasonable in relation to disclosure, we will allow you to set the precise standards yourselves. If you deviate from the broad outlines that we have in mind, we may be compelled to intervene and establish standards of our own." As in *Natanson*, courts do from time to time assume the power to establish reasonable standards of professional or commercial practice when they believe that an entire profession or industry has been derelict in monitoring its practices (57,58). Despite the failure of the court in *Natanson* to acknowledge this approach, it is clear that this is the course it took.

Another type of mixed standard should be mentioned as well. Some courts combine the professional and patient-oriented standards by explicitly requiring disclosure to meet both standards (59,60). That is, if information were withheld that either professional practices or the desires of a reasonable patient would indicate should be disclosed, liability could be imposed. Although Theodore LeBlang calls this a "hybrid" standard (61), it seems likely that in practice it would have the same effect as the more demanding of its components, the patient-oriented standard. Most courts would likely subsume the professional standard under the patient-oriented standard—that is, anything physicians ordinarily disclose would be deemed material to the decision of a reasonable person.

To some extent, these types of debates about different standards of disclosure may be academic. A comparison of states employing a professional standard versus those employing a "materiality" or patient-centered standard did not reveal great differences in physician disclosures (62). At least one court has held that concerns about the professional standard undermining patient autonomy are no longer justified, since professional standards of full disclosure are well established (63). On the other hand, there is some empirical evidence that the standards would require disclosure of different information (64).

Even if there are differences in disclosure based on the standards, they may not be the most significant concern. Instead, the failure to obtain informed consent and to involve patients in decision making is a persistent and more serious problem. Lack of informed consent, when there is no other allegation of negligence, is not a frequent cause of lawsuits, and an even less frequent basis for recovery (65). Without effective enforcement mechanisms or other incentives, physicians may be likely to ignore informed consent requirements regardless of the standard applied, perhaps rationalizing that they are acting in the patient's best interests. There is some evidence of this (66,67). As Katz has noted, "the idea of physicians making decisions *for*, rather than *with*, patients is still deeply embedded in the ideology of medical professionalism" (68, p. 290). One survey found that although most physicians are aware of legal consent standards, they do not apply them properly (69). The authors suggest that while this may be due to lack of understanding of how to apply the law, it may also result from physicians' reluctance to allow even competent patients to refuse medically indicated treatment.

Elements of Disclosure: Further Guidance for Physicians

Standards of disclosure are intended to address the question: How much information must patients be given? If the answers to this question provided by courts and legislatures are not helpful in assisting physicians to understand the extent of their obligations to reveal information to patients, this omission may be explained in part by the fact that these standards are derived from the litigation process. They are devised not to aid physicians in performing their legal duty to inform patients, but to instruct juries that must decide, in retrospect, whether or not a particular physician-defendant had adequately informed the patient-plaintiff.

Judicial opinions and legislative enactments have addressed a related question: What information must patients be given? The answer frequently provided has been that for a patient to be informed adequately according to legal standards, information must be given about the nature and purpose of the proposed treatment, its risks and benefits, and any available alternatives. These have come to be known as the *elements* of disclosure. Again, the goal of the courts in addressing this issue has largely been to assist juries rather than to instruct physicians.

Nonetheless, these are not unrelated goals, and it is possible to glean from the enormous body of case law and statutes some basic guidelines for the proper scope of physicians' disclosures. Although differences among states cannot be ignored, certain generalizations can be extracted from the opinions and statutes that should be useful to all clinicians. Inevitably, there will be courts that disagree with these generalizations. The following discussion attempts to identify the types of elements that are commonly required, as well as some less commonly required elements that physicians should be aware may be required in particular jurisdictions.

Under either a professional standard or a patient-oriented standard the physician must still determine which elements of information should be disclosed. Too much information can be as harmful as too little. Patients can become overwhelmed by vast amounts of information, or by information that is not put into context. Physicians need to determine not only what to tell patients but also how to tell them; in particular, physicians must decipher technical information and interpret it in light of the needs of the particular patient.

A physician is unlikely to be sued successfully for providing too much information (70), unless that information is given in such a way as to be incomprehensible. In fact, studies show that lack of communication and collaboration with the patient are more likely to lead to a malpractice suit (71–73). Thus, where there is a question, a physician may be better off from a liability prevention standpoint erring on the side of disclosure, rather than of withholding information. Although physicians may argue that from a patient welfare standpoint more information is harmful, since it may cause the patient to become unduly agitated or to refuse medically necessary treatment, this theory is not borne out in practice. Studies suggest that sharing information with patients generally does not lead to their refusing necessary treatment (74), nor is information usually "toxic" or harmful (75).

Nature of the Procedure

Almost all courts and statutes require that the physician provide the patient with an explanation of the nature of the procedure or treatment, that is, what is going to happen. This requirement stems historically from simple consent law, since even it necessitates that the patient be apprised of the nature of the procedure. Frequently the requirement is coupled with one to disclose the "character" of the treatment (76), or its "purpose" (77). Sometimes there is the qualification that the patient must have a "true understanding" of the nature of the procedure (78).

There are several different ways in which the nature of a medical procedure may be conceptualized. When a procedure is diagnostic (e.g., biopsy) rather than therapeutic (e.g., appendectomy), that fact ought to be explained, since the ordinary expectation of patients is likely to be that physicians' ministrations are meant to bring relief from suffering. Moreover, the differences between the two should be explained with particular emphasis on the fact that a diagnostic procedure is intended to provide the physician with more information to aid development of a future course of action, not directly to alleviate the symptoms or to cure the patient's illness. Furthermore, patients should be told whether procedures are invasive (i.e., involve physical entry into the body) and how invasive—for example, will there be blood drawn or a section of an organ removed, or will the procedure simply entail external manipulations such as an X-ray or CT scan.

Some states explicitly limit the scope of informed consent to invasive procedures (50,79). This stems from the original cause of action in battery for which the plaintiff must prove that he or she was "touched" without consent. In Pennsylvania, for example, where a battery cause of action is still used, there is no need for informed consent for radiation treatment or drug therapy (80,81). A patient who voluntarily takes the medication would be de facto consenting. From a practical standpoint, physicians would do better to focus less on whether a procedure is technically covered by law, and more on giving the patient sufficient information to make an informed choice. In part this is because in most jurisdictions the doctrine of informed consent has been expanded to include informed *refusals* of treatment, and also to require that physicians disclose alternatives. Thus, the mere fact that the treatment the physician recommends is not invasive does not necessarily address the question of the degree of information that should be disclosed (e.g., the physician may recommend a non-invasive procedure but one of the alternatives may be surgical). As a general rule, physicians should explain what they intend to do to patients, even where formal informed consent is not legally required. Thus, although a long dialogue regarding the risks and benefits of taking antibiotics for a bacterial infection is generally not required for routine office visits, physicians should still explain what they are prescribing and why.

In addition to the type of procedure, relevant information also includes the duration of the procedure, where it will take place (the physician's office or a hospital), the need for anesthesia, the type of instruments to be used, and an explanation of the bodily parts affected by the procedure. Since many patients are concerned with exposure to radiation, the use of radiation and some rough way of quantifying its magnitude (e.g., about as much as a chest X-ray) may be an important part of describing some procedures. Likewise, given many patients' fears about infectious disease, information about blood transfusions or exposure to blood-borne pathogens may also be important (82,83).

Finally, the physician should clarify whether the procedure is considered experimental, and whether the patient will be participating in a research protocol (see Chapters 12 and 13 on informed consent to research). At least one court has held that failure to disclose the investigational status of a device automatically constitutes negligence as a matter of law (*negligence per se*) (59). But the regulatory status of a drug or device alone does not provide comprehensive information about the treatment's safety or potential benefit (see 84). Generally physicians should disclose any uncertainty about risks or benefits, and investigational status may serve as a relevant indicator.

Risks

In addition to the nature of the procedure, disclosure of risk information is most likely to be stressed by the courts or legislatures. In fact, much litigation focuses on the physician's duty to warn of risks, and in practice informed consent often and unfortunately reduces merely to risk disclosure (28). The judicial focus on risks is not surprising. Under simple consent law, disclosure of risk information was not necessary. Physicians evaluated the risks and benefits of procedures before they suggested a treatment, and patients' only role was to agree to the recommended procedure. Although physicians may have chosen to impart the risk of no treatment (e.g., "If you do not have surgery you will die"), the risks involved in treatment were rarely discussed. With the development of modern informed consent law, courts focused on this element as being crucial to the patient's exercise of an autonomous choice. Since the locus of decisionmaking control shifted to the patients, they needed an understanding of the risks entailed for a particular procedure. The physician's recommendation alone was not considered sufficient; even though the medical benefits may outweigh the risks (which in effect is what the physician implies when she recommends a treatment), each patient must evaluate those risks for himself.

Case law generally refers to risks that must be disclosed as "material," "substantial," "probable," or "significant" (85,86). These terms are not easily applied, and the physician must walk a fine line between providing pertinent risk information and overwhelming the patient with frightening statistics. Providing too much extraneous information may be as likely to impair informed decision making as providing too little information. Some recent state statutes (87) have described in detail the requirements of disclosure, but in the absence of such guidance physicians should keep in mind the following.

There are four elements of risk information that the physician needs to consider regarding disclosure: (*1*) the nature of the risk, (*2*) the magnitude of the risk, (*3*) the probability that the risk might materialize, and (*4*) the imminence of risk materialization. Each of these factors affects whether the particular risk should be disclosed to the patient. Once it is established that a risk must be disclosed, the physician should convey information about all four elements.

First, for example, if the risk of a particular procedure is that it may sever nerves that control movement of a limb, the *nature of the risk* is just that: the loss of motion in that appendage. The nature of a risk is important in determining whether or not a patient contemplating the procedure in question should be told about it, but it will not resolve the issue.

The *magnitude*, or seriousness, of the risk is a closely related factor. Analysis of the magnitude is often straightforward—loss of movement in a limb, blindness, or death are serious sequelae for any patient. Sometimes, on the other hand, one must consider the interaction between the nature of the risk and the situation of a particular patient. A minor loss of sensation in the hand may not be terribly serious for a retiree whose main occupation is watching television, but could be critical to a retiree who is an amateur sculptor.

The *probability* of a risk being manifested must also be taken into account. The fact that a risk is serious does not necessarily mean that it must be disclosed (88). If a risk is fairly likely to occur but relatively minor, non-disclosure may be justified. Similarly, if the probability of serious risk is extremely low, non-disclosure may again be justifiable. On the other hand, as a practical matter to prepare patients for likely, albeit minor sequelae, disclosure may be advisable. Moreover, most severe risks (e.g., paralysis, death), even those that are unlikely to occur, should be disclosed to the patient. In some sense this serves as liability protection for the physician. If more minor risks are disclosed, a patient may assume that the physician would have explained any serious risks and, in the absence of such disclosure, erroneously assume no serious risks exist. Similarly, there are some drugs and procedures that entail unknown effects or unknown probabilities of side effects. In these cases, the greater uncertainty should be explained to the patient.

Finally, a patient may wish to consider the *imminence* of the risk—that is, when the risk might materialize, if it will materialize at all. A risk that is likely to occur immediately postoperatively, for example, may be considered more serious by some patients than a risk that materializes gradually or one that materializes after the passage of a substantial period of time.

Another related matter is the problem of *lesser included* risks. A physician may believe that because patients have been informed about a particularly serious risk of a procedure, there is no need to inform them about less serious risks. The difficulty with this apparently logical view, particularly in a jurisdiction applying a patient-oriented standard, is that what is more or less serious is supposed to be determined according to the patient's perspective. A physician may believe that because a patient has been told the removal of a spinal tumor could lead to death, there is no need to discuss the possibility that it may also lead to paraplegia. However, the patient in question may fear the latter far more than the former, and a jury may conclude that a reasonable person informed about the possibility of death would wish to know about the possibility of paraplegia as well (89–92).

In some jurisdictions, risks that are "remote," "minor," "known," or "common" are exempt from mandatory disclosure (86). Commonly known risks are excluded on the rationale that patients possess common sense and should be required to exercise it for their own well-being. Some courts have used a subjective test to determine whether a risk is commonly known; thus, the judge or jury must consider whether the risk in question was "in fact known to the patient usually because of a past experience with the procedure in question" (45). Other jurisdictions apply an objective test, questioning whether a reasonable person would have known of the risk. In addition to commonly known risks, so-called minor or remote risks may not need to be disclosed. The term *remote* seems to refer to those risks bearing a low probability, or in more conventional legal terminology, those risks that are not reasonably foreseeable. In contrast, the term *minor* seems to refer to the nature or magnitude of harm, rather than likelihood. Minor risks are those that, if they materialize, will not cause the patient substantial harm, pain, or discomfort.

We refer to these types of information that need not be disclosed—common, known, remote, or minor risks—as negative elements of disclosure. Alternatively, they may be viewed merely as concrete applications of the standard of disclosure. That is, the negative elements need not be disclosed under a lay standard because, as a matter of law, a reasonable patient would not find them material to medical decision making simply because they are remote, minor, or known. Under a professional standard they need not be disclosed because it is not customary for physicians to tell patients about risks of which, for example, the patient is already aware (i.e., known risks). Thus, even in those jurisdictions that do not specifically recognize the negative elements, it can be said with a high degree of certainty that they need not be disclosed.

In some states, statutes are very specific and require that only certain risks, such as those of "brain damage, quadriplegia, paraplegia, the loss or loss of function of any organ or limb, or disfiguring scars" be enumerated, even though they may have very low probability of occurring (86, p. 430). In these states the physician need not disclose other risks to meet the legal requirements for informed consent. In effect, those enumerated are deemed material as a matter of law. However, a physician still may be concerned from an ethical standpoint with ensuring that the patient is fully informed and thus choose greater disclosure.

A few states authorize medical panels to identify which treatments and procedures require informed consent, as well as the degree and form of disclosure (50,93–97). Texas adopted this checklist approach to the fullest extent. A panel of physicians and lawyers was statutorily established to develop a list of procedures and the risks that must be disclosed for each, and another list of procedures for which no disclosure need be made (97). The Hawaii statutory scheme relies upon an administrative agency to establish the scope of the required disclosure, defined as "reasonable medical standards, applicable to specific treatment and surgical procedures" (96). Louisiana created the "Medical Disclosure Panel," which has developed a suggested informed consent form and a list of material risks for over 100 procedures (98). Use of the form and list are not mandatory but do provide additional protection from malpractice awards.

Such systems may lend greater precision to the task of disclosure, but they are contrary to the spirit of the informed consent doctrine. Their effect is to depersonalize the physician–patient relationship rather than to emphasize the necessity for increased communication in the name of enhancing patient autonomy. This is a serious problem. The practice of medicine has itself become increasingly technological and impersonal. If communication between physician and patient is to be based on the same model, patients may wind up with even less knowledge about and control over the care they receive. Under a wooden approach, it might be possible to have a computer make the necessary disclosure to the patient, in much the same way that computers are now being programmed to make medical diagnoses (99). In fact, after a computer makes a diagnosis, it could also be programmed to make the appropriate disclosure for the recommended procedure (100). Although electronic media may offer new and better ways to educate patients, physicians should take care not to abdicate their responsibilities to engage in direct communication and dialogue with patients (101).

Alternatives or Options

Risks and benefits of the recommended procedure are not the only information necessary to make an informed choice. A patient's knowledge of alternatives to the recommended treatment is crucial to medical decision making (102,103). Informed consent was less of an issue in the past when there were few choices regarding treatments. Today, patients often have a number of alternatives from which to select. Furthermore, there is always the alternative of no treatment. At the time of simple consent, the fact that the patient chose to visit the physician (or stayed for the administration of the treatment) could be taken as evidence of consent. Now there is more emphasis on allowing patients to determine the extent to which they want to undergo treatment, if at all, once they have discovered what ails them. As one court stated, it is simply common sense that a physician should disclose the alternative of no treatment—"how can a patient give an informed consent to treatment for a condition if the patient is not informed that the condition might resolve itself without any treatment at all?" (104,105). In addition, patients may choose not to pursue any medical intervention because of the potential harms and side effects of many treatments.

The term "alternatives" suggests that the physician has already determined what is best for the patient, and that any other procedures are secondary in value. In one sense, this is true. Physicians ought to suggest what they deem to be the medically preferable course of action. However, if decision making about care were simply a matter of what is preferable on medical grounds alone, there would be no need for the informed consent doctrine; simple consent would do just as well if not better. The physician would propose the medically preferable course of treatment, and the patient would decide to have it or not.

In many cases, however, the choice among options cannot be made on the basis of objective criteria—the recommended treatment may be merely a matter of medical taste and may be influenced by the specialty of a particular doctor (106). Informing the patient about alternatives permits the patient to make a decision in light of his values, preferences, goals, and needs. Although the basis for selection may have medical components (different treatments have different side effects and outcomes), the patient must weigh the risks and benefits of any alternatives against the goals he is trying to achieve. For example, the choice between a medical or a surgical treatment approach involves a qualitative assessment of risks and benefits, which depends on the patient's personal values and not just on health values. The treatment that the physician (or even the patient) believes is the optimal one for the patient's medical health may not be the best choice when other factors are considered.

When viewed in this light, a treatment decision involves choosing among medically acceptable options (including the option of no treatment), not simply accepting or rejecting the medically preferable options (32). For patients to make such choices, they must be informed about the nature and purpose of options, as well as their risks and benefits. They will then presumably be able to evaluate the comparative medical risks and benefits in light of their personal considerations. For these reasons it may make more sense to speak of "options" than "alternatives," although the terms are often used interchangeably.

Although most treatment options should be disclosed, it is unclear whether physicians have a duty to disclose non-readily available alternatives—for example, options that are only available in another institution, state, or country; options that are beyond the financial means of a patient (but see discussion in Chapter 10); or treatments that are experimental. In some cases (e.g., AIDS treatment) "experimental" treatments have become standard therapy and should certainly be disclosed to the patient. One author suggests that a physician is obligated to inform patients about the possibility of participation in a research protocol (107). As a legal requirement this obligation would be problematic for a number of reasons. First, there already exists a great deal of confusion about the difference between treatment and research; participation in a research protocol is not a "treatment" alternative. Second, patients often interpret physicians' disclosure of research as a recommendation of participation (why else would the physician suggest it as a possibility?). Finally, physicians cannot keep up-to-date on all research trials that are being conducted; would a disclosure requirement include only research about which the physician is already aware, all research being conducted at the institution, or all research conducted in the country? A better policy is to have physicians evaluate the appropriateness of disclosure of research options on a case-by-case basis.

Although non-readily available alternatives may not be a required part of disclosure, physicians may want to take into account the obtainability of an option for the particular patient (e.g., consider the patient's insurance coverage and general financial situation, mobility, and geographic location) (108). For example, a patient who has access to large financial resources may well want to be told about an option available overseas. But on the reverse side, physicians must be cautious not to withhold information about standard treatment options from patients who lack funds or patients whose insurance does not cover alternatives (see Chapter 10).

Despite the importance of the concept of alternatives in informed decision making, the requirement that they be disclosed is sometimes absent in case law and statutes (102), and there are few cases that hold a physician liable merely for the failure to disclose alternatives (109). Some courts define the notion of alternatives narrowly—to include only entirely different courses of treatment, rather than variation in a particular course of treatment, for example, whether to employ secondary additional measures (109). New York and Maine, however, have mandated disclosure of alternatives for some surgical procedures (110,111). And other states require disclosure of alternatives to sterilization (112) or breast cancer treatments (113,114).

Benefits

Occasionally a court or legislature has stated that in making proper disclosure a physician is obliged to enumerate the treatment's expected benefits. In most instances, the anticipated benefits are self-evident and probably the same as the purpose of the procedure— to relieve or remove the problem that occasioned the patient's seeking treatment. The patient usually is suffering from some illness or injury and anticipates that the proposed procedure will relieve that suffering. In such an instance, failure to disclose expressly the anticipated benefits is not so important. However, physicians should take care in all cases to disclose the likelihood of the anticipated benefit, especially when this benefit is uncertain.

There are, however, two situations in which benefit disclosure is crucial. First, when the procedure is diagnostic rather than therapeutic, the patient should be explicitly informed that it is not intended to relieve suffering directly, but only to provide information as to whether and how therapeutic procedures might be initiated. Second, in all instances in which the anticipated benefits are something less than full relief of the patient's suffering, the physician should inform the patient of that limitation. In this regard, the concept of benefits bears a close relationship to that of risks, the risk being the probability of a less-than-complete cure (see, e.g., 49). Thus, the provision of information with a negative connotation, rather than the positive connotation we ordinarily associate with the term benefits, may also be required in order to fulfill the duty of disclosure.

Physician-Specific Information

Informed consent disclosure is often thought to apply only to information about the therapy or alternative therapies. But a patient also consents to treatment by a particular physician. In fact, a number of cases have held physicians liable when one surgeon has been substituted for another without the patient's consent (115, pp. 189–90). How much information should a physician disclose about herself as part of the informed consent process? For example, should a physician be required to disclose how many times she has done a procedure (116,117), her success rate, pecuniary interests in a particular procedure (118), financial incentives to limit services (119,120), or HIV status (121)? Clearly these are all things that a reasonable patient may find material to making an informed decision.

The state of the law regarding disclosure of physician information is unclear. Information about a physician's general physical or mental state is somewhat removed from the focus of traditional informed consent. For example, it may seem odd to require a physician to disclose details of a turbulent personal life, or that she is sleep-deprived before a procedure that requires a high level of concentration (an everyday reality for residents), but both situations may affect patient care. The lack of disclosure of such information is explained in part because the risks involved are neither well documented nor entirely clear, at least not to the extent that such a general disclosure would likely help the patient make a decision. Moreover, in many of these cases there is an assumption that the physician in question will use his best judgment as to whether to proceed, and basic malpractice doctrine will shape physician behavior. But even in those cases where the physician does not exercise good judgment, courts have been unwilling to expand the doctrine of informed consent to encompass such information. For example, in a 2000 case the Georgia Supreme Court held that "absent inquiry by the patient . . . [physicians need not] disclose unspecified life factors which might be subjectively considered to adversely affect the professional's performance" (122). The physician in the case was sued for not disclosing drug use. In rejecting the patient's claim of lack of informed consent, the court stressed both the availability of a general malpractice suit and the difficulty in defining which life factors would be subject to an affirmative duty to disclose.

Specific information about the physician's physical health, such as whether she has a communicable disease, may be treated differently. Where the information in question should not directly influence a patient's decision (e.g., HIV status when the treatment is non-invasive, such as the administration of medication), a physician is not obligated to disclose. But HIV status may indeed be deemed material when the procedure is invasive. Yet there has been only one case to date of documented transmission of HIV from surgeon to patient (123). In fact, the statistical risk of injury by an HIV-positive physician is probably less than the risk of injury from a severely sleep-deprived surgeon. Even so, HIV status is clearly an issue many patients consider material. Moreover, at least one court has awarded damages for the psychological distress experienced between the time a patient found out that a physician was HIV-positive and the patient tested HIV-negative (124). Potentially material information about the physician's physical health is not limited to HIV status; there are a number of other diseases that pose a greater risk of transmission and thus harm to the patient. Although in theory this type of information should be treated like any other risk information (i.e., with consideration of the magnitude and the probability of the harm), courts may be unsympathetic to physicians who are aware that they are infected and continue to perform procedures without disclosing the risk to their patients.

Information about pecuniary interests or financial incentives is more difficult to analyze (see complete discussion Chapter 10). Rather than rely on informed consent to alleviate the conflict, it may be more prudent to take the position that some financial conflicts, such as physician self-referral, are not appropriate (115, Opinion 8.032).

Some authors have proposed that physicians should disclose quality of care statistics along with financial incentives (125). One case arose when a patient sued claiming lack of informed consent on the grounds that he was not informed that the physician who would do his biopsy had never done one previously (126). This lack of experience may be extreme, and other courts have held that there is no duty to disclose non-treatment-related facts and thus no duty to disclose physician experience or lack thereof (84,127,128). However, a 1999 Louisiana court stated that a physician who was not qualified to perform a procedure and failed to disclose that fact to the patient may be liable for lack of informed consent (129). Moreover, the Wisconsin highest court held that information relating to the physician's lack of experience and competence, relative to other physicians, were correctly considered part of informed consent disclosure (116). The court stressed that the general risk of paralysis from the procedure in question (clipping a brain aneurysm) rose from 10 percent for an experienced surgeon to 40 percent for an inexperienced one (116, p. 507). Some commentators have argued that these decisions signal a new trend in informed consent disclosure requirements (130).

The issue of experience is a serious one for teaching hospitals, where it is often the case that the individual actually doing the procedure is inexperienced, although a more experienced physician oversees the work. But, even if such information is required, it is not clear what this would mean in practice. How is a physician supposed to calculate experience or relative competence? Disclosure of "quality" statistics may not be very helpful to patients; people are notoriously bad at understanding statistical information. Moreover, it is not clear what type of information would be most useful. For example, the number of malpractice suits or awards says nothing about the physician's skill or expertise, since suits may be brought for a number of reasons (131), and are often settled by an insurance company regardless of the physician's culpability.

On the other hand, the reasonable patient is likely to consider experience-related information integral to making a healthcare decision. Although it is unclear whether physicians need to volunteer such information under the current legal framework, there are some guidelines physicians should follow. In teaching hospitals, patients should be told that students and residents are part of the treatment team and informed of the extent to which they participate, with supervision, in a procedure. When asked specifically about experience or success rates, physicians should disclose appropriate information and avoid misleading patients (117). For example, a physician who has performed a procedure once or twice before should not inform patients that she has a 100 percent success rate, unless she also makes clear the number of cases involved. Moreover, a physician who clearly lacks experience in a particular area, or is not competent to perform a procedure, should inform the patient of this fact.

Disclosure of physician-specific information is one of the most controversial areas of informed consent, in part because it runs counter to other disclosure requirements. With respect to treatment options, the patient may rely on the physician's recommendation to be focused on the patient's best medical interests. But disclosure of physician-specific information may place the physician in an odd position. Part of the confusion is due to the conceptual difficulty of thinking about the physician as part of the *risk* of a procedure, rather than the person who will bring about a benefit. Although it is clear that who performs a procedure is important, since this factor may have a significant effect on outcome, it is not clear how to provide relevant physician-specific information to patients making a decision. Nor is it completely clear how to disclose alternatives in this context. At least one court rejected the notion that a physician must disclose the fact that there were more qualified doctors available, since there was no evidence that the physician in question was not qualified to do the procedure (129).

Nevertheless, disclosure of some physician-specific information is justified on the basis of a rationale that elevates patient preferences over other considerations that might be relevant in judging materiality of information. For example, a physician's HIV status can be viewed as material primarily because typical patients deem it to be, not because there is documented evidence of a correlation between physicians' HIV status and negative patient outcomes. A standard of disclosure that looks to the aggregate of "reasonable patients" to inform the standard opens the ideal of the reasonably prudent patient to prejudices, as well as norms of prudence.

Summary of the Requirements of Disclosure

The law of informed consent has developed almost exclusively from cases in which injured patients have claimed that a physician failed to inform them adequately before they consented to treatment. The opinions in these cases serve to educate lawyers and judges about how future cases are to be litigated and decided. They indicate, for example, what the plaintiff-patient must prove and how it must be proved, in order to recover damages from the defendant-physician, as well as what affirmative defenses might be available to the physician if, in fact, adequate information was not conveyed to the patient. Only secondarily have the courts been concerned with instructing physicians on how informed consent is to be obtained.

Even those parts of judicial opinions that deal with the broader aspects of informed consent are not particularly helpful in instructing physicians, because of the sweeping generalities of the opinions. When courts do attend more specifically to explaining what constitutes adequate disclosure of information, they tend to offer a vague checklist of subjects to be addressed, which has not been particularly helpful.

Ironically, then, despite the large number of court decisions and varying formulae, there is a lack of clear definition of the scope of required disclosure. The legal requirements for informed consent remain unclear, and probably inherently so, given the development of judicially created rules from particular cases with idiosyncratic factual settings. Therefore, clinicians are probably best advised to fall back on the spirit of the informed consent doctrine for guidance. Sufficient information should be disclosed to provide patients with a genuine opportunity to consider risks and benefits and to participate fully in the selection among appropriate options. Regardless of the formal legal standard, physicians who satisfy their patients' desires for information in this regard are most unlikely to be sued for failure to obtain informed consent (73). (A method of accomplishing this goal is described in Chapter 8.) This informal information disclosure may even satisfy legal requirements. The advantages gained in increased trust, decreased likelihood of lawsuits, and patient compliance far outweigh the costs in time and effort expended by physicians.

The Requirement of Consent

The duty of disclosure, or the duty to inform, is the truly distinguishing and innovative aspect of contemporary informed consent doctrine. So much emphasis may be placed on it that one can easily lose sight of the other long-standing duty—that of obtaining consent to treatment.

Consent is not merely the simple matter of the patient's agreement to undergo treatment. Certainly a decision (we prefer this term to "consent," since it does not imply whether the patient will agree to a proposed treatment or not) of some sort is essential, but it is only the beginning of the matter. There are two other essential features of a legally valid decision besides assent to or dissent from treatment, to use traditional legal terminology (1). One is understanding, the other is voluntariness (132).

Understanding

People are often told things they do not understand, and there is no reason why this phenomenon should not occur at least occasionally, perhaps even frequently, in conversations between doctors and patients. In fact, empirical studies suggest that patients frequently fail to understand the information they are told or are expected to read (133) (see Chapter 7). It has been clear since long before there was any full-scale duty of disclosure that a patient incapable of understanding the nature and consequences of a proposed treatment was deemed incompetent to consent (22,134; see also Chapter 5). But it is uncertain whether an apparently competent patient who fails to understand the disclosure for some other reason— perhaps a failure to attend to certain information or confusion based on conflicting information obtained elsewhere—may render a legally valid consent.

In the landmark *Canterbury* opinion, Judge Robinson noted two different ways in which the term informed consent is used:

> The doctrine that a consent effective as authority to form [*sic*; perform(?)] therapy can arise only from the patient's understanding of alternatives to and risks of the therapy is commonly denominated "informed consent." . . . The same appellation is frequently assigned to the doctrine requiring physicians, as a matter of duty to patients to communicate information as to such alternatives and risks. (32)

In other words, the term informed consent might denote either the giving of information to a patient, or the understanding of information by that patient, or both. (See also discussion of the multiple senses of informed consent in Chapter 2; 135) The duty of disclosure is fulfilled merely by giving information. The meaning of the word consent as it is used in law generally suggests that there may be an additional requirement of patient understanding. But even after almost half a century of judicial opinions and legislation on informed consent, it remains unclear whether the physician is obligated not to render treatment unless the patient understands that information (beyond the basic requirement that the patient not be incompetent), and if so, how that obligation is to be fulfilled.

There are several sources of this uncertainty. First is the use of loose language in judicial opinions. Many courts have failed to distinguish between the physician's giving of information and the patient's receiving of it. Judicial opinions often use words like *inform, disclose, tell, know,* and *understand* interchangeably without any apparent realization that disclosure of information does not assure the patient's understanding of that information (55,136). This confusion in terminology betrays a deeper uncertainty on the part of the courts as to the true nature of the obligations imposed by the legal requirements of informed consent.

Second, and even more fundamentally, the courts appear uncertain as to the underlying purpose of the legal requirement of informed consent. If the function of the informed consent doctrine is to safeguard the individual's right of choice—however imprudently exercised—the proper concern is exclusively with the information disclosed by the physician. Of course, this in no way prohibits the state from adopting means of encouraging patient understanding. If, however, the function of the doctrine is to assure that the decisionmaking process is based on adequate understanding, then the patient's comprehension must also be a focus of judicial concern.

Third, there is uncertainty about the definition of incompetence and the scope of the competence requirement (see Chapter 5). Although most informed consent cases do not expressly hold that patients must understand the information disclosed to them before their decision will be considered valid, there is some support for this view in dictum[1] in the case law regarding incompetence. Justice Cardozo's statement that "every human being of adult years and sound mind has a right to determine what shall be done with his own body" (22) is often echoed in later informed consent cases (32,43). The judicial statements acknowledging that the decision of a person of unsound mind is legally ineffective do not appear to be geared toward requiring that patients consistently be tested to determine whether *in fact* they understand the information that is provided to them. Instead, the courts seem merely to be establishing a requirement of general competence.

---

[1]Dictum is a statement in a judicial opinion that is not necessary to the holding of the case. Thus, it is not binding as law but is often cited as evidence of a court's reasoning on a particular matter.

However, this conclusion is not at all certain, because the courts have not expressly addressed the issue.

A small group of cases more directly suggests that assent to medical care given by a patient who actually has not understood disclosed information does not constitute valid authorization for treatment, because the patient was incompetent. In each of these cases the patient claimed that he was under the influence of some therapeutically administered sedative medication that compromised his cognitive faculties. The courts have held that if it can be established that the sedative was administered and that the patient was thereby disabled from understanding information, the patient's authorization of care is not legally valid (9,137,138). However, there is disagreement as to whether the burden is on the plaintiff to establish lack of understanding, or whether the fiduciary nature of the doctor–patient relationship requires the physician to attempt to ascertain the patient's level of understanding and to refrain from proceeding with treatment when comprehension is compromised.

Thus—although there is considerable uncertainty—even if a patient is competent and has been provided adequate information, his subsequent decision about medical care may not be legally valid. It may be that the duty of disclosure or the duty to obtain consent, or both, imply a concomitant duty on the part of the physician to ascertain that the patient substantially understands the information. Whether or not the law requires understanding, the patient's actual understanding seems to be an integral component of the idea of informed consent. Regardless of the extent of disclosure, patients cannot participate meaningfully in decision making without an understanding of the facts. Physicians dedicated to the principles underlying the law of informed consent should take steps to ensure patient understanding even in the absence of a legal requirement.

Voluntariness

There is no doubt that a patient's decision about treatment is not legally valid if the patient has not given it voluntarily. The Restatement of Torts tersely states in this regard that "consent is not effective if it is given under duress" (132). To state the rule is far simpler than to apply it. There has been virtually no litigation in this context concerning what constitutes duress or illegitimate pressure. However, since the concept of voluntariness plays a role in a number of other areas of law, some analogical guidance can be derived from them.

First, it is difficult to define coercion. Alan Wertheimer notes that inducements, persuasion, and authority are all forms of pressure that may be considered coercive in certain circumstances (139). In fact, individual perception appears to play a significant role in determining what constitutes coercion (140). Wertheimer attempts to provide some clarity by distinguishing between a "threat" that is coercive and an "offer" that is not; a proposal that makes a person worse off (judged against the relevant baseline) is a threat, whereas one that does not is an offer (139). The classic proposal of "your money or your life" is a threat because the individual's baseline immediately prior included both money and life, and the choice limits the individual's options. Others have attempted to map influences along a spectrum ranging from persuasion, to inducements, to threats, to force (135,140,141). Although persuasion by appeals to reason seems quite appropriate, a decision obtained by the use of physical force or the threatened or attempted use of force is highly suspect in its legal and ethical validity. There are circumstances in which a patient may be treated against his or her will, but (as we discuss in the next two chapters) such situations constitute exceptions to the requirement of informed consent, rather than valid instances of obtaining it. Moreover, although actual force is clear-cut, it is likely to be rare in practice.

More troublesome are the varieties of verbal pressures that may be imposed on patients, compromising the degree to which they are able freely to consent to or refuse treatment (139). Human interaction can never be free of pressures that one person consciously or unconsciously places on another. Many pressures are inherent in human interaction and constitute a normal and often desirable part of relationships. Such pressures are often intended to and do in fact influence the behavior of the person to whom they are directed—for example, when a physician strongly recommends a particular form of treatment. These pressures form a necessary component of socialization and education.

All human behavior involves such pressures, but sometimes they affect behavior so extremely as to deprive it of some of the legal consequences it might otherwise have had. For example, wills are voided if the testator was subjected to undue influence (142), criminal confessions are void if coerced (143), and contracts entered into under duress are voidable (144). So too with consent to medical care; choice based upon illegitimate pressure would not constitute valid informed consent.

It is important to recognize that the legal discussion of voluntariness focuses on pressures and threats imposed by others. Being ill brings with it a multitude of pressures, and a patient suffering from a life-threatening disease may feel as though she has little choice regarding treatment (145). Physicians should be aware of how vulnerable patients may be to the coercive influence of unrealistic hope, especially those suffering from chronic, life-threatening disorders. However, consent to treatment under such circumstances should not be considered involuntary. In addition, imagined outside pressures also may not invalidate consent. The United States Supreme Court has held that a confession is not involuntary when the defendant disclosed information to law enforcement authorities after being directed to do so by voices in his head (143). Patients who make choices based on imagined pressures may lack capacity to make decisions (see Chapter 5), but the choices are not likely to be deemed involuntary.

Although it is difficult to specify exhaustively the kinds of conduct that will render consent invalid, some general rules may be derived (132). One concern in this area is whether the pressure is based on legitimate authority (146). For example, suppose the pressure consisted of a threat that the physician or family member would whip the patient until he agreed. A decision made in response to this pressure would not be considered legitimate because neither the physician nor the family member has the legal (or ethical) right to make such a threat. It is less clear how to construe a threat that an individual does have a legal right to make, but which may be impossible to carry out. For example, may a physician legitimately "threaten" with involuntary commitment a patient with mental illness who is non-compliant if he continues to fail to take his medication? Although the physician knows that the patient is likely to decompensate and thus meet legal commitment criteria, the patient may not satisfy such criteria at the time of the "threat." It is extremely difficult in such cases to draw lines between providing important information ("if you do not take your medication you will eventually be hospitalized") and threats ("take your medication or I will commit you") (146). Moreover, we might be comfortable allowing, and perhaps even encouraging, physicians to use their authority or inducements to get patients to make particular decisions about health care. There is nothing in the doctrine of informed consent that says the physician must function as a neutral bystander in medical decision making.

Alternatively, where the nature of a pressure is not inherently illegitimate, it may become illegitimate because of its source. The doctrine of informed consent is intended to regulate primarily, if not solely, the relationship between physicians (or more broadly conceived, healthcare providers) and patients, not that between other private parties and patients. Thus, there is a significant difference between a situation in which a physician threatens to break off relations with a patient if the recommended surgery is not agreed to, and a situation in which a spouse issues the same threat. From a legal perspective, as long as the spouse's threat is legitimate, the patient's choice based in whole or in part on that threat should not be overturned. On the other hand, the physician's legal (and ethical) right to carry out this same threat is limited to a certain extent by rules preventing abandonment of patients.

Even in situations where the private party exerting pressure on a patient has acted illegitimately, or unethically, the patient should not necessarily have recourse against a healthcare provider who administers treatment on the basis of the patient's pressured decision. Health care providers have committed a wrong against the patient only if they have been a party to the private coercion. Conversely, a physician who enlists a private party to pressure a patient, or who collaborates with a private party in pressuring a patient, is clearly not free from wrongdoing. More difficult is the case of a physician who knows of a private source of coercion but does not actively enlist, cooperate with, or encourage it. Such situations may make some physicians uncomfortable in administering treatment and equally uncomfortable about withholding treatment or intervening in family disputes.

Voluntariness is a critical, though ill-defined, concept. To date, it stands almost alone among issues raised by informed consent in the paucity of analytic thinking being directed to it. While courts have enthusiastically endorsed the dictum that to be effective informed consent must be freely given, they have shied away from the onerous task of giving content and meaning to this concept. This task will become more, rather than less, difficult in the years to come, as physicians are increasingly called on to take into consideration costs and benefits of alternative therapeutic courses when making recommendations to patients.

References

1. Harper, F. and James, F. (1956) *The Law of Torts.* Boston: Little, Brown.
2. Keeton, W., Dobbs, D., Keeton, R., and Owen, D. (1984) *Prosser and Keeton on the Law of Torts.* St. Paul: West.
3. Cruzan v. Director, Missouri Dep't of Health, 497 U.S. 261 (1990).
4. Meisel, A., Roth, L., and Lidz, C. (1977) Toward a model of the legal doctrine of informed consent. *Am J Psychiatry*, 134:285–289.
5. Slater v. Baker & Stapleton, 95 Eng. Rep. 860 (K.B. 1767).
6. Rolater v. Strain, 137 Pac. 96 (Okla. 1913).
7. Perry v. Hodgson, 140 S.E. 396 (Ga. 1927).
8. Dicenzo v. Berg, 16 A.2d 15 (Pa. 1940).
9. Demmers v. Gerety, 515 P.2d 645 (N.M. Ct. App. 1973).
10. Meek v. City of Loveland, 276 Pac. 30 (Colo. 1929).
11. Markart v. Zeimer, 227 Pac. 683 (Cal. Ct. App. 1924).
12. Corn v. French, 289 P.2d 173 (Nev. 1955).
13. Kinkead, E. (1903) *Commentaries on the Law of Torts: A Phlosophic Discussion of the General Principles Underlying Civil Wrongs Ex Delicto.* San Francisco: Bancroft Whitney.
14. Waynick v. Reardon, 72 S.E.2d 4 (N.C. 1952).
15. Wall v. Brim, 138 F.2d 478 (5th Cir. 1943).
16. Paulsen v. Gundersen, 260 N.W. 448 (Wis. 1935).
17. Hunt v. Bradshaw, 88 S.E. 2d 762 (N.C. 1955).
18. Nolan v. Kechijian, 64 A.2d 866 (R.I. 1949).
19. State ex rel. Janney v. Housekeeper, 16 Atl. 382 (Md. 1889).
20. Kenny v. Lockwood, [1932] 1 D.L.R. 507 (Ont. Ct. App. 1931).
21. Hunter v. Burroughs, 96 S.E. 360 (Va. 1918).
22. Schloendorff v. Society of New York Hospital, 105 N.E. 92 (N.Y. 1914).
23. Bang v. Chas. T. Miller Hosp., 88 N.W.2d 186 (Minn. 1958).
24. Salgo v. Leland Standford Jr. Univ. Bd. of Trustees, 317 P.2d 170 (Cal. Ct. App. 1957).
25. Woods v. Pommerening, 271 P.2d 705 (Wash. 1954).
26. Hall v. United States, 136 F. Supp. 187 (W.D. La. 1955).
27. Ferrara v. Galluchio, 152 N.E.2d 249 (N.Y. 1958).

28. Katz, J. (1977) Informed consent— a fairy tale? *University of Pittsburgh Law Review*, 39:137–174.
29. Natanson v. Kline, 350 P.2d 1093 (Kan. 1960).
30. Mitchell v. Robinson, 334 S.W.2d 11 (Mo. 1960).
31. Louisell, D. and Williams, H. (eds) (1985) *Medical Malpractice.* New York: Mathew Bender.
32. Canterbury v. Spence, 464 F.2d 772 (D.C. Cir. 1972).
33. Meisel, A. (1977) The expansion of liability for medical accidents: from negligence to strict liability by way of informed consent. *Nebraska Law Review*, 56:51–152.
34. Bly v. Rhoads, 222 S.E.2d 783 (Va. 1976).
35. Belli, M. (1956) An ancient therapy still applied: the silent medical treatment. *Villanova Law Review*, 1:250–289.
36. Waltz, J. (1969) The rise and fall of the locality rule in medical malpractice litigation. *DePaul Law Review*, 18:408–420.
37. Ala. Code § 6-5-484 (2000 LEXIS).
38. Idaho Code § 6-1012 (2000 LEXIS).
39. Louisiana Rev. Stat. Ann. 9:2794.
40. Pearson, J. (1980) Modern status of "locality rule" in malpractice action against physician who is not a specialist. *American Law Reports 3rd*, 99:1133.
41. Turner v. Temple, 602 So.2d 817 (1992).
42. Grice v. Atkinson, 826 S.W.2d 810 (1992).
43. Cobbs v. Grant, 502 P.2d 1 (Cal. 1972).
44. Cooper v. Roberts, 286 A.2d 647 (Pa. Super. 1971).
45. Wilkinson v. Vesey, 295 .2d 676 (R.I. 1972).
46. Waltz, J. and Scheuneman, T. (1970) Informed consent to therapy. *Northwestern University Law Review*, 64:628–650.
47. Katz, J. (1984) *The Silent World of Doctor and Patient.* New York: Free Press.
48. Rozovsky, F. (1990) *Consent to Treatment: A Practical Guide.* Boston: Little, Brown.
49. Hartman v. D'Ambrosia, 665 So.2d 1206 (La. App. 4th Cir. 1995).
50. Szczygiel, A. (1994) Beyond informed consent. *Ohio Northern University Law Review*, 21:171–262.
51. Minnow, M. (1997) *Not Only for Myself: Identity, Politics and the Law.* New York: The New Press.
52. Cooper, E.B. (1999) Testing for genetic traits: the need for a new legal doctrine of informed consent. *Maryland Law Review*, 58:346–422.
53. Napoli, L. (1996) The doctrine of informed consent and women: the achievement of equal value and equal exercise of autonomy. *Am J Gender Law*, 4:335–358.
54. Gatter, R. (2000) Informed consent law and the forgotten duty of physician inquiry. *Loyola University Chicago Law Journal*, 31:557–597.
55. Wyandt, C. (1965–1966) Valid consent to medical treatment: need the patient know? *Duquesne University Law Review*, 4:450–462.
56. Miller, L. (1980) Informed consent. *JAMA*, 244:2100–2103.
57. Helling v. Carey, 519 P.2d 981 (Wash. 1974).
58. The T.J. Hooper, 60 F.2d 737 (2nd Cir. 1932).
59. Daum v. Spinecare Medical Group, 52 Cal. App. 4th 1285 (1997).
60. Jambazian v. Borden, 25 Cal. App. 4th 835 (1994).
61. LeBlang, T. (1983) Informed consent—duty and causation: a survey of current developments. *The Forum*, 2:280–289.

62. Rosoff, A. (1981) *Informed Consent. A Guide for Health Care Providers.* Rockville: Aspen Systems.

63. Culbertson v. Mernitz, 602 N.E.2d 98 (Ind. 1992).

64. Feldman-Stewart, D., Chammas, S., Hayter, C., Pater, J., and Mackillop, W. (1996) An empirical approach to informed consent in ovarian cancer. *J Clin Epidemiol,* 49:1259–1269.

65. Hudson, T. (1991) Informed consent problems becoming more complicated. *Hospitals,* 65:38–40.

66. Lidz, C.W. and Meisel, A. (1982) Informed consent and the structure of medical care. In President's Commission for the Study of Ethical Problems in Medicine and Biomedical and Behavioral Research, *Making Health Care Decisions: The Ethical and Legal Implications of Informed Consent in the Patient-Practitioner Relationship,* Volume 2, Appendices. Washington, D.C.: U.S. Government Printing Office.

67. Lidz, C.W., Meisel, A., Zerubavel, E., et al. (1984) *Informed Consent: A Study of Decisionmaking in Psychiatry.* New York: Guilford.

68. Katz, J. (1996) Informed consent to medical entrepreneurialism. In Speece, R.G., Shimm, D., Buchanan, A.E. (eds) *Conflicts of Interest in Clinical Practice and Research.* New York: Oxford University Press.

69. Markson, L., Kern, D., Annas, G., and Glantz, L.H. (1994) Physician assessment of patient competence. *J Am Geriatr Soc,* 42:1074–1080.

70. Rosoff, A. (1994) Commentary: Truce on the battlefield: a proposal for a different approach to medical informed consent. *J Law Med Ethics,* 22:314–317.

71. Hickson, G.B., Clayton, E.W., Githens, P.B., and Sloan, F.A. (1992) Factors that prompted families to file medical malpractice claims following perinatal injuries. *JAMA,* 267:1359–1363.

72. Beckman, H.B., Markakis, K.M., Cuchman, A.L., and Frankel, R.M. (1994) The doctor-patient relationship and malpractice. *Arch Intern Med,* 154:1365–1370.

73. Levinson, W., Roter, D., Mullooly, J., Dull, V., and Frankel, R. (1997) Physician-patient communication: the relationship with malpractice claims among primary care physicians and surgeons. *JAMA,* 277:553–559.

74. Meisel, A. and Roth, L. (1983) Toward an informed discussion of informed consent: a review and critique of the empirical studies. *Arizona Law Review,* 25:265–346.

75. President's Commission for the Study of Ethical Problems in Medicine and Biomedical and Behavioral Research (1982) *Making Health Care Decisions:The Ethical and Legal Implications of Informed Consent in the Patient-Practitioner Relationship.* Washington, D.C.: U.S. Government Printing Office.

76. Wash. Rev. Code Ann. § 7.70.050(3)(a) (Supp. 1985).

77. Ohio Rev. Code Ann. § 2317.54(A) (Page 1981).

78. Gray v. Grunnagle, 223 A.2d 663 (Pa. 1966).

79. N.Y. Pub. Health Law § 2805-d(4)(b) (McKinney 1977).

80. Dible v. Vagley, 612 A.2d 493 (Pa. Super Ct. 1992).

81. Wu v. Spence, 605 A.2d 395 (Pa. Super Ct. 1992).

82. Lusford v. University of California Regents, No. 837936 (Sup. Ct., San Franscisco County, Cal., April 19, 1990).

83. Ashcraft v. King, 278 Cal. Rptr. 900 (Ct. App. 1991).

84. Beck, J. and Azari, E. (1998) FDA, off-label use, and informed consent: debunking myths and misconceptions. *Food and Drug Law Journal,* 53:71–104.

85. (1982) Studies on foundations of informed consent. In President's Commission for the Study of Ethical Problems in Medicine and Biomedical and Behavioral Research,

Making Health Care Decisions:The Ethical and Legal Implications of Informed Consent in the Patient-Practitioner Relationship, Volume 3, Appendices. Washington, D.C.: U.S. Government Printing Office.

86. Meisel, A. and Kabnick, L. (1980) Informed consent to medical treatment: an analysis of recent legislation. *University of Pittsburgh Law Review*, 41:407–564.
87. Utah Code Ann. § 78-14-5 (1997).
88. Feely v. Baer, 679 N.E.2d 180 (Ma. 1997).
89. Archer v. Galbraith, 567 P.2d 1155 (Wash. App. 1977).
90. MacDonald v. Ortho Pharmaceutical Corp., 475 N.E.2d 65 (Mass. 1985).
91. Petty v. United States, 740 F.2d 1428 (8th Cir. 1984).
92. Unthank v. United States, 732 F.2d 1517 (10th Cir. 1984).
93. Fla. Stat. ch. 458.324 (1994).
94. Mich. Comp. Laws Ann. § 14.15(17013) (West 1993).
95. La. Admin. Code tit. 40 § 1299.40 (1992).
96. Hawaii Rev. Stat. § 671-3(a)(b) (Supp. 1995).
97. Texas Rev. Civ. Stat. Ann. Art. 4590I §§ 6.03(a), 6.04(a) and (d) (Vernon Cum. Supp. 1985).
98. Louisiana Rev. Stat. Ann. 9:2794.
99. Gawande, A. (1998) No mistake. *The New Yorker*, March 30, 74–81.
100. Stillman, R., Cohen, D., Mitchell, W., et al. (1977) ICBM—A solution to the problem of informed consent. *J Clin Engineering*, 2:127–132.
101. Rosoff, A.J. (1999) Informed consent in the electronic age. *Am J Law Med*, 25:367–386.
102. Derrick, J. (1985) Medical malpractice: liability for failure of physician to inform patient of alternative modes of diagnosis or treatment. *American Law Reports 4th*, 38:901–915.
103. Logan v. Greenwich Hosp. Assoc., 465 A.2d 294 (Cann. 1983).
104. Caputa v. Antiles, 1997 N.J. Super LEXIS 186.
105. Wecker v. Amend, 918 P.2d 658, 661 (Ka Ct. App. 1996).
106. Fowler, F.J., Collins, M.M., Albertsen, P.C., Zietman, A., Elliott, D., and Barry, M.J. (2000) Comparison of recommendations by urologists and radiation oncologists for treatment of clinically localized prostate cancer. *JAMA*, 283:3217–3222.
107. Daugherty, C.K. (1996) Commentary. *Hastings Cent Rep*, 25:20–21.
108. Terrion, H. (1993) Informed choice: physician's duty to disclose nonreadily available alternatives. *Case Western Reserve Law Review*, 43:491–523.
109. Hall, M. (1997) A theory of economic informed consent. *Georgia Law Review*, 31:511–586.
110. N.Y. Pub. Health Law § 2404 (McKinney 1994).
111. Me. Rev. Stat. Ann. tit. 24 § 2905-A (West 1994).
112. Oregon Rev. Stat. § 436.225 (1997).
113. Cal. Health. Saf. Code § 109275 (1997).
114. 24 Maine Rev. Stat. § 2905-A (1997).
115. American Medical Association Council on Ethical and Judicial Affairs (2000) *Code of Medical Ethics*. Chicago: AMA.
116. Johnson v. Kokemoor, 545 N.W.2d (Wis. 1996).
117. Duttry v. Patterson, 741 A.2d 199 (Pa. 1999).
118. Moore v. Regents of the University of California, 793 P2d 479 (Cal. 1990).
119. Shea v. Esensten, 107 F.3d 625 (1997).
120. McGraw, D. (1995) Financial incentives to limit services: should physicians

be required to disclose these to patients? *Georgetown Law Journal*, 83:1821–1847.

121. Doe v. Noe, 690 N.E. 2d 1012 (Ill. App. Ct. 1st Dist: 1997).
122. Albany Urology Clinic PC v. Cleveland, 2000 Ga. LEXIS 214.
123. Simons, M. (1997) French doctor with AIDS reportedly infected patients in surgery. *New York Times*, January, 17, A5.
124. Faya v. Almaraz, 620 A.2d 327 (Md. Ct. App. 1993).
125. Brennan, T.A. (1993) An ethical perspective on health care insurance reform. *Am J Law Med*, 19:36–74.
126. Hofmann, P.B. (1996) Physician experience as a measure of competency: implications for informed consent. *Camb Q Healthc Ethics*, 5:458–466.
127. Ditto v. McCurdy, 947 P.2d 952 (Hawaii 1997).
128. Whiteside v. Lukson, 947 P.2d 1263 (Wash. Ct. App. 1997).
129. Leger v. Louisiana Medical Mutual Insurance, 732 So.2d 654 (La. Ct. App. 1999).
130. Twerski, A. and Cohen, N. (1999) The second revolution in informed consent: comparing physicians to each other. *Northwestern University Law Review*, 94:1–75.
131. Ely, J., Dawson, J., Young, P., et al. (1999) Malpractice claims against family physicians: are the best doctors sued more? *J Fam Pract*, 48:23–30.
132. American Law Institute (1979) *Restatement (Second) of the Law of Torts*. St. Paul: ALI
133. Williams, M., Parker, R., Baker, D., et al. (1995) Inadequate functional health literacy among patients at two public hospitals. *JAMA*, 274: 1677–82.
134. Pratt v. Davis, 118 Ill. App. 161 (1905), *aff'd* 79 N.E. 562 (Ill. 1906).
135. Faden, R.R. and Beauchamp, T.L. (1986) *A History and Theory of Informed Consent*. New York: Oxford University Press.
136. Dunham v. Wright, 423 F.2d 940 (3rd Cir. 1970).
137. Gravis v. Physicians and Surgeons Hosp., 427 S.W.2d 310 (Tex. 1968).
138. Frannum v. Berard, 422 P.2d 812 (Wash. 1967).
139. Wertheimer, A. (1993) A philosophical examination of coercion for mental health issues. *Behav Sci Law*, 11:239–258.
140. Monahan, J., Hoge, S., Lidz, C., et al. (1996) Coercion to inpatient treatment: initial results and implications for assertive treatment in the community. In Dennis, D., Monahan, J. (eds) *Coercion and Aggressive Community Treatment*. New York: Plenum.
141. Carroll, J.S. (1991) Consent to mental health treatment: a theoretical analysis of coercion, freedom, and control. *Behav Sci Law*, 9:129, 131–136.
142. Page, W. (1960) *Wills*. Bowe, W.J., Parker D.H. (eds) Cincinnati: W.H. Anderson.
143. Colorado v. Connelly, 497 U.S. 157 (1986).
144. American Law Institute (1981) *Restatement (Second) of the Law of Contracts*. St. Paul: American Law Institute.
145. Draft Memorandum to Members of the PDIA Task Force on the Ethics of Human Experimentation on Persons Near the End of Life, October 7, 1996 (on file with authors).
146. Berg, J.W. and Bonnie, R.J. (1996) When push comes to shove: aggressive community treatment and the law. In Dennis, D., Monahan, J. (eds) *Coercion and Aggressive Community Treatment: A New Frontier in Mental Health Law*. New York: Plenum.

4

Exceptions to the Legal Requirements:
Emergency, Waiver, Therapeutic Privilege,
and Compulsory Treatment

In the preceding chapter we spoke of the requirement for informed consent in absolute terms, as something that was an invariable component of medical decision making. Over the years, courts have come to recognize that there are a number of situations in which physicians are permitted to render treatment without patients' informed consent. Even under the earlier simple consent requirement, consent to treatment was not required in all situations.

There are different kinds of situations in which requiring disclosure and obtaining consent could be detrimental to the patient, such as in an emergency or when the disclosure itself would harm the patient, and therefore in these situations informed consent is not required. Patients may also waive, or give up, the right to be informed and/or to consent. Here the concern is not with promoting health values but with promoting autonomy. Informed consent may also be dispensed with in a fourth set of cases, those of legally required treatment, in which the harm from requiring informed consent is not necessarily to the patient (or the patient alone) but to other important societal interests (e.g., civil commitment of the dangerous mentally ill—see Chapter 11—or forced treatment of patients with infectious disease). In addition, informed consent requirements are modified when a patient is incompetent (see Chapter 5).

Each of these exceptions contains the potential for undermining the values sought to be implemented by the informed consent doctrine: self-determination and informed decision making. Exceptions that are too broadly defined and applied are a threat to these values. On the other hand, these exceptions are an important vehicle for the interjection into the decisionmaking process of another set of values, society's interest in promoting the health of individuals. When judiciously defined and applied, the exceptions accord health-related values their due. However, the exceptions can be, and sometimes have been, defined so broadly as to dilute, if not dissolve, the fundamental duties imposed by the doctrine and to undermine its essential purpose of assuring patient participation in medical decision making (1).

Since the informed consent requirement imposes not a single duty but two, making disclosure and obtaining consent, exceptions are more complicated than they were under the simple consent requirement. In fact, there is a threshold question that needs to be addressed—namely, exceptions to what? Since there are two duties, it is possible that circumstances will justify a physician's noncompliance with one duty but not the other. That is, in some circumstances a physician may be required to obtain consent but not make disclosure, or vice versa. In other situations, the circumstances may justify omitting both duties.

The Emergency Exception

As a general rule, in an emergency a doctor may render treatment without the patient's consent; consent is said to be implied. The rationale for this rule is that since reasonable persons would consent to treatment in an emergency if they were able to do so, it is presumed that any particular patient would consent under the same circumstances (2, §18). In addition, if no treatment is rendered, the patient will experience irreparable harm or possibly death, thus making later decision making moot.

The definition of the term *emergency* is not clear-cut, though admittedly there is an intuitive or commonsense notion of what it means in a medical context. Many courts have refrained from attempting to define an emergency while still finding one to exist. The few definitions that courts have provided are scattered along a very broad spectrum. At one extreme, an emergency has been said to exist when there was an immediate, serious, and definite threat to life or limb (3). For example, a California Court stated that:

> [a]n emergency exists when there is a sudden marked change in the patient's condition so the action is immediately necessary for the preservation of life, or the prevention of serious bodily harm to the patient or others, and it is impractical to first obtain consent. (4)

This sort of standard establishes a very high threshold for finding that an emergency exists. Other courts have been far more lenient in recognizing the existence of an emergency. For instance, an emergency sufficient to excuse the failure to obtain consent has been found to exist merely when "suffering or pain [would] be alleviated" by treatment (5). At least fifteen states have incorporated some language into their informed consent statute allowing for treatment in an emergency (6).

What should the definition of an emergency be for the purpose of determining when informed consent should be suspended? The answer to this question must take into consideration the extent to which the abandonment or relaxation of informed consent requirements both undermines the values the doctrine seeks to promote and furthers the competing value of health. If informed consent is suspended in an emergency, it should be because the time it would take to make disclosure and elicit patients' decisions would work to the disadvantage of some compelling interest of patients. Thus, the urgency of the need for medical care is a prime determinant of whether a particular situation should be classified as an emergency. How urgent a situation is depends primarily upon the consequences to the patient of delay in the rendering of treatment. One court noted that an emergency exists when the "harm from a failure to treat is imminent and outweighs harm threatened by proposed treatment" (7).

The possible consequences of delayed or withheld treatment range from an extreme of death at one end of the spectrum to no deleterious consequences at the other. The intermediate consequences vary in nature, degree, and duration. They may involve physical harm, emotional harm, economic harm, or some combination of the three. The harm may be to the patient or to other persons. For instance, in the case of a highly contagious disease, the harm posed is clearly to others as well as to the patient. The psychological harm from delay could conceivably affect members of the patient's family, as could the economic consequences. The degree of harm involved could range from serious to slight, and the duration of harm may vary from momentary to permanent.

If a patient's condition is such that the time necessary for disclosure and consent would be so great that health or life would be seriously jeopardized (e.g., choking or myocardial infarction), none of the interests promoted by the informed consent doctrine are served.

As a result, the applicability of the exception should vary according to the particular case at hand. In general, courts are unwilling to second-guess a physician's determination that a medical emergency exists. However, there are some limits to the physician's discretion. For example, only reasonable treatment as necessary within the confines of the emergency is allowed. Thus, a patient who comes in bleeding profusely should be stabilized, but if informed consent can then be obtained for further treatment it should be sought. Likewise, even if an initial procedure is undertaken without consent, subsequent procedures or follow-up work must be consented to if possible. The initial emergency does not constitute continuing authorization to do whatever procedures the physician deems appropriate. In addition, an initial consent does not constitute authorization for additional interventions the physician decides are medically beneficial (Compare reference 8 with reference 9). For example, if during the course of an unrelated surgery, the physician discovers potentially cancerous growths on the patient's ovaries, he may be justified in taking a biopsy for analysis. The harm to the patient is minimal, and most reasonable patients would agree to the procedure under these circumstances. However, unless the situation is so grave as to warrant immediate action (i.e., an emergency exists), the physician must wait until the patient recovers and obtain a separate informed consent for removal of the ovaries. The initial consent for surgery is probably broad enough to cover the biopsy, because a reasonable patient expects that while the physician is "inside" he will take notice of other problems. This does not mean that the patient will assume that the physician will perform all other surgeries (unless, of course, this was discussed during the initial consent process). Where the harm is not imminent, no emergency exists.

Finally, it is not appropriate for a physician to wait until an emergency occurs in order to avoid the need to obtain informed consent. There is, however, a fine line between anticipating future problems and delaying consent until an emergency situation. Thus, one court found no negligence occurred when consent was not obtained from a woman who was admitted to a hospital three days before her condition worsened to the point of needing an emergency amputation (10). It is likely that a court would overrule the physician's judgment under these circumstances only when the avoidance of informed consent requirements appears intentional. For example, a physician who is aware that a patient does not want a procedure and waits until harm to the patient is imminent cannot justify proceeding without consent on the basis of an emergency. Likewise, an emergency does not abrogate a patient's previous refusal to give informed consent nor invalidate a legally executed advance directive. The emergency exception assumes that the patient would have consented if he had been fully informed. When there is strong evidence to the contrary, the physician may not override the patient's wishes.

Effect of Invoking the Emergency Exception

Because the disclosure obligation is the most time-consuming part of the informed consent requirement (except in the simplest of cases) and is therefore most likely to cause detrimental delay, the emergency exception should ordinarily suspend disclosure. The applicability of the exception is not as clear, however, in the case of the consent requirement. It is easy to imagine situations so urgent that full disclosure would be counterproductive but not so urgent that consent, possibly following a highly abbreviated disclosure, could not be obtained. For example, a patient who has suffered a severed finger in an accident and who is conscious when brought to the hospital should be asked whether the doctors should attempt to reattach it, and the decision usually should be honored. Minimal disclosure would seem to make sense in such a situation, at least to the extent that the patient might want to know about the probability of success and whether the consequences of failure were grave or minimal. Of course, as stated earlier, where time is of such essence that there will be a grave threat to the patient's life or health if the time is taken to obtain consent, the consent requirement should be suspended too.

When the patient is incapable of giving informed consent, but there is time to obtain consent from a proxy, no emergency exception applies, and physicians must obtain surrogate consent (11,12; but see 13). Thus, one court noted that where a patient's parents were present at the hospital, and the physician had time to drink a cup of coffee before conducting the procedure, the emergency exception did not apply, and the physician was obligated to get informed consent from the parents (11). As with cases involving patient consent, there may be situations allowing only abbreviated disclosure to proxies. In such situations, the physician should disclose as much information as possible given the time constraints.

Therapeutic Privilege

Physicians may, in appropriate circumstances, withhold information they would otherwise be obliged to disclose, if disclosure would be harmful to a patient. Like the emergency exception, therapeutic privilege is based on the promotion of health values over patient self-determination. A number of states include such an exception in their informed consent statutes, allowing physicians the discretion to withhold information that would have a substantially adverse impact on the patient's condition (6). Of all the exceptions to the informed consent doctrine this is the best known and most discussed, despite the fact that the outcome of very few cases turns on its application.

Although the contours of therapeutic privilege are uncertain, its general purpose is clear: to "free physicians from a legal requirement which would force them to violate their 'primary duty' to do what is beneficial for the patient" (14). Others have said that the privilege permits doctors to uphold their professional, ethical obligation to "do no harm" (15). The source of this obligation in the informed consent context is unclear, and its existence in case law appears mostly in dictum (16,17). Moreover, the basis for the exception is problematic, since physicians often harm patients in pursuit of a greater good. For example, some treatments, like chemotherapy, are extremely harmful to the patient but may achieve the greater good of destroying cancer cells. Often diagnostic interventions cause harm, such as a spinal tap (headache), or bone marrow biopsy (pain). Thus, the possible small harm that may result from disclosing upsetting information to a patient may be outweighed by the greater good to be achieved by having the patient participate in the decisionmaking process. In fact, there do not appear to be any cases that have held a physician liable for causing an injury to the patient by disclosing upsetting information.

In practice, it is likely that the privilege serves to lend false legitimacy to the natural aversion of physicians to disclose information to patients (18–20). The President's Commission for the Study of Ethical Problems in Medicine stated that "there is much to suggest that therapeutic privilege has been vastly overused as an excuse for not informing patients of facts they are entitled to know"(21, p. 92). If the scope of the privilege is not severely circumscribed, it contains the potential to swallow the general obligation of disclosure. Viewing the harm to patients from disclosure broadly, as it occasionally has been by the courts (22), to include the risk that patients may choose to reject medical care, would, in effect, permit physicians to substitute their judgment for patients' in every instance of medical decision making. Therefore, it should be made clear that "[t]he privilege does not accept the paternalistic notion that the physician may remain silent simply because divulgence might prompt the patient to forego therapy the physician feels the patient really needs" (23). The boundaries of the privilege ought to be defined in terms of the primary functions of the informed consent doctrine, rather than by reference to the harm that may be done to the patient by disclosure. Thus, if the doctrine exists primarily to promote patient participation in medical decision making and to promote informed decision making, information should only be permitted to be withheld if its disclosure would thwart one of these objectives.

Judicial Formulations

In one of the few cases whose result actually turned on the therapeutic privilege, *Nishi v. Hartwell*, the court did not confine itself to a restrictive definition of the privilege and formulated its definition so as to permit physicians extensive leeway in withholding information. The court stated that because

> the doctrine [of informed consent] recognizes that the primary duty of a physician is to do what is best for his patient . . . a physician may withhold disclosure of information regarding any untoward consequences of a treatment where full disclosure will be detrimental to the patient's total care and best interest. (24)

At another point, the court suggested that information might be properly withheld from the patient if its disclosure "might induce an adverse psychosomatic reaction in a patient highly apprehensive of his condition" (24). Patients might conceivably have mild, transitory "psychosomatic reactions" (e.g., anxiety reactions characterized by increased pulse, rapid breathing, flushing) to the disclosure of risk information, yet it is questionable whether these would interfere with their decisionmaking ability. Such a standard is not functionally related to patients' abilities to participate in decision making and, moreover, emphasizes the value of patients' health almost to the exclusion of the right to choose. Nevertheless, the privilege continues to be recognized. For example, in a 1993 case the California Supreme Court refused to require disclosure of specific types of risk information (mortality rates), noting both the uncertainty inherent in risk calculations as well as the physician's discretion in deciding what information is appropriate to disclose (16).

In the landmark informed consent case of *Canterbury v. Spence*, the court seemed to have adopted a more restrictive approach than one based upon physician discretion when it stated that information about the possible untoward consequences of the treatment may be withheld from patients because "[i]t is recognized that patients occasionally become so ill or emotionally distraught on disclosure as to foreclose a rational decision" (23). That is, information may be withheld when its disclosure would so upset patients that they would be unable to engage in decision making in a rational way or at all (25).

In addition to its stringent formulation of the privilege, the *Canterbury* case also contains language suggesting that there are less restrictive circumstances in which it should properly apply. In fact, the court's most general statement is that the privilege applies "when risk disclosure poses such a threat of detriment to the patient as to become unfeasible or contraindicated from a medical point of view" (23). However, the court took pains to explain that it did not intend that the privilege be framed so broadly

> that the physician may remain silent simply because divulgence might prompt the patient to forego therapy the physician feels the patient really needs. That attitude presumes instability or perversity for even the normal patient, and runs counter to the foundation principle that the patient should and ordinarily can make the choice for himself. (23)

The privilege is to operate only "where the patient's reaction to risk information, as reasonabl[y] foreseen by the physician, is menacing" (23). Yet the court did not limit the operation of the privilege merely to those situations in which disclosure would so upset the patient as to preclude participation in decision making. It would also permit the privilege to operate when risk disclosure would "complicate or hinder the treatment" or "pose psychological damage to the patient" (23).

The discussion of the privilege in *Canterbury* is confused by the use of some language suggesting a strict formulation and other language suggesting a looser formulation. Because of this conflict, the case nicely exemplifies the disparate values sought to be reconciled by the general rule of informed consent and the exception for therapeutic reasons. Although disclosure of treatment information and patient decision making are important, if not compelling, goals, they should not be pursued so single-mindedly that they become self-defeating. When disclosure clearly threatens to impede rather than promote patient decision making, consideration must be given to dispensing with it. In fact, there is some authority suggesting that disclosure must be suspended when it poses an unreasonable threat of harm to patients (26–28).

When properly invoked, the therapeutic privilege does not necessarily contemplate complete non-disclosure. The *Canterbury* formulation of the privilege indicates that it is primarily, if not exclusively, information about the risks of treatment that may be withheld, although if the disclosure of information about the purpose, benefits, or alternatives would interfere substantially with patients' decisionmaking capacity, it is reasonable to assume that such disclosure should be also dispensed with or abbreviated.

Whether or not the privilege contemplates that the duties of both disclosure and consent are suspended is not clear. Since the discussion of the privilege in *Canterbury* is framed primarily in terms of relieving physicians of the duty to disclose risk information, the implication is that physicians are still obligated to disclose all other relevant information and to obtain consent as well. In fact, it is difficult to see how giving consent to treatment would ever seriously "menace" (23) a patient's physical or psychological well-being. Yet the court in *Canterbury* ends its discussion of the therapeutic privilege with the suggestion that when the privilege is invoked, disclosure should be made to a close relative "with a view to securing consent to the proposed treatment" (23). Although the court does not clearly address the issue, a fair reading is that the consent of the relative is to be obtained in lieu of the patient's consent and not in addition to it (29,30). *Nishi* explicitly states, on the other hand, that disclosure need not have been made to the patient's wife, because only the patient's own consent, and not his wife's, was necessary to authorize treatment (24). We believe that the duty to obtain consent should not be abrogated by the invocation of the therapeutic privilege. To do so would unnecessarily compromise patients' right to decide, without any corresponding gain to their health. In cases where the therapeutic privilege might operate and serious doubt exists regarding the patient's ability to give an adequately informed consent because of the information withheld, physicians should disclose the information and seek input from appropriate family or other proxy decision makers. In this sense the therapeutic privilege would work much the same as the incompetence exception described in Chapter 5.

The Therapeutic Privilege in Perspective

To the extent that it merely dispenses with the disclosure of some, but not necessarily all, risk information while continuing to require physicians to disclose all other information and to obtain patients' consent to treatment, the privilege still permits patients a measure of decisional authority. If the need for patients' consent is dispensed with, but the consent of close relatives is still required, some protection is provided against excessive medical zeal, and some room is made for the interjection of non-medical values into the decisionmaking process.

As stated previously, a stringently formulated privilege is most consistent with the individualistic values sought to be promoted by the informed consent doctrine. Yet the effect of even a stringently formulated privilege may be easily undercut by rules related to its application. Whether a lay or professional standard is applied to determine whether disclosure would have harmed a patient, whether expert testimony other than that of the defendant is necessary to show that a patient would have been harmed by full disclosure, and whether the burden of proof is on physicians or patients will critically affect how the balance is struck between individualism and health.

Some commentators believe that the therapeutic privilege poses so great a danger to self-determination in medical decision making that its abolition should seriously be considered. To do so would not be as revolutionary as it might seem at first because of the overlap between the therapeutic privilege and two of the other exceptions: waiver (discussed later) and incompetence (addressed in Chapter 5). The waiver exception might serve as sufficient means of reconciling patients' right to and need for information with the obligation of physicians to do no harm. To reduce the risk of upsetting patients, while avoiding the substantially reduced disclosure consequent to the application of the therapeutic privilege, physicians might tell patients something like the following: "There is some information about your treatment that you should know before making a decision. There's a chance that this information may upset you, and if you'd rather that I not go into detail, please say so. If you'd like, I'll discuss it with your spouse [or other family member] instead." Such a statement shifts the responsibility for halting harmful disclosure to patients, keeping them, not their physicians, in control of their right of self-determination. However, as we note later in the context of the discussion of waiver, the physician should not begin an encounter with this type of statement. Only when the physician has reason to believe that a patient will have an extreme adverse reaction to the disclosure, or the patient has indicated a desire not to participate in the decisionmaking process should the physician propose such an option. If there are no indications, physicians run the risk of convincing patients that (*1*) the information will be more than they can deal with, and/or (*2*) that they should waive their right to informed consent.

As currently conceived, the therapeutic privilege overlooks the possibility that if patients were asked to make a prospective determination, they might decide that they prefer to risk being harmed by being informed than be harmed by having to make choices without full disclosure. In contrast, waiver—operating in the manner previously described—permits patients to make this very determination. It is possible that even the limited disclosure that "this information may upset you" will harm patients (31), although this is not likely. But to require this minimal preparatory disclosure does not seem an unreasonable compromise between the competing interests of patients' rights to disclosure and consent, and physicians' ethical obligation to do no harm.

In some cases in which the therapeutic privilege might be invoked there is also room for the operation of the incompetence exception, depending in part on how that exception is defined. This is especially so when a physician has experience with a particular patient and can more reasonably predict how the patient will react to frightening information (19). Patients whose emotional states are so fragile that risk disclosure might seriously harm them or prevent them from participating in decision making might be considered incompetent, depending on what standard for determining incompetence is applied. (See Chapter 5 for a full discussion of incompetence.)

The abolition of the therapeutic privilege might have another salutary effect on the physician–patient relationship. Although physicians may not know of the privilege by name, they probably have a general understanding that the law permits them to withhold information that might harm patients. The therapeutic privilege has been extensively discussed in medical journals, and it is reasonable to assume that physicians have at least a passing acquaintance with the concept. There is equally good reason to believe that most people suspect that physicians withhold information from patients, thus undermining the trust that is thought to be highly desirable in promoting good therapeutic results (32). The affirmative act of abolishing the privilege might be viewed as a withdrawal of the legitimation of physicians' natural reticence to disclose information.

At the present time, there is insufficient empirical evidence to validate the basis for the therapeutic privilege—that is, that patients can be harmed by disclosure of information per se, or even that they will refuse potentially beneficial treatment because of risk disclosure. Studies suggest just the opposite (33). In fact, there is evidence that physicians routinely underestimate the degree to which patients would like to be informed, but, paradoxically, overestimate patients' eagerness to make decisions (33–35). Significantly, one study found that terminally ill patients who initially stated that they did not want much input into the decisionmaking process desired greater involvement as they acquired more information about their condition (36). If it is true that physicians underestimate patient preferences to be informed and that those preferences themselves might change as patients learn more about their conditions, then the therapeutic privilege should be replaced by the waiver exception. Patients should be given all relevant information but be allowed to rely on physician recommendations as to final choice of treatment if they so choose.

Unusual cases where the therapeutic privilege may apply can be imagined (e.g., a patient with an unstable cardiac arrhythmia being asked to consent to its treatment, the explanation of which might heighten anxiety and thus increase the risk of sudden death). However, even if the privilege were retained to take these cases into account, there is still no valid reason to preserve a privilege that is so

loosely defined. Clearly a diagnosis of HIV-positive status can be extremely upsetting, but individuals can now receive their test results over the telephone.
Other diagnoses, like cancer or positive results of a genetic test for the Hunt-
ington disease gene, may also upset patients, often to a high degree, but withholding the information causes harm in itself. Most patients want to know what
is happening to them. This often is the reason they sought the physician's services in the first place. Unless the patient has indicated that he does not want to be
told information, withholding information may actually cause more harm than
disclosure (33).

The bottom line is that physicians need to consider how best to inform patients
about bad news. Often problems can be avoided by taking more time and not
"dumping" bad news on a patient all at once. When there is no additional time,
the emergency exception might kick in, modifying the disclosure and/or consent
requirements. If there is any room at all for a therapeutic privilege, it must be
framed narrowly in terms of interference with patients' decisionmaking capabilities and be applied only in extreme cases.

Waiver

Another exception to the requirements of informed consent is known as waiver.
Unlike the emergency and therapeutic privilege exceptions, the waiver exception
is focused on promoting the same value as the doctrine of informed consent
itself—autonomy. A small number of cases (37–40) and some statutes (6,41,42)
acknowledge that patients may waive their right to give an informed consent to
treatment. The statutes and the cases to date, however, do little more than recognize the existence of waiver, leaving some important problems of definition and
application unexplained. Nonetheless, reasoning by analogy from other areas of
the law in which waiver of individual rights has been an issue leads to some conclusions as to what constitutes a valid waiver of informed consent. For at least
four decades, the Supreme Court has defined "waiver" as a voluntary and intentional relinquishment of a known right, a definition with substantial common-law
precedent (43). This provides a useful starting point.

The Elements of Waiver

In order for patients to waive their right to render informed consent, they must
know that they have that right. That is, they must know that (*1*) physicians have a
duty to disclose information to them about treatment, (*2*) patients have a legal
right to make decisions about treatment, (*3*) physicians cannot render treatment
without their consent, and (*4*) the right of decision includes a right to consent to
or to refuse treatment. Unless a particular patient is far more knowledgeable than

most, she is unlikely to know all this without being told by the physician. Yet if an obligation were imposed upon physicians to explain patients' rights not to have information disclosed, there is a risk that patients might infer that they ought not to want information or that the physician does not want it disclosed, when as a matter of law patients are entitled to it. There is a very fine line between cases in which patients express a desire not to participate and cases in which physicians subtly suggest that they do not care to have patients participate. This fact is a major flaw in suggestions that doctors, in lieu of an affirmative duty of disclosure, inform patients generally that all procedures carry risks and then shift the burden to patients to ask for additional information (32,44,45).

Thus, physicians should have no absolute obligation to inform patients of their rights in an initial encounter. Physicians may assume that their act of disclosing information and requesting patient consent implies that a patient has the right to the information and a corresponding right to make a decision about treatment. However, when patients express a desire not to participate in the decisionmaking process, a conditional obligation arises to inform them of their rights. Patients may express such a desire either by indicating that they do not want information, or that they do not want to decide, or both. Statements like, "Please don't tell me about that, it will only upset me" (the functional equivalent of relinquishment of the right to be informed), or "Doctor, you decide what's best for me, I don't know" (the functional equivalent of relinquishment of the right to decide), should activate the duty to tell patients that they have a right to the information and a right to decide, but also a right to waive. One way of putting this might be for the physician to say, for example, "I'd be glad to stop here if you like, but I want you to know that the final decision about treatment is yours, if you choose to make it, and you have the right to hear as much information as you need to make a decision."

Although physicians may not have an *apriori* obligation to inform patients of their rights, in part because we are concerned that it may send the wrong message to patients, and in part because requiring such disclosure at the outset may impair the physician–patient relationship, healthcare organizations may be obligated to take on this responsibility. Thus, patient rights with respect to informed consent may be posted in waiting rooms, incorporated into pamphlets that are distributed, or explained during general intake procedures. Although it may be odd (or set an adversarial tone) for a physician to begin an encounter by laying out the patient's legal and ethical rights, it is entirely appropriate for an institution to ensure that patients are fully informed in this respect. However, this additional education should not be presumed, and physicians still have an obligation to make sure that a patient who expresses a desire not to participate in the decisionmaking process is aware of the rights he is waiving.

Not only must physicians assure that patients are aware of their rights in this context, but they must convey accurate information. Thus, physicians may not make material misrepresentations of fact to patients, such as facts about the nature of the treatment (e.g., risks, benefits, or alternatives). For example, a physician who does not wish to disclose information to patients and wishes to be absolved of the disclosure duty by obtaining a patient's waiver might inform a patient that the contemplated procedures are very simple and that the patient should not be concerned about them, when in fact they are complicated and risky (see, e.g., 46 and 47). If misrepresentation of facts induces patients to relinquish their rights, the resulting waiver would be invalid.

The knowledge requirement raises the issue of capacity. A patient must be competent to waive a right as well as to exercise one. The law regarding capacity to make medical decisions is not settled (see Chapter 5). And there has been virtually no discussion of the level of capacity necessary to waive the right to make medical decisions. Drawing from other areas of law, for example, waiver of Fifth or Sixth Amendment rights, we might argue that the level of capacity needed to waive informed consent is equivalent to the level of capacity needed to exercise informed consent (48). But the criminal context is vastly different from the informed consent context. We might be much less concerned about the harm of letting a patient with dubious capacity waive her right to informed consent.

If an individual lacks capacity to waive informed consent, he most certainly lacks capacity to make the medical decision. So allowing a possibly incapacitated individual to waive decisionmaking authority has an end result of allowing that person to control, at least to a certain degree, what happens to him—in this case deciding to grant decisionmaking authority to another person. This, in itself, might be a good we want to encourage. Thus, we might require a lower level of capacity to waive informed consent than to make a medical decision. Alternatively, the issue may not be one of lesser capacity in the sense of using a lower threshold or a less stringent test (see Chapter 5), but lower in the sense that the information in question is simply easier to understand. For example, a patient who waives his right to decide whether to undergo surgery does not need to understand aspects of the surgery or possible alternative treatments, but merely that he has the right to get this information and to make a decision.

The Issue of Voluntariness

Waivers also must be freely and voluntarily given in order to be valid. The issue of voluntariness in the context of waiver of informed consent is closely related to, and as unclear as, the same issue in the context of consent itself. In other words, both consent and waiver of informed consent are subtypes of the same general action, which we might call making a decision. In the case of consent (or informed consent), patients decide about treatment; in the case of waiver, patients decide either that they do not want information, or that they do not want to decide, or both. Both situations affect patients' decisional rights. Thus, as in consent to treatment, a waiver certainly would not be voluntary if physical force were applied by physicians to compel patients' relinquishment of their rights. Of course, it would be highly unusual for such a situation to occur.

As noted previously, inducements, persuasion, and authority are all forms of pressure that may be considered coercive in certain circumstances, depending on individual perception (49,50). Once again we are stuck trying to draw fine lines. To what degree is a physician justified in saying, "Do this because it is good for you," and to what extent are we concerned that an overt use of authority will induce a patient to give up decisionmaking rights? Since we have already acknowledged that the scope of the exceptions involves a balance between the right of self-determination and society's interest in promoting the health of the individual, we can draw lines between physician actions that constitute impermissible coercion and actions that constitute permissible pressure. Thus, a physician should be aware of the potential influence she has on a patient and use it judiciously. Although a patient should not be ordered to comply with a treatment recommendation, or pressured into waiving decisionmaking rights, a physician should feel comfortable advocating for a particular treatment option and attempting to convince a patient to exercise his decisionmaking rights to consent. In fact, disclosure of information without any recommendations is an abdication of physician responsibility. Patients who request help in decision making should not be viewed as waiving their rights, but as asking the physician to discharge her duty.

The Waiver Exception in Perspective

Because the doctrine of informed consent is designed to permit patients to make decisions and to provide them with information so that they may make them rationally, an exception that denies them this information seems to undermine these goals. However, effectuating decision making is not the sole or ultimate goal of the doctrine of informed consent. Rather, the primary objective of the doctrine is to promote individual self-determination. Permitting patients to make healthcare decisions is one way of fostering self-determination. On the other hand, compelling them to receive information they do not want or to make decisions they do not wish to make is a denial of the right of self-determination, even though in this case the consequence is that patients will not participate fully (or at all) in decision making. Thus, a waiver, properly given, is in keeping with the values sought to be promoted by informed consent, because the patient remains the ultimate decision maker.

Patients should be able to waive either or both of the duties imposed upon physicians. They should be able to give up the right to information without relinquishing the right to decide, or vice versa. Alternatively, they might determine that they wish neither to be informed nor to decide. Each of these has different implications for informed consent.

Patients who decide to waive the *consent* aspect but maintain that they want to receive all information are the easiest to deal with. Essentially the patient may be saying that she will acquiesce in whatever the physician's final recommendation is, but that she wants to remain informed. One way to look at this is to understand the patient as actually making a choice between treatments, but basing that choice on the physician's recommendation. Alternatively, the patient may want to waive her right to decide and, instead, have a family member make the decision. Here, too, one might say that the patient is making the choice based on what the family member recommends.

But in both cases there may be difficulty in documenting legally valid informed consent. A patient who waives her right to decide may not want to sign a consent form, and may not even want to be asked what her decision is in a particular case. These are things she may prefer to have handled by the person chosen to make the decision. But most healthcare proxies are designed to take effect only when a patient is incompetent (51). Thus, it remains unclear whether a proxy would have legal authority to make decisions for a competent patient. In part this is an artifact of the surrogate statutes that are designed to allow designation of a proxy in anticipation of later incapacity, as opposed to traditional proxy statutes that permit immediate assumption of decisionmaking authority. An additional problem is that most of the statutes do not allow physicians to assume surrogate decisionmaking authority, and thus a waiver that essentially entails the patient saying, "Choose whichever treatment you think is best, doctor," may not represent a valid transfer of decisionmaking authority.

Patients who waive the *information* element, but not decisionmaking authority, present additional difficulties. Essentially these individuals are making a decision without full information and thus fail to meet the understanding requirement of informed consent. For example, a patient who does not want to hear about the risks of treatment before making a decision arguably is making an incompetent decision. There is disagreement about whether competence requires patients actually to understand information, or whether it simply requires that patients demonstrate that they have capacity to understand, regardless of whether understanding exists in the case at hand (see Chapter 5). Even if the capacity requirement does not require actual understanding, the notion of consent may have a built-in understanding requirement (see Chapter 3). It makes no sense to argue that a patient who fails to understand the nature and consequences of a particular treatment is making an informed choice and thus exercising self-determination, regardless of whether that patient has the capacity to understand.

On the other hand, compelling patients to receive information that they do not want would also deny self-determination. The answer to this problem might lie in how much understanding is necessary to make a decision an effective demonstration of self-determination. One possibility is to allow patients to waive information, but only if they are aware at least of the nature of the information they are waiving. Thus, a patient who waives information about risks must be aware that the treatment in question involves risk, and perhaps even serious risk, but would be allowed to make a decision without knowing the exact nature of the risks.

But unlike a waiver of a particular type of information, such as risk information, a wholesale waiver that included all information about a treatment, for example, the patient says, "Just tell me the names of the treatments and I'll pick one," would not meet the understanding requirement. Physicians justifiably may be wary of relying on the patient's choice under such circumstances. The solution in these situations may be the same as the solution in the case where patients waive both information and decisionmaking authority. Ideally patients should be encouraged to identify a third party who can both receive information and make decisions. Again, we face some of the problems outlined previously, since many state statutes are not set up to accommodate competent patients who want to transfer decisionmaking authority. But this is likely to be a technical problem only. Competent patients in these circumstances should be treated as patients who have some capacity, but not full capacity, to make the medical decision at hand. In these cases, patient assent rather than consent would be sought. The assent requirement allows the patient to participate in the decision but enables the physician to receive legally valid consent from a fully informed third party.

Waiver permits patients to be protected from any harmful impact they believe disclosure might have upon them or from the possible anxiety that may accompany the decisionmaking process. In contrast to therapeutic privilege, patients, not doctors, determine that disclosure or decision making will be harmful.

Compulsory Treatment

Informed consent may also be dispensed with in certain cases of legally compelled treatment. The overriding justification is not solely the individual's health (although this clearly plays a role), but also society's interest in protecting others. Thus, treatment may be ordered for the dangerous mentally ill (see Chapter 11), patients with infectious diseases [e.g., tuberculosis (52,53) or AIDS (54)], alcohol or drug abusers, prisoners (55,56), and (more controversially) pregnant women (57,58). Often compulsory treatment follows refusal of treatment, a topic addressed in more detail in Chapter 11. Because compulsory treatment threatens the basic premise upon which informed consent is based, and the justification is societal interests in conjunction with individual interests, the scope of this exception must be carefully constrained.

With therapeutic privilege a physician makes a determination of what treatment is most appropriate and presumably acts, even when withholding information, in the patient's best interest. The same cannot necessarily be said of compulsory treatment. The treatment in question must be potentially beneficial for the patient, but it may not be in the patient's best interests as the patient defines them. On the other hand, unlike the scope of the waiver exception, which is determined by patients, and the therapeutic exception, which is determined by physicians, the compulsory treatment exception applies only where there is a valid court order or statute authorizing treatment. Thus, there appears to be less likelihood of abuse or misapplication.

Compulsory treatment is not usually thought of as an exception to informed consent and this is probably appropriate. In almost all situations of compulsory treatment, a patient's informed consent should be sought initially for recommended treatment, and only in exceptional cases should legal action be taken. Many decisions by patients have consequences, some harmful, to other people, and compulsory treatment is not appropriate in most of these cases. For example, a young father's decision to discontinue dialysis (or to refuse kidney transplantation) in the case of chronic renal failure may "harm" his children by leaving them with one parent. The courts often use this rationale when they order treatment over a patient's religious objections (see Chapter 11). Even decisions to consent to treatment can have deleterious effects on third parties because of financial or emotional strain. Recognizing that most individual actions have an effect on a number of people may be a good reason to include close family in treatment decision making, but it is not sufficient in most circumstances to override the competent patient's right to make the final choice about what will happen to himself.

Conclusion

The exceptions of emergency, therapeutic privilege, and waiver play an important role in the theoretical and day-to-day functioning of the legal doctrine of informed consent. Compulsory treatment, on the other hand, does not play as prominent a role, since its parameters require judicial intervention. As intricate and subject to dispute as the issues raised in this chapter are, the other major exception to the requirement for informed consent, incompetence, is far more complex and controversial. It is discussed in detail in the following chapter.

References

1. Meisel, A. (1979) The "exceptions" to the informed consent doctrine: striking a balance between competing values in medical decisionmaking. *Wisconsin Law Review*, 413–488.
2. Keeton, W., Dobbs, D., Keeton, R., and Owen, D. (1984) *Prosser and Keeton on the Law of Torts*. St. Paul: West.
3. Cunningham v. Yankton Clinic, P.A., 262 N.W.2d 508 (S.D. 1978).
4. (1983) California consent decree gives patients the right to refuse antipsychotic medication. *Mental Disability Law Reporter*, 7:436–439.

5. Sullivan v. Montgomery, 279 N.Y.S. 575 (City Ct. 1935).
6. LeBlang, T. (1993) Informed consent. In *Medical Liability Issues for Lawyers, Physicians, and Insurers: Current Trends and Future Directions*. Chicago: ABA Section of Tort and Insurance Law.
7. Hondroulis v. Schumacher, 546 So.2d 466,470 (La. 1989).
8. Millard v. Nagle, 587 A.2d 10 (Pa. Super. 1990).
9. Douget v. Touro Infirmary, 527 So.2d 251 (La. App. 1988).
10. Stafford v. Louisiana State Univ., 448 So.2d 852 (La. Ct. App. 1984).
11. Dewes v. Indian Health Service, 504 F.Supp. 203 (1980).
12. Miller v. Rhode Island Hospital, 625 A.2d 778 (R.I. 1993).
13. Aikins v. St. Helene Hospital, 843 F. Supp. 1329, (N.D. California 1994).
14. (1974) Informed consent: the illusion of patient choice. *Emory Law Journal*, 23: 503–522.
15. Lund, C. (1946) The doctor, the patient, and the truth. *Tennessee Law Review*, 344–348.
16. Arato v. Avedon, 858 P.2d 598 (Cal. 1993).
17. Salgo v. Leland Standford Jr. Univ. Bd. of Trustees, 317 P2d 170 (Cal. Ct. App. 1957).
18. Schneyer, T. (1976) Informed consent and the danger of bias in the formation of medical disclosure practices. *Wisconsin Law Review*, 124–170.
19. Meisel, A. and Roth, L. (1983) Toward an informed dicussion of informed consent: a review and critique of the empirical studies. *Arizona Law Review*, 25:265–346.
20. Glass, E. (1970) Restructuring informed consent: legal therapy for the doctor-patient relationship. *Yale Law Journal*, 179:1533–1576.
21. President's Commission for the Study of Ethical Problems in Medicine and Biomedical and Behavioral Research (1982) *Making Health Care Decisions: The Ethical and Legal Implications of Informed Consent in the Patient-Practitioner Relationship.* Washington D.C.: U.S. Government Printing Office.
22. Barclay v. Campbell, 683 S.W.2d 498 (Tex. Civ. App. 1984).
23. Canterbury v. Spence, 464 F.2d 772 (D.C. Cir. 1972).
24. Nishi v. Hartwell, 473 P.2d 116 (Haw. 1970).
25. Pluger v. Physicians Insurance Co. of Wisconsin, Inc, 549 N.W.2d 286 (Wis. App. 1996).
26. Ferrara v. Galluchio, 152 N.E.2d 249 (N.Y. 1958).
27. Kraus v. Spielberg, 236 N.Y.S.2d 143 (Sup. Ct. 1962).
28. Williams v. Menehan, 379 P.2d 292, 294 (Kan. 1963).
29. Cornfeldt v. Tongen, 262 N.W.2d 684, 701 n.14 (Minn. 1977).
30. Cal. Code Regs. Tit. 22 § 72528.
31. Blumenfield, M., Levy, N., and Kaufinan, D. (1978) Do patients want to be told? *N Engl J Med*, 299: 1128.
32. Alfidi, R. (1975) Controversy, alternatives, and decisions in complying with the legal doctrine of informed consent. *Radiology*, 114:231–234.
33. Andrews, L. (1984) Informed consent statutes and the decisionmaking process. *J Leg Med*, 5:163–217.
34. Harris, L., Boyle, J., and Brounstein, P. (1982) Views of informed consent and decisionmaking: parallel surveys of physicians and the public. In President's Commission for the Study of Ethical Problems in Medicine and Biomedical and Behavioral Research, *Empirical Studies of Informed Consent*, Volume 2, Appendices. Washington D.C.: U.S. Goverment Printing Office.
35. Patients opt for medical information but prefer physician decision making. (1984) *Medical World News,* March 26, p. 70.

36. Barry, B. and Henderson, A. (1996) Nature of decision making in the terminally ill patient. *Cancer Nurs*, 19:384–391.
37. Cobbs v. Grant, 502 P.2d 1 (Cal. 1972).
38. Kaimowitz v. Michigan Dep't of Mental Health, 1 Ment. Dis. Law Rprt. 147 (Cir. Ct. Wayne County Mich. 1976).
39. Putensen v. Clay Adams, Inc., 12 Cal. App.3d 1062 (1970).
40. Holt v. Nelson, 523 P.2d 211 (Wash. App. 1974).
41. N.Y. Pub. Health Law § 2805-d(4)(b) (McKinney 1977).
42. Utah Code Ann. § 78-14-5.2(c) (1977).
43. (1966) Estoppel and Waiver § 154. *American Jurisprudence 2d*, Vol. 28.
44. Or. Rev. Stat. § 677.097 (1977).
45. Lankton, J., Batchelder, B., and Ominsky, A. (1977) Emotional responses to detailed risk disclosure for anesthesia—a prospective randomized study. *Anesthesiology*, 46:294–296.
46. Campbell v. Oliva, 424 F.2d 1244 (6th Cir. 1970).
47. Paulsen v. Gundersen, 260 N.W. 448 (Wis. 1935).
48. Godinez v. Moran, 509 U.S. 389 (1993).
49. Wertheimer, A. (1993) A philosophical examination of coercion for mental health Iisues. *Behav Sci Law*, 11:239–258.
50. Monahan, J., Hoge, S., Lidz, C. , et al. (1996) Coercion to inpatient treatment: initial results and implications for assertive treatment in the community. In Dennis, D., Monahan, J. (eds) *Coercion and Aggressive Community Treatment*. New York: Plenum.
51. Sabatino, C. (1994) Legislative trends in health-care decisionmaking. *ABA Bioethics Bulletin*, 3:10–11.
52. Gostin, L.O. (1995) The resurgent tuberculosis epidemic in the era of AIDS: reflections on public health, law, and society. *Maryland Law Review*, 54:1–131.
53. California Health & Safety Code Sec. 3531 (West 1993).
54. Gostin, L. and Curran, W.J. (1987) Legal control measures for AIDS: reporting requirements, surveillance, quarantine, and regulation of public meeting places. *Am J Public Health*, 77:214–218.
55. Washington v. Harper, 494 U.S. 210 (1990).
56. Zimring, F.E. (1993) Drug treatment as a criminal sanction. *University of Colorado Law Review*, 64:809–825.
57. Linden, P.M. (1995) Drug addiction during pregnancy: a call for increased social responsibility. *Am U J Gender Law*, 4:105–139.
58. Chavkin, D.F. (1992) For their own good: civil commitment of alcohol and drug-dependent pregnant women. *South Dakota Law Review*, 37:224–288.

5

Exceptions to the Legal Requirements: Incompetence

It might seem strange to locate discussion of incompetence under the heading of "exceptions." Although patient competence serves as a prerequisite for informed consent, surely patient *in*competence cannot serve to relieve physicians of all obligations, either ethical or legal, under the doctrine of informed consent. The goals of informed consent—safeguarding patient welfare and autonomy—apply no less to incompetent patients, although they must be pursued differently.[1] The

---

[1]It may seem strange to speak of promoting the autonomy of incompetent patients. Yet some patients are only temporarily incompetent and non-autonomous, as when they are briefly unconscious or are infants. These patients will regain consciousness or mature; decisions made on their behalf should, therefore, safeguard their future autonomy and their opportunities to make future autonomous decisions (1). For this reason, for example, parents generally may not elect to sterilize their children; to do so would infringe on the future reproductive autonomy of their children. The patient who is delirious with sepsis may recover; decisions made on his behalf should respect his past autonomy (e.g., should be in accordance with his values or express wishes) and protect his future autonomy (i.e., should not unnecessarily foreclose future options for him). In contrast, some patients who are incompetent to decide about a particular medical decision may be permanently incapable of acting autonomously with respect not only to similar decisions but to all of life's choices. Some of these patients will never have been competent or able to act autonomously, such as severely neurologically impaired infants. Others have been autonomous in the past, such as a patient with advanced Alzheimer disease, and decisions made on her behalf should respect her past autonomy. (Some theorists, for example, Rebecca Dresser and John Robertson, question why the past autonomy-values or preferences of a currently incompetent patient should trump the patient's current best interests (2).

goals of informed consent are pursued on behalf of an incompetent patient by a
process of surrogate decision making. A surrogate or proxy participates in the informed consent process on behalf of the incompetent patient. Yet, from the perspective of the physician, the patient's incompetence constitutes an exception to
the usual process of informed consent. A determination of incompetence alters
the legal requirements for physician disclosure and for patient consent and thus it
is properly regarded as an exception in this sense. This chapter, like the previous
two, focuses on the legal doctrine of informed consent and addresses the variation in the legal requirements occasioned by a patient's incompetence. We leave
to others to examine in greater detail the ethical justifications for the legal framework surrounding treatment of incompetent patients (3).

It has been recognized since the earliest legal cases dealing with consent that
certain individuals are incompetent to consent to treatment and that they may be
treated without their consent (4,5). One alternative to treatment without the patient's consent would be no treatment at all (6), a result that would make a fetish
of consent, for it would mean that those lacking the ability to make medical decisions would be required to forgo medical care. The exception for incompetent
patients is closely related to the emergency exception. In fact, many situations
involve an overlap of the two exceptions, since a number of cases of genuine
emergency treatment involve unconscious (and thus incompetent) patients. However, the class of incompetent patients includes more than just those who are unconscious, and situations arise involving the treatment of incompetent patients
that are not emergencies.

Making medical decisions in cases involving incompetent patients has been an
area of great confusion, although the fog may be slowly beginning to lift. The
first step in clarifying the matter is to understand that there are a number of different but interrelated issues embedded in the problem of decision making for incompetent patients. These issues need to be sorted out before they can be intelli-
gently addressed.

First, there is the substantive issue of defining the scope of the problem itself,
which in this case means defining what is meant by an incompetent patient. Until
that is done, the boundaries of the problem cannot even be established. This
threshold issue, unfortunately, is in a state of great confusion (7). Although we
can go on to talk about the other issues, and in clinical settings can follow a set of
procedures for decision making with patients deemed incompetent, we may still
be left with a nagging doubt about whether a particular patient actually is incompetent. Part of this difficulty stems from the terminology employed. Patient *capacity* is determined by medical or mental health professionals. But *incompe-*

Refuting their arguments is beyond the scope of our project; let it suffice to say that, instead, we believe that competent people should have the ethical and legal right to make effective advance directives governing their future care.)

tence is a legal construct— a determination that the patient does not have the requisite capacities to make a medical decision. Which capacities are relevant to which decisions, and identifying ways to measure such capacity, are both philosophical and empirical questions beyond the scope of this chapter. But assuming we have some agreement on the type of capacities required for making choices (such as an understanding of the different options presented), we must still determine from a legal standpoint which of these, and evidenced at what level, will be sufficient for exercising the right of informed consent.

Second, a closely related issue is also largely unsettled, or at least there is often a large gulf between legal doctrine and clinical practice. Who is or ought to be empowered to determine whether a patient is incompetent? Taken together, we might characterize these two threshold issues in the incompetence conundrum as: By what standards should a person be declared incompetent, and who should make that decision?

Assuming for argument's sake that these issues can be satisfactorily resolved— and in practice they usually are—the remaining issues are largely procedural. Who should decide for the incompetent patient? Must informed consent be obtained from this surrogate? By what standards should the surrogate decide? Should there be any review of such a decision, if so by whom, and utilizing what criteria? The remainder of the chapter addresses these questions in turn.

Global Versus Specific Incompetence

Strictly speaking, persons are legally incompetent if they are minors or, if adults, they have been determined by a court (adjudicated) to be incompetent. A person who is incompetent suffers certain legal disabilities. In the past, an adjudication of incompetence placed an individual under total legal disability, and a guardian was appointed to make all decisions on the individual's behalf. In practice, such incompetence affected primarily financial matters. In recent years, increasing attention has been paid to whether the adjudication of incompetence and appointment of a guardian should render the person incompetent for all purposes. Some states have dealt with this problem through the enactment of statutes, others through judicial decisions, in both situations distinguishing between general and specific incompetence.

Although an adjudication of general incompetence continues to render the person incompetent for all purposes, an adjudication of specific incompetence, as the term suggests, renders the person incompetent only for limited purposes, which are indicated in the court order. Competence to make medical decisions is now almost always considered distinct from competence to perform other tasks, and thus is dealt with through adjudication of specific incompetence. For example, recent judicial decisions have noted that simply because an individual is adjudicated incompetent to stand trial does not mean he is necessarily incompetent to make medical decisions (8, 9). Even in cases where the individual is deemed incompetent for multiple purposes, these usually are considered and listed separately. Moreover, when a general guardianship order is entered, many states restrict the guardian's ability to make certain medical decisions unless specifically authorized by the court.

Minors

In the case of minors, even age does not necessarily render a person incompetent for all purposes. In many states, statutes exist permitting older children validly to authorize the administration of certain limited kinds of medical care (e.g., treatment for mental illness, substance abuse, venereal disease, pregnancy), or there may be a common law basis for permitting mature minors to consent to medical care (10–13). It is not clear why a child who is deemed competent to consent to treatment in one context (e.g., treating a sexually transmitted disease) should be considered incompetent to consent to treatment in another context. Competence may vary according to the importance or difficulty of the decision but surely does not rest on treatment categories. Indeed, these particular exceptions are made to promote the welfare of minor patients and the public's health and are based on the rationale that minors will be less likely to seek medical care for these particular conditions if parental consent were required, rather than on any belief in minors' greater competence with respect to particular treatment categories.

Most authors in this area agree that age cut-offs should not be used as automatic determinants of de facto capacity for any type of decision but may function as an indicator to shift presumptions. Thus, individuals below the age of consent are presumed to lack capacity unless shown otherwise, and those above the age of consent are presumed to have capacity until shown otherwise. In fact, studies of cognitive development and decision making in juveniles show that, according to the measures used, children above age fourteen are, in general, as capable as adults of making decisions (14), while children below age eleven lack many capacities thought necessary to make decisions (15). Some children in the middle group (ages eleven to fourteen) have the capacity to make decisions, while others do not (15,16). However, it is worth noting that, on average, children will have less background knowledge about medicine than adults and thus may require considerably more instruction to achieve adequate understanding. In addition, they may lack a general context of life experiences by which to judge the risks and benefits of the proposed treatment.

There have been various proposals either to allow minors to make medical decisions, or to ensure their involvement in decision making (17). Many of these proposals acknowledge that children have differing levels of capacity and should be involved to the extent that they are able to participate in decision making. The American Academy of Pediatrics, for example, has recently stated that if a child is judged to have decisional capacity his consent should be sufficient (18). In situations where consent is not appropriate, the academy notes that information may still be provided and the child's *assent*[2] to treatment may be sought. While some states require that minors be informed of their legal rights regarding psychiatric hospitalization and other mental health treatments (19), at present assent is legally required only for research purposes (20).

Despite the extensive literature on minors' decision making, there has been little discussion of standards by which to judge their capacity. Although a full analysis of the rights and interests of children and parents is beyond the scope of this book, we can at least offer some assistance in this area. The standards identified in the following section are not limited to adults and can be used to evaluate children's capacity either to assent or to consent to medical treatment.

Standards for Determining Incompetence

As noted previously, the threshold problem raised by the incompetence exception is that of defining what is meant by incompetence. The courts have spoken in vague generalities, and no comprehensive judicial exegesis of the subject has yet appeared (7). In determining which standards should be applied in particular cases, physicians should keep in mind that the criteria selected for the determination of incompetence ought to promote the values sought to be achieved by the doctrine of informed consent (individual self-determination through decision making in accordance with the patient's values) balanced against the general goal of medicine, which is the preservation or promotion of the patient's health.

There is considerable confusion as to the appropriate procedures for making such a determination (see later under *Who Makes the Determination?*). Although the courts are available to make such determinations (at least in theory, since such recourse frequently may not be practical), it is customary practice in the medical profession for a patient's attending physician to do so. In any event, of necessity, clinicians must provide the first level of screening for incompetence, since the initial decision as to whether to seek or to accept a patient's decision rests with

[2]"Assent" in this context refers to the child's agreement to participate in the treatment, after being provided with information appropriate to her age and cognitive abilities. Authorization, or "consent," is obtained from parents or guardians.

them. Thus, clinicians require guidance as to what standards courts may employ in judging incompetence.

General Standards

A general incompetence standard attempts to predict specific incompetence for medical decision making on the basis of particular characteristics of the patient. Under this standard, it is assumed that if patients are intoxicated, developmentally disabled, demented, or psychotic, and disclosure were made, they could not understand, make rational decisions, or participate in a rational way, and so they are not given the opportunity to do so. Thus, competence is determined by the patient's *potential* inability to meet one or more of the specific standards described in the following section.

A general standard of incompetence focuses on certain qualities of persons whose competence is in question as persons rather than specifically as patients— that is, as they function outside the medical decisionmaking context rather than within it. For example, individuals whose overall functioning is impaired by permanent conditions, such as severe developmental disabilities, or temporary conditions, such as alcohol or drug intoxication, could be viewed as incompetent just on the basis of their diagnosis or intoxication (21–29). Other conditions, such as certain psychiatric illnesses or symptoms, or advanced age (30) might also impair an individual's overall functioning. This approach might be made slightly more specific by looking not at general ability to function but at the ability to make decisions in general, as opposed to the ability to make medical decisions (see, e.g., 31). In some respects the general incompetence standard could be viewed as encompassing each of the specific tests discussed later, because it attempts to infer a person's capacity for participation in medical decision making from his overall ability to function, rather than determining it in a limited way in the medical context.

Although it is clear that some people are globally incompetent (e.g., persons with moderate to advanced dementia), the problems with a general incompetence standard are twofold. First, there may be little correspondence between a determination of general incompetence and a patient's ability to participate in medical decision making, however that ability may be determined (32). A patient who falls into one of the categories of general incompetence (e.g., advanced dementia or mental illness) actually may be capable of making decisions if a reasonable amount of time and energy are spent by the physician attempting to facilitate understanding. Second, this standard can only be applied either mechanically or subjectively. A mechanical standard would deem incompetent any individual who could be reasonably characterized as, for example, intoxicated or psychotic. Although a mechanical standard has administrative convenience, has the potential to save enormous amounts of time, and frees physicians from being second-guessed by juries, it suffers from the serious deficiency of not necessarily being functionally related to actual decisionmaking ability. For example, if all persons with IQs less that 75 were deemed incompetent to make medical decisions by virtue of their IQ, it would be relatively simple to determine who is competent and who is not. However, there are persons with IQs greater than 75 who may not be capable of making medical decisions. Conversely, there are probably people with IQs less than 75 who are capable of understanding the relevant information, at least about certain medical procedures that may be recommended for them. A subjective application, on the other hand, undermines much of the purpose of applying the general standard in the first place. It does not lend itself to consistency and is more likely to be challenged in court (thus adding time and expense to the process of determining capacity).

Specific Incompetence

Unlike general incompetence, specific incompetence focuses on particular abilities or capacities. The determination of specific incompetence can be approached in several different ways. A review of the legal, ethical, and medical literature reveals a distinct group of standards, composed of a relatively small number of components of competence (7). Although different standards may be found in different statutes and cases, the basic components from which these standards are constructed remain the same.

Presence of Decision

One standard for incompetence focuses on the mere presence (or absence) of a patient's decision. This is also referred to as "evidencing a choice" (33). That is, the patient who chooses one treatment rather than another, or no treatment at all, could be deemed competent without regard to the manner in which the choice was made and without regard to the nature of the choice itself. On the other hand, a patient who is unable effectively to make known her wishes regarding treatment is deemed incompetent. The mere failure to manifest a choice is determinative of the issue. A number of courts have implicitly adopted this criterion by holding that an uncommunicative patient is incompetent (23).

This component of a standard potentially offers the greatest protection for individual decisionmaking rights because it focuses simply on communication and disregards the decisionmaking process. On the other hand, if used as the sole criterion, it would allow a number of patients with poor capacity to make decisions. Although patients who fail to manifest a decision should be treated as incompetent, the opposite is not always true. Whether patients who manifest a choice should be automatically considered competent depends upon the particular understanding of self-determination and the weight to be accorded to it at the expense of competing values. Mere manifestation of a choice may not be indicative of the exercise of autonomy in any meaningful sense if, for example, the person manifesting a choice did not understand the options being presented; therefore, it is not clear that this criterion of competence, taken by itself, actually protects patients' rights of self-determination. Moreover, this criterion is troubling from the perspective of protecting patients' welfare, because if the ability merely to manifest a decision is accepted as the standard for competence, persons who have no ability to comprehend what they are deciding about, but object nonetheless, will be able to thwart the administration of treatments, some of which may be highly beneficial and relatively risk-free.

In addition to communicating a choice, the "presence of decision" criterion may also address situations where patients vacillate to such a degree that it is impossible to implement a treatment choice. Many patients change their mind about treatments, perhaps even multiple times. The application of the idea that a patient who fails to commit to one treatment choice for any significant period of time is incompetent can be controversial. Should such an individual be determined to be incompetent, decisionmaking authority may be taken away and given to a third party. Although it may be unclear how much vacillation is necessary before deeming a patient incompetent, it is clear that merely changing one's mind about treatment should not suffice. In fact, one 1999 court decision held that a patient's decision to withdraw consent, even in the middle of a procedure, as long as there are still viable treatment options available, simply triggers the need for a new informed consent discussion (34).

Understanding

Competence is universally viewed as incorporating the requirement that a patient have the ability to understand the information required to be disclosed by the informed consent doctrine. A patient who does not know or comprehend the requisite elements of disclosure could be considered incompetent (33). No inquiry would be needed into how the patient arrives at the ultimate treatment decision or into the nature of the decision itself.

To be competent, patients have to understand the factual basis for their decision. Conversely, failing to grasp essential information would render one incompetent. But the values of the individual evaluating capacity will play an insidious and probably unavoidable role in the attempt to gauge the patient's understanding. Not only does the evaluator's view of what constitutes understanding affect the determination, but the initial selection of the information on which the patient is to be tested reflects the importance the evaluator attaches to that information. If the evaluator is a physician or other clinician, health values may receive great weight.

A further problem with this component of a standard is that large numbers of persons may be found incompetent if a high level of understanding is expected. The level of understanding that a reasonable person could be expected to have is an appropriate measure, but physicians may have difficulty recognizing just how low this level may be. Courts routinely focus on patients' capacity to understand the elements of the informed consent disclosure, for example, nature of the intervention, risks, potential benefit, and alternatives and their corresponding risks and benefits. In practice, however, patients must demonstrate actual understanding (see, e.g., 35). Although the law generally presumes that a competent person, when given information, will understand the information and be able to reach a decision (36), in practice this does not always happen (37). Empirical studies of informed consent demonstrate that a number of patients do not understand that to which they have consented, even though their capacity is not necessarily suspect (38,39).

Understanding is the most common standard of decisionmaking competence. Like ability to evidence a choice, a patient who fails to understand information is likely to be considered incompetent. Pure or simple understanding alone may not be sufficient. A more complex form of understanding, usually referred to as appreciation, may also be required.

Appreciation

A patient may understand in an abstract sense the risk of a particular treatment but fail to understand how those risks will affect her. Thus, another component of competence is ability to appreciate the information in the informed consent disclosure. This element is sometimes referred to as "deep" understanding. At issue is whether the patient comprehends, or appreciates, the nature and consequences of the various treatment choices when applied to her situation. For example, understanding that full-leg amputation involves removal of the appendage is different from appreciating that the removal will result in the patient's requiring some type of prosthesis to walk without aid.

As with understanding, a patient must have the capacity to appreciate the information, as well as actually to appreciate the consequences. Delusions, hallucinations, or thought disorders may hinder actual appreciation. Thus, if the patient in the prior example believes that "magic" powder will make her leg grow back, she fails actually to appreciate the implications of amputation (but see 40). In addition, patients who deny illness in the face of objective evidence to the contrary, or who deny the likely effectiveness of treatment, would fail to meet the appreciation standard.

An understanding criterion focuses on a patient's ability to acquire information, while appreciation focuses on the patient's ability to evaluate information. There is another standard of competence that shifts the focus once more, to the nature of the decisionmaking process itself.

The Nature of the Decisionmaking Process

A more complex standard for incompetence examines the nature of the decision-making process employed by a patient. After patients are provided with, and presumably understand, the requisite information about treatment options, inquiry is made into the manner in which they make their decisions. At issue is whether the patient employs logical thought processes to compare the risks and benefits of treatment options. Because people do not necessarily employ a logical thought process when making choices, the standard is best thought of as requiring a patient to be able to explain his decision in a manner that demonstrates a logical thought process. For example, the patient who elects medical outpatient treatment instead of inpatient surgical treatment would need to describe the considerations that entered into that choice and how they were weighed. A patient who can communicate, understand, and appreciate still may be incompetent because he is unable to process information logically, in accordance with his preferences. Conversely, a patient may employ logical thought processes but base them on impaired understanding.

This approach to the determination of incompetence, like the appreciation standard, honors health values more than tests that merely look to the presence of a decision on the part of the patient, or even the patient's understanding.[3] If the patient makes a decision, but fails to make it in the proper manner, then one might argue that the decision is less of an autonomous decision and thus deserves less to be honored. The unstated premise is that there is a greater chance that if the decision is made improperly, reliance on it will be detrimental to the patient's medical well-being. By not obligating the physician to honor such a decision, both society's interest in advancing health and the profession's interest in ameliorating illness are promoted. Moreover, since an incompetent decision is not an autonomous decision, we are justifiably less concerned with protecting such a choice. Many people, however, are uncomfortable with the degree of discretion this standard lodges in the medical profession. In fact, much of the concern surrounding this standard is due to the fear that it will be confused with a standard that looks not at the patient's decisionmaking process, but at the decision itself.

The Nature of the Decision

Rather than focusing on characteristics of the patient or how the patient makes a decision, another alternative is to examine the nature of the decision itself. It might be thought that a patient who chooses no treatment over treatment, or one who chooses a risky treatment over a less risky one could be said to be incompetent. One problem with this approach is that it is difficult, if not impossible, objectively to rank the seriousness of various kinds of hazards and benefits. For

---

[3]If emphasis is placed on the decision's adherence to the patient's values, rather than some abstract notion of "logic," then the standard also serves to protect patient autonomy, as with the compound standard described later under *Compound Standards*.

example, which is the greater hazard, paralysis or blindness? The answer depends not only on circumstances that vary from situation to situation but also on personal values, ultimately making the resolution highly subjective. Another problem is that a treatment rarely has only one material hazard associated with it. Thus, a patient must weigh combinations of hazards, or of hazards and benefits, substantially complicating any sort of ranking. More problematic is the possibility that a patient's decision simply will be termed wrong, unreasonable, irrational, and so forth, and on this purely subjective basis found incompetent (7).

The most fundamental problem with this approach is that a standard by which the nature of the decision determines whether the patient is incompetent seriously undermines individual autonomy. Such a determination is paternalistic to an extreme and, in fact, is not an element of capacity at all, but a judgment about the patient's choice of treatment. It does not even maintain a pretense of seeking to achieve a balance between competing values, but instead completely eliminates the role of patient self-determination and denies the relevance of patients' own values and treatment preferences. Another serious although less fundamental problem is that this test is probably biased in favor of decisions by patients to accept treatment, even when the consent is given by a patient who does not understand any of the information disclosed or is unable to weigh the risks and benefits. If the patient consents, the physician's bias in favor of treatment (especially one that the physician has taken the time to inform the patient about and presumably recommends) will cause the physician to judge the patient competent merely because the patient has agreed with the favored recommendation (41).

Compound Standards

From a legal standpoint, precisely which standard of specific incompetence is employed should be a function of the law in a particular jurisdiction. The vast majority of states apply the choice and understanding criteria, and many also add on the appreciation and/or reasoning components (7). But the law in some states may be so vague as to provide no guidance, and physicians will be in the position of selecting the standard themselves. Moreover, despite guidance on which standards to apply, there are many questions left unanswered regarding how to apply the standards (see later under *Procedural Issues*). Ideally, providers likely to face questions of competence should arrive in advance at agreement on the standard to be employed; this process can involve clinicians, administrators, and legal counsel. In any event, confusion in this area makes it essential that clinicians have a clear idea in their own minds of which standard(s) they are applying and be able to explicate them if the issue comes to court. Some commentators have suggested that the standard to be employed could vary with the consequences of the patient's decision (42). Others have favored use of a stable set of criteria regardless of the situation, perhaps combining the presence-of-decision, understanding, appreciation, and a process-of-decision-making test (7,43).

Formulation of a standard will depend on balancing the extent to which a failure to demonstrate the ability measured by a test indicates impaired decisionmaking ability against whether such a failure is a sufficient basis for limiting a patient's decisionmaking authority (7). Although seriously impaired people should be protected, the right to make decisions for oneself should not be restricted more than is absolutely necessary. In addition, care should be taken in crafting and applying the standard so that it results in people correctly (according to whichever measure chosen) being identified as competent or incompetent.

Three aspects of formulating a standard need to be taken into account. First, the choice of components is important, since different standards may result in different people and/or different numbers of people being identified as impaired. Second, the required level of performance in a quantitative sense must be specified (e.g., if an understanding component is used, how much information must the patient understand—50 percent, 75 percent, 90 percent?). Third, necessary qualitative aspects of performance must be identified (e.g., what elements of information must the patient understand?). In some situations the patient may have a better understanding if she grasps only one key item (e.g., that the treatment has an 80 percent chance of preventing certain death) than if she understands many details about the treatment but misses the big picture. Additional empirical work may be necessary before settling on an authoritative standard for incompetence.

Finally, from an ethical perspective, the standard of specific competence that is most justifiable is the one that best serves the goals of informed consent and health care in general, and that may be applied fairly. In short, it would be a standard that promotes autonomy, enables patients to protect their health-related welfare, and may be employed by practitioners with a minimum of bias. Thus, ethical considerations seem to advocate a standard that focuses on the *process* of decision making and that requires that in order to be deemed competent, the decision maker must first understand and appreciate the risks and benefits of options presented and then weigh those options to make a decision in light of her own values. Such a standard would maximally promote patient autonomy and patient well-being as patients themselves define their well-being. Admittedly, this standard would sometimes permit patients to choose to sacrifice their health interests for the sake of other values (3).

A Conjunctive Approach

Although the general incompetence standard may be viewed as an alternative to using a specific incompetence standard, the two can and should operate in conjunction. The general incompetence standard should be used as a threshold standard for incompetence. Because most patients are in fact competent to make medical decisions and because of the legal presumption of competence, if there is to be a more formal inquiry into incompetence, something must trigger it. One possibility is the presence of some of the factors of general incompetence described previously. Another possible trigger is patient refusal of a recommended treatment. This does not mean that refusal equals incompetence, merely that it may trigger additional scrutiny (7).

If patients are determined to be generally competent (which they are legally presumed to be above the age of majority), physicians are obligated to attempt disclosure. After an effort to disclose and obtain consent has begun, it may become apparent that the patient is specifically incompetent by reference to one or more of the criteria described before: the patient (*1*) does not manifest a decision, (*2*) does not understand the disclosure, (*3*) does not appreciate the nature and consequences of the treatment options, or (*4*) does not engage in the proper sort of decisionmaking process.

Thus, the determination of incompetence is a two-step process, which has a varied effect upon the obligations imposed by the informed consent doctrine. First, the physician should be alert for warning signs, which should prompt increased scrutiny of the patient's capacity. Second, where no warning signs are initially apparent, the physician should begin disclosure, and only if the patient fails to demonstrate specific capacity is the consent requirement suspended. Practically, physicians should begin disclosure in all but the most obvious cases of general incompetence. Thus disclosure is ordinarily suspended for patients who are clearly delirious, severely intoxicated, or unconscious. However, all other "warning" signs should indicate that the physician needs to be sensitive to the additional time and effort needed to accomplish the disclosure, but not that disclosure should be bypassed. Only by beginning the informed consent disclosure can the physician evaluate the patient's specific capacities to understand, appreciate, and engage in a rational decisionmaking process.

From a legal perspective, if the patient fails to meet the criteria adopted for determining competence, the physician's obligation to obtain consent from the *patient* is suspended. The patient's decision (if any is rendered) need not be honored, and the decision as to whether and how the patient is to be treated may be made without his further participation, although legal proceedings, depending on the treatment and the jurisdiction, may be required. It is still legally obligatory, and from an ethical perspective highly desirable, that the goals of informed consent be pursued on behalf of the incompetent patient through a process of surrogate decision making.

Who Makes the Determination?

In theory, the determination of incompetence requires an official legal act known as adjudication. An adjudicated incompetent is referred to as de jure incompetent. In practice, however, many people who have not been subjected to an adjudication of incompetence are deemed incompetent to manage their financial affairs and/or make personal decisions. Such people are called de facto incompetent; they are incompetent in fact, but have not by legal procedures been determined to be so. Some people have suggested that the term "incapacitated" be used instead of "incompetent," to differentiate situations where an individual has be adjudicated incompetent from those in which a physician or mental health professional has determined the patient lacks the capacity to make decisions.

Consideration of persons who are incompetent to manage their financial affairs sheds light on related problems with medical decision making. In many cases, the absence of wealth and complicated financial problems militates against invoking so formal, cumbersome, and potentially expensive a proceeding as an adjudication of incompetence and the concurrent appointment of a guardian to manage the incompetent's estate. Family members often make less formal arrangements for an incompetent person's financial affairs. For example, if a person is having difficulty remembering to pay utility bills, a relative may take over the job by means of a joint checking account. Or if an elderly person suddenly starts to give away to strangers all of the money needed for living, arrangements can be made with the Social Security Administration to have a relative named representative payee (44), to whom Social Security checks are then sent to be used for the elderly person's living expenses.

In practice, determinations of incompetence to make medical decisions proceed much the same way as determinations of incompetence to handle financial affairs, despite assertions by some commentators that medical decisions can or should be made for an incompetent patient only by a court-appointed guardian (45,46). Most cases simply do not warrant the invocation of legal proceedings. The issues often are not complex, and the cost of legal proceedings is great. The delay attendant to seeking an adjudication of incompetence might add substantially to the cost of care or might sometimes be injurious to the patient's health (47). Ordinarily, family members make decisions about medical care for de facto incompetent persons in much the same way as they take over their financial affairs (45). We will refer to such family members as surrogates. The number of states that have codified the informal next-of-kin decisionmaking hierarchies in this context reinforces the legality of such practice (see discussion later under *Choosing a Surrogate*). Only in a small proportion of cases is an adjudication of incompetence sought: when there is no family member to make decisions, when the family member makes a decision that the attending physician believes to be detrimental to the well-being of the patient, when there is intractable conflict among family members over what course to pursue, or when it is unclear whether legal liability (either criminal or civil) might be incurred as a result of the particular kind of decision that needs to be made.

An important distinction between the informal mechanisms of de facto incompetence and the more formal appointment of a guardian concerns accountability.

In the financial context, court-appointed guardians must account to the court on a regular basis for the assets of the incompetent that have been entrusted to them. Although legal remedies do exist to call to account a person who has failed to use a de facto incompetent's assets for the benefit of the incompetent, these remedies are expensive and unwieldy. Furthermore, they will not operate at all unless the incompetent individual or someone else is aware that the incompetent's assets are being misused and is willing to assert the incompetent person's rights. By contrast, in medical decision making, there is an additional safeguard in that there are other persons besides the surrogate (e.g., medical personnel) focused on the patient's welfare. Thus, if the surrogate makes a decision out of improper motives or reaches a decision that will be harmful to the patient, at least some other party will know of it. Although this situation does not guarantee that action will be taken to prevent harm to the patient, there is a greater likelihood of protection than with respect to financial matters.

In terms of law, it has not been settled whether the final determination of incompetence must be made by a court or whether it may be made in the clinical setting without judicial participation. However, there is a long tradition in medical practice of physicians relying upon family members to make decisions on behalf of patients unable to do so themselves (48). The practice of obtaining consent from a family member, notes Alexander Capron, "is so well known in society at large that any individual who finds the prospect particularly odious has ample warning to make other arrangements better suited to protecting his own ends or interests" (49).

In other words, determinations that a patient is incompetent are frequently—indeed, overwhelmingly—made by physicians. Such determinations have been made not only routinely but sometimes without a conscious awareness on the part of the participants of what they were doing. To call such a process a determination is to accord it far too much formality. It is usually only an implicit by-product of the physician's more overt decision to engage in medical decision making not with the patient, but with the patient's family.

Doubt about the legitimacy of this informal process lingers because of a number of factors. First, there is some question about whether all health professionals are qualified to make determinations regarding capacity or whether this is a role for mental health professionals (51).[4] Nothing in the law suggests the latter, but courts do seem to give additional credence to psychiatrists' assessments of decisionmaking capacity when they are available. Second, all states have statutory procedures for the determination of incompetence through the judicial process (52). A court may determine that such a statute identifies the sole legally valid means for making such a determination in that jurisdiction. Such a ruling, how-

---

[4]One study, for example, showed that residents' and nurses' informal assessments of patient capacity correlated highly with mental status testing (50).

ever, in the face of the long-standing practice of physician determinations of capacity seems unlikely. Moreover, the increasing number of states that have put in place proxy decision making statutes and decisionmaker hierarchies (see later under *Choosing a Surrogate*) belies such an interpretation. But there are reported cases in many, if not all, jurisdictions in which physicians, or hospital administrators acting at their behest, have sought an adjudication of incompetence. Only rarely has a court suggested that resort to the judicial process for such a determination was unwarranted (53). The very fact that courts do make such adjudications indicates that the professional custom is not entirely clear-cut.

There are no clear guidelines to distinguish the cases in which physicians should make their own determinations from the cases in which they should not. Whether a judicial determination of incompetence is necessary is part of the larger issue of whether to resort to the courts at a number of possible points in the medical decisionmaking process. Given the high costs of requiring judicial intervention in all cases, it is likely that the responsibility for making informal capacity judgments will remain with physicians (54). This may, in fact, be most appropriate (54). But if this is indeed how most cases of decisionmaking incapacity are to be handled, it is increasingly important that physicians become aware of the legal standards of competence and also of the fact that there may be some states that require judicial authorization in specific types of cases.

Procedural Issues

Choosing a Surrogate

Once a patient is determined to be incompetent, whether the determination is made clinically or judicially, someone must be selected to make decisions for the patient. This person is referred to generically as a surrogate (54). All states permit some form of surrogate decision making for incompetent patients (55). Particular kinds of surrogates include a guardian, who is a court-appointed surrogate, and a proxy, who is a surrogate selected by the patient himself. The term "proxy" is sometimes used specifically to denote a surrogate selected by the patient using an advance care document (e.g., advance directive, living will, or durable power of attorney), whereas a "surrogate" often refers to an informal designation. The two terms, however, are often used interchangeably. The phrases "legal representative" or "legally authorized representative" are sometimes used in the same general way as the term surrogate (56). Occasionally, the terms "committee" or "conservator" are used to indicate a court appointed surrogate. To further confuse the matter, sometimes the term surrogate denotes someone who is court-appointed. When there is so much inconsistency over matters as simple as terminology, it is no wonder that there is so much uncertainty about a matter as important as who may serve as a surrogate and how the surrogate is to be chosen.

Courts making the determination of incompetence may ask healthcare personnel to recommend a guardian, if no likely person is immediately in evidence, such as a close and concerned family member. The preference for family members is based on a number of factors. There is some evidence that relatives are better able to judge patient preferences accurately (see, e.g., 57), although this has not held true in all circumstances, especially in the absence of any previous discussion between the family member and patient regarding treatment choices (58). Moreover, close family members are likely to be in a better position to judge what action would be in the patient's best interests (3). But some commentators have raised questions about family decision makers, particularly when these individuals may have conflicting interests (59). In most cases, one family member may have been more involved than others in caring for the patient, dealing with health care personnel, and expressing concern. This person may have been making decisions for the patient before hospitalization or care was needed and continues naturally to do so when the need for more formal decisionmaking arises.

There is some question concerning the authority of physicians unilaterally to identify a surrogate. Since all states have some mechanism allowing a patient to designate a proxy, as well as a method of judicially appointing a guardian, allowing physician appointment may be inappropriate. However, common law authority supports the notion that an informal next-of-kin surrogate can make treatment decisions (48). Physicians often make an effort to include all close family members in the decisionmaking process, and this is likely to be the safest route and is ethically commendable. One author suggests that the legal requirements should be changed explicitly to require that the physician gather all relevant decision makers—those with "some personal tie to the patient"—and discuss possible options until a consensus is reached, in his terms a position "to which no one strongly objects and the group generally supports" (60). Although such a legal requirement seems impracticable given the difficulty of identifying who has such relevant personal ties, from a practical standpoint when all family members agree on the appropriate treatment it is unlikely that any of them will bring a subsequent court challenge. Moreover, even when a suit is brought, a judge is likely to defer to physicians' determination of competence. Since a family member would in all likelihood have been appointed as the surrogate, a court is likely to ratify the decision unless there is clear evidence of misconduct either on the part of the family or the physician.

In some states, statutes specify a hierarchy of family members who are empowered to consent on behalf of incompetent patients; some even include close friends (61). Such hierarchies reflect the informed next-of-kin hierarchy used in most other decisionmaking situations. Where such legislation exists, there is ordinarily no need for court appointment of a guardian, unless there is serious conflict among family members of equal degree of relationship and the statute fails to differentiate among the possible decision makers. Presumably it is the responsibility of the attending physician, with guidance from the hospital administration, to determine which particular person qualifies under the statutory requirements in given cases. Stressing the benefits of such legislation, one author noted that "[a]ll states have intestacy laws to provide for the distribution of the decedent's property without a will. A comparable alternative is needed to provide for those individuals who fail to execute a living will or a durable power of attorney" (62). Others have voiced concern that the use of such hierarchies will result in wooden application of the list without consideration for who actually might be the most appropriate decision maker.

As noted before, there is one other way in which a surrogate may be selected, and that is by the patient before becoming incompetent. Through the use of legal instruments such as a durable power of attorney, living will, or advance directive, patients may designate another person to make medical decisions should they become incompetent (63). The term "advance directive"—specifically, proxy directives, because through them patients appoint proxies—is often used to refer to these types of documents. (Another kind of advance directive, an instruction directive, is discussed later under *Standards of Surrogate Decisionmaking*.) In all cases, the patient can limit the proxy's decisionmaking power. In addition, some states specifically limit the proxy's authority to make decisions about certain types of treatments, for example, life-sustaining treatment, experimental treatment, psychosurgery, and sterilization.

Increasingly, many healthcare institutions actually have formal procedures governing these matters, including issues such as whether it is the responsibility of the attending physician or of other hospital personnel, such as nursing or social services, to identify a surrogate. Two forces are pushing healthcare institutions to adopt more formal policies for surrogate selection and incompetence determinations (64). The first stems from demographic trends. There are increasing numbers of elderly persons who, though not incompetent simply because of age, are more likely in fact to be incompetent due to chronic illness and to require a series of decisions to be made on their behalf over an extended period of time (13). The second force is legal. Increasing attention is being paid by courts, legislatures, regulators, and possibly prosecutors to procedures and standards for decision making, especially with regard to life-sustaining treatment.

Institutions developing formal policies should address the question of who within the institutional structure should have the responsibility to designate formally a surrogate, as well as the problem of how that person should make the designation. In the absence of legal requirements, institutions should develop guidelines, which should then be clearly articulated to the individuals responsible for identifying a surrogate. Although no precise formula can be established, these guidelines may focus on factors such as the absence or presence of a family relationship, the closeness of that relationship according to law, and the closeness of that relationship in fact. Attention must also be given to situations in which either patients have no family or there are no readily available or concerned family members. In the absence of other alternatives, the policy should specify whether a friend, if one exists, may serve as a surrogate or whether in such a case judicial guidance will be sought.

For those situations in which there is no readily available person, either family or friend, guidelines should be established to determine who should be appointed as a surrogate. It is generally thought to be inappropriate to appoint the patient's physician, nurse, or social worker, or anyone directly involved in the patient's care or even affiliated with the hospital, since the possibilities for a conflict of interest are obvious. Many state statutes explicitly bar such individuals from serving as a surrogate. Nonetheless, in many cases there is no one else who can or will serve as a surrogate. Governmental and nonprofit health and welfare agencies, which often are considered other likely candidates for providing surrogates, in fact rarely have the resources or inclination to do so. Bank trust departments, the traditional source of guardians of an incompetent person's estate, are similarly reluctant and ill equipped to become involved in making medical decisions. New York, for example, dealt with this problem by creating "surrogate decision-making committees and panels" that are authorized to make treatment decisions for mentally disabled persons who lack decisionmaking capacity and have no available family members (65). The panels are made up of at least twelve persons, including members of each of the following groups: licensed healthcare professionals (physicians, nurses, psychologists, etc.); licensed attorneys; former patients, or family or advocates of mentally disabled persons; and other persons with expertise or interest in the care of the mentally disabled.

How Should the Surrogate Decide?

Once a surrogate has been selected, by whatever means, the decisionmaking process should proceed much as it would if the patient were competent, but with the surrogate participating in place of the patient. The ideal embodied in the spirit of informed consent remains: collaborative decision making, in this case between surrogate and physician. The role of the physician is to provide the surrogate with information about the medical options, their risks, and their potential benefits. The ideal role of the surrogate is to interject the patient's values into the decision-making process, to the extent that they are known or knowable. Thus, an added responsibility of the surrogate, especially one who does not know the patient very well or at all, is to attempt to learn more about the patient. In the case of a patient who is incompetent but not uncommunicative, the surrogate may carry on conversations with the patient, as well as talk with others—friends and family—who knew or know the patient well. The goal is to learn about the patient's values, goals, hopes, and fears in general, as well as with particular reference to the patient's medical condition, its prognosis, and the available treatments. The argument that family members are best suited for surrogate decision making stems from the belief that they will be best able to ascertain the patient's values and preferences (62), and also, when those values cannot be known or applied, best able to determine the patient's best interests (3). Thus, the question of who should be the surrogate is closely linked with the issue of what the surrogate should take into consideration in making the decision.

The result of this system of surrogate decision making is that the decisionmaking process for incompetent patients ought to look very much as it should when the patient is competent, with the obvious exception that the surrogate plays the patient's role. Nevertheless, there is still the problem of substantive standards for decision making. Two basic questions remain to be answered: (*1*) what standard should the surrogate apply (e.g., subjective or objective), and (*2*) what level of certainty is needed?

Standards of Surrogate Decisionmaking

When competent patients make decisions for themselves, by definition they do so in accordance with their own sense of what is best. This is not to say that others will agree that the decision is best, or even good. Nor is it to say that if faced with the same decision at a different time, the patient would necessarily make the same decision, or that if there were a succession of decisions the logical consistency among them would be apparent. People's goals, values, preferences, and desires are not so certain, consistent, and known even to themselves that rationality of this kind often will be achieved.

Most commentators contend that the goal of decision making by surrogates should be to replicate the decision that patients would make for themselves if they were competent to do so (54,66). This ideal is far more easily stated than achieved, if only because many people cannot even say with much precision how they themselves would act in the future should a certain set of circumstances arise, let alone how someone else would. Nonetheless, people can and do leave evidence of their wishes so that others may attempt to carry them out, at least in a general sort of way.

Decision making by a surrogate on behalf of an incompetent patient that attempts to replicate the patient's own decision, guided by the patient's own values, goals, preferences, and wishes, is called a subjective approach (54). It can be implemented in several ways. The simplest and most unequivocal is for patients, while competent, to leave written instructions about the kind of care they would wish to have in the event that they become incompetent. This is known as an advance directive, specifically an instruction directive. Instruction directives, however, need not be made in writing. A number of courts have enforced oral instructions from patients who have stated, while competent, that they would not wish to have certain kinds of life-sustaining treatment administered should they become incompetent and incurably ill (48,67–71). When the patient has specifically indicated what she would want in a particular situation, the surrogate's role is to (*1*) ensure that the facts of the patient's present situation match the anticipated situation of the advance directive, and (2) implement the advance directive.

While useful, instruction directives have limitations. The more general they are, the less useful they may be. On the other hand, if they are too specific, they may not contemplate the particular decision with which the surrogate is faced. Moreover, it may be unrealistic to think that patients can make specific treatment decisions significantly in advance of particular healthcare needs (72). The value of an instruction directive thus can be enhanced if combined with a proxy directive—that is, the naming of a particular person to act as surrogate. If the proxy both knows the patient and has the benefit of the instruction directive, the patient's wishes may be more closely approximated than with an instruction directive alone. When the surrogate must interpret the advance instructions, or when there are no specific advance instructions, the standard that should be applied is called "substituted judgment" (3).

The substituted judgment approach is a subjective one; its aim is to implement the subjective preferences of the patient about and for whom decisions must be made. As such, it is most consonant with the goals of the informed consent doctrine itself. However, in many cases—indeed, probably most—patients have not given either written or oral instructions. In these situations surrogates cannot be guided by the patient's express wishes. Some other standard must be applied.

Historically the doctrine of substituted judgment appears to have been borrowed from English common law where it developed as a legal fiction allowing courts to distribute parts of a "lunatic's" estate to relatives that were not owed any legal duty of support (73). Although it initially started out with no constraints, it quickly became dependent upon evidence of what the incompetent person would have wanted (or done) were he competent. But even in this format the substituted judgment standard may be a type of legal fiction if there is little or no evidence of the incompetent person's preferences. Thus, in some cases it is more appropriate (and honest) to apply a traditional best interests standard. This standard requires the surrogate to decide according to her views of what would benefit the patient most. It is common in medical decision making and in law, and used to be the sole standard by which decisions were made on behalf of incompetent patients. Only in the last half-century or so, roughly the same period in which the informed consent doctrine was born and matured, has the best interests standard increasingly received competition from the substituted judgment approach.

The conflict between the two standards may be greater in theory than in practice. All surrogate decision makers are, in a general way, under a duty to act in the best interests of the incompetent patient. The difficulty with the best interests standard is not in the statement of it but in giving content to it. The substituted judgment approach is, in fact, one way of doing so. That is, a surrogate who makes a decision for an incompetent patient on the basis of that patient's instructions—written or oral, express or implied—is seeking to implement the patient's best interests *as that patient would have defined them*. The forces that have served as an impetus to obtaining informed consent from competent patients have acted similarly in regard to decision making for incompetent patients, who presumably would wish to have decisions made for them in accordance with their values rather than someone else's.

In the absence of advance directives from patients, content must be given to the best interests standard through the application of objective standards. Even if patients do not leave express directions about their health care, the patterns of their lives provide some, possibly substantial, information about their values, goals, preferences, and wishes that may prove useful to a surrogate. A decision based on such information can be called a limited-objective approach (64), or subjective best interests (although this label may be confusing in light of the prior discussion). Because there is often no bright line between one's express directives, especially when cast in a general way, and one's religious beliefs, ethical values, or lifestyle, the substituted judgment and the limited-objective best interest approaches shade into each other.

The limited-objective approach, in turn, stands in contrast to a pure-objective approach to determining best interests, which is used when the surrogate has no information whatsoever available about the patient that can serve as a guide, or when there is substantial reason to doubt the competence of the patient's previous choices. In such cases surrogates must make determinations based entirely on objective criteria; that is, they must make decisions that reasonable people would want made for them (64). But the application of this standard is not truly neutral, nor should it be. Even in the usual tort cases in which such a construct is applied, it is almost impossible to imagine the hypothetical reasonable person who exists without any background identity. Especially in the context of informed consent to medical care it seems ludicrous to make decisions discounting all evidence of the individual's background and experiences. Thus, even the purely objective standard is subject to evaluation by the surrogate.

It is worth noting that application of these standards by family members (as opposed to some theoretically neutral third party) raises another problem: the individuals making decisions are likely to have relevant interests of their own that will be affected by the choice (59). The extent to which family members should take into account these interests has never been clear. To a great degree the deference courts show to family decision making stems from the reluctance to interfere within a family unit—a tacit acknowledgment that even competent patients do not make decisions in a vacuum, with only themselves in mind. Sometimes courts allow family members' interests to be considered under either the substituted judgment or best interests standards. For example, one might determine that a particular patient would have wanted the financial impact on her children to be taken into account in deciding about life-sustaining treatment. Other courts have simply stretched the meaning of "best interests" to include interests in maintaining family relationships, as one court did in holding that a guardian could decide in favor of donating a kidney from an incompetent individual to his brother, based on the benefit that the incompetent individual derived from his relationship with his brother (22).

Level of Certainty

Most of the judicial discussions about applying the different standards of surrogate decision making revolve around the level of certainty needed to enforce a patient's advance instructions. There are a number of possibilities, but courts generally have focused on three evidentiary standards: preponderance of the evidence (greater than 50 percent probability), clear and convincing evidence (greater than 75 percent probability), and beyond a reasonable doubt (greater than 95 percent to 99 percent probability). The latter is reserved for criminal cases and thought to be inappropriate for this setting. Although most other civil actions require a preponderance of the evidence to succeed, civil commitment proceedings use the more stringent clear and convincing evidence standard.

In *Cruzan v. Director, Missouri Department of Health* (48), the United States Supreme Court held that a state may require clear and convincing evidence of a patient's wishes in the context of withdrawal of life-sustaining treatment. Thus, although the court recognized the validity of advance instructions, it held that states may require a high level of certainty as to what the patient would have wanted. Written instructions are likely to meet this standard, while oral instructions must be evaluated on a case-by-case basis. Certainty is needed not only as to what the patient would have wanted but also as to whether the patient considered the situation he is currently in. Thus, an advance directive may clearly state that the patient does not want ventilator support if in a persistent vegetative state, but it may be unclear whether those same instructions apply if the patient is in a coma, or bedridden and dependent on multiple life-support machines. At least one state's highest court has noted that where the evidence has not met the clear and convincing standard, life-support measures must be continued, despite the proxy's belief that the patient would not want treatment (74).

An increasing number of states have shifted toward the clear and convincing evidence standard, at least where the issue is the withdrawal of life-sustaining treatment. But what this actually means in practice appears to vary considerably, and evidence that meets the standard in one case may not meet it in another. Not surprisingly, whether or not disagreement exists between family members seems to be the best indicator of whether evidence of the patient's wishes to decline treatment is deemed sufficient. In those cases where disagreement exists, courts appear more likely to err on the side of continuing life-sustaining treatment, especially in cases where the patient does not appear to be in any pain (see, e.g., 74). The trend to require a higher standard of evidence, coupled with a few recent decisions that have declined to assess damages against physicians or other medical personnel for providing treatment against a patient's *explicit* wishes (see, e.g., 75), have created a situation that threatens to undermine the usefulness of advance directives. There is evidence that along with the continued difficulty in getting people to complete advance care documents (76,77), physicians are not necessarily following the preferences expressed in these documents, especially in end-of-life situations (78). Therefore, although there is widespread agreement about the benefits of proxy directives, there continues to be controversy over the best form and content of instruction directions.

The Role of the Courts

There are a number of points in the process of decision making for incompetent patients when consideration might be given to seeking judicial guidance. Among the reasons for doing so are the fear of civil or criminal liability for an action taken without judicial sanction, a desire to protect patient autonomy, and a genuine desire for help in making the right decision.

The first point at which the courts might be consulted is in the determination of incompetence. If there is no serious question about a patient's competence, it may not be necessary to go to court, depending upon the precise statutory requirements and case law of the particular jurisdiction. In any event, customary practice is not to seek an adjudication of incompetence when a patient is clearly incompetent, for example, comatose.

The second point where judicial guidance may be sought is in the appointment of a surrogate. If an adjudication of incompetence has been sought and obtained, the surrogate will be appointed by the court. If incompetence is determined in the clinical setting, a surrogate will ordinarily be selected in that setting. Only when special circumstances arise, such as substantial and intractable conflict among potential candidates for the role of surrogate, or if there is no one at all to serve as surrogate, will judicial guidance be sought for the appointment of a surrogate, if it was not previously sought for the determination of incompetence.

Even if there has been no resort to the judicial process either for a determination of incompetence or the appointment of a surrogate, the existence of an advance directive from the incompetent patient may create a need for judicial guidance. Questions about the formal validity of the directive (e.g., whether a written document is a forgery) or its substantive validity (e.g., whether it requests an act that is illegal) may prompt the seeking of judicial review. Judicial review may also be needed to help interpret directives that are vague, confusing, or internally conflicting, or that are in conflict with the wishes of the surrogate or with the current expressed wishes of the patient, incompetent though she may be.

Assuming that none of the foregoing events has prompted recourse to the courts, a hearing may still be sought to review the substance of the decision made by the surrogate, especially if that decision is in serious conflict with what the attending physician or other professional staff believes to be medically or ethically appropriate. Even if there is no such disagreement, there may still be a legal requirement for judicial review in some cases, or if not a requirement, at least some concern to assure that the chosen course of action is legally sound.

The courts have infrequently addressed the question of when resort to the judicial process in medical decision making for incompetent patients is required. The issue rarely arises largely because the medical profession has tacit customs governing decision making for incompetent patients that ordinarily operate smoothly. Only when some difficulty with customary practice occurs is guidance from courts sought.

Although in theory there are a number of discrete points at which judicial review might be sought, in practice they tend to overlap or collapse into a single question. The questions of adjudication of incompetence and selection of a surrogate, though conceptually distinct, are usually resolved as a single issue. From the perspective of the participants in the decisionmaking process, the question to be addressed, to which all other questions are subordinate is: what treatment, if any, should be provided? If this overriding question can be resolved without intractable conflict among the interested parties (patients, family, friends, attending physician, house staff, nurses, social workers, technicians, and administrators, some or all of whom may have a say in a particular case) the issue of judicial review is unlikely to arise. Such recourse is sought when some apparent complication develops, for example: a patient who is not clearly incompetent and is refusing medically indicated treatment (40,79–81), conflict between the family's and the patient's wishes (40), conflict among family members about the proper course of treatment (74), concern that the patient's surrogate is not acting in the patient's best interests (82–84), fear of civil or criminal liability (85, 86), a conflict between the surrogate's decision and the ethical precepts of the attending physician, or confusion over what a patient's substituted judgment would be (87).

Such problems are most likely to occur, it seems, in cases involving decisions about life-sustaining treatment and about involuntarily hospitalized psychiatric patients. In these areas a number of pitched battles have been fought since the late 1970s. The debates continue, though resolution seems to be slowly coming. The New Jersey Supreme Court has explicitly required that incompetence be determined judicially in cases involving the forgoing of life-sustaining treatment (88). In the context both of life-sustaining treatment and psychiatric treatment, the Massachusetts Supreme Court has required that the decisions of surrogates either consenting to or refusing treatment be subjected to judicial review (23, 89,90). At the same time, in cases involving life-sustaining treatment, that court has also transformed what had originally seemed to be an ironclad rule of judicial review into a more flexible one, thereby creating uncertainty about precisely when review is required (91). By and large, the few courts that have made any mention of the issue of judicial participation seem to take the position of being available for judicial review, but not requiring it (25,67,88,92–95).

The Advantages and Disadvantages of Judicial Review

The question of when judicial guidance should be sought has occasioned a great deal of debate in the courts and especially in the medical and legal literatures. Much of the controversy stems from the fact that to have judicial guidance, oversight, or review—whichever name is used—of medical decision making is substantially at odds with long-standing professional custom. Consequently, such guidance has the potential to cause considerable resentment and discomfort among physicians who believe that their prerogatives are being eroded or eliminated. In fact, in many respects judicial review of medical decision making for incompetent patients engenders adverse reactions from the medical profession similar to its reactions to the requirement to obtain informed consent from competent patients. Both informed consent and judicial review are perceived to threaten physicians' freedom to make decisions about what kinds of treatment patients will receive. Because both interject non-medical values (and non-physicians) into the decisionmaking process they are perceived to undermine the authority of individual physicians and of the medical profession itself.

In addition, judicial participation in the process moves the locus of decision making out of a forum where physicians not only largely control the process but also can shield it from any substantial scrutiny by others. In fact, decision making within the clinical setting is all but invisible, whereas a judicial forum not only opens the content of the decisionmaking process to review but also exposes the very fact that such decisions are made at all.

Although attempting to avoid legal liability is one of the motivations for seeking judicial review, it will not absolutely confer immunity (88,91). In fact, absolute immunity will never be conferred on physicians or other health-care personnel when they are making a decision that involves the exercise of professional judgment. A judicial determination of incompetence will assure that a physician may rely upon the decisions of a judicially appointed guardian without incurring liability for battery for unauthorized treatment, as long as the guardian has consented. This does not constitute an absolute grant of immunity from liability, because physicians will still be liable, criminally or civilly, to the same extent they would have been had they dealt directly with a competent patient. That is, if the physician fails to use reasonable care in making a diagnosis, recommends improper treatment, or fails to use reasonable care in providing treatment, there can still be liability for negligence if the patient is harmed as a result of the physician's conduct, regardless of the fact that the guardian may have consented to the conduct.

Similarly, physicians who disclose inadequate information to surrogates may be liable for failing to obtain informed consent. If they fail altogether to obtain consent from surrogates, they may be liable for battery for unauthorized administration of medical care. Additionally, physicians must ensure that the surrogate has the capacity to make a decision; a decision from an incompetent surrogate is as invalid as one from an incompetent patient. Finally, any conduct that would be criminal even if performed by a physician with the consent of the patient will likewise be criminal if performed with the consent of the surrogate; any criminal omission to treat will similarly be grounds for liability even if the surrogate consents to it.

Apart from questions of liability, there are other arguments for seeking or avoiding judicial review of surrogates' decisions. First, the logistics of obtaining judicial review argue against it (7). If a situation is not labeled an emergency, the case is likely to be considered by the courts as a routine matter, which means that some delay, perhaps a great deal, may occur. Delay may not threaten a patient's life or health, but it may impose physical pain, emotional suffering, and added cost, as well as contribute to the demoralization of professionals, patients, and families. (If the situation is an emergency, a determination of incompetence is not needed, since in the absence of a surrogate decision maker or an advance directive, the emergency exception will authorize the physician to provide necessary treatment at least to maintain the status quo.) Judicial review also involves a significant loss of privacy. Decisions made in a healthcare setting with the involvement of the minimum number of relevant, concerned parties better protect patients' interests in privacy and confidentiality, which are considered to be intimately connected to both autonomy and well-being.

Resort to the courts can also impose financial costs, sometimes substantial, for both the hospital and the patient or family (7). In some jurisdictions legal counsel for both parties will be mandatory, and where it is not mandatory it will usually be desirable. If the issue is serious enough to require judicial attention, it would be unwise to enter judicial proceedings unrepresented by an attorney. Furthermore, even if judicial review is relatively simple to obtain in a particular case, the judicial system is probably not well equipped to handle the large number of cases that would arise if all such cases were subjected to judicial review.

Beyond these logistical matters is the question of whether courts are well suited to decision making of this kind. A good theoretical argument can be made that the business of courts is to make decisions, but in practice judges often feel uneasy and insecure about their own ability to make medical decisions (53). The result is substantial deference to professional medical judgment. If courts merely rubber-stamp professional decisions, much of the value of judicial review is lost (7,96). Another problem is the nature of the adversary process. Courts may seek to appoint an opposing party with a contrary view, even when there is no disagreement between families and healthcare professionals (62, p. 166).

However, the judicial forum does have some value. What appears in the vast majority of cases to be rubber-stamping of professional decisions may be an acknowledgment that the time-honored method of decision making involving physician and family usually does result in decisions that are in an incompetent patient's best interests. But usually does not mean always. If the courts exist to identify those cases in which professional judgment or family inclinations have gone astray, then this identification can only be accomplished by the review of all cases, which is impractical for reasons outlined before. Although judicial hearings do have strong symbolic value and may lead to a more accurate reflection of the patient's preferences (7), the costs imposed by review of all cases in order to identify a few incorrectly decided ones are too high a price to pay. There may be other ways of identifying such cases at lower cost. New York State, for example, established a quasi-judicial hearing board to determine patient capacity to consent to or refuse medical treatment (65).

Ethics Committees

The inadequacies of the existing method of making decisions for incompetent patients have long been apparent. The primary deficiency is that the process is riddled with uncertainty about two issues. First, what substantive decisions are legally and ethically acceptable? Second, assuming that a decision is a legitimate one, what are the appropriate procedures for making it? Physicians, and the hospital or nursing home administrators to whom they usually turn for advice in such matters, are unclear about when they are entitled to rely on decisions to terminate care made by competent patients, or family members of incompetent patients, without fear of legal liability and without violating professional ethics. Their concerns prompt the simple question they often ask: do we have to go to court? Hospital attorneys often advise that when in doubt, it is either best to play it safe and go to court, or to continue to provide treatment even if patients or their families object. However, the latter course may be not only unethical, but in some cases illegal.

Judicial resolution of these kinds of questions rarely occurred prior to recent times, and such recourse has not always been well received by the courts. In 1966, a New York trial court judge, presented with the question of whether the gangrenous limb of an eighty-year-old woman should be amputated at the request of her lawyer son, over the objection of her physician son, opined against

> the current practice of members of the medical profession and their associated hospitals of shifting the burden of their responsibilities to the courts, to determine, in effect, whether doctors should proceed with certain medical procedures [and against the] ultra-legalistic maze we have created to the extent that society and the individual have become enmeshed and paralyzed by its unrealistic entanglements!(53)

Although somewhat intemperate, the judge's remarks are not hard to understand when viewed as a symptom of his frustration, born of uncertainty as to what the law really requires. Physicians, hospital administrators, and their lawyers are not the only ones who are uncertain about how decisions should be made and what decisions are acceptable. Indeed, they are in the dark as much as they are largely because of the absence of legislative guidance or authoritative judicial precedents.

The exasperation expressed by the New York judge was not repeated in recorded legal annals for another decade, until the *Quinlan* case in 1976. Again, a court was confronted with the problem of how decisions should be made for incompetent patients. In more measured tones, the New Jersey Supreme Court recommended that a hospital ethics committee review such decision making rather than requiring judicial review:

> We consider that a practice of applying to a court to confirm such decisions would generally be inappropriate, not only because that would be a gratuitous encroachment upon the medical profession's field of competence, but because it would be impossibly cumbersome. (85)

The court based its recommendation for the use of an ethics committee on a law review article (97). The court obviously believed that such committees existed; however, in fact they did not. Furthermore, the term ethics committee was somewhat of a misnomer in light of the function that the court assigned to it— namely, confirmation of the patient's prognosis.

Nonetheless, the idea of using ethics committees instead of courts to make such decisions captured the imagination of many physicians and hospital administrators, who saw recourse to such committees as a way of avoiding having "the law" telling them how to practice medicine, as well as the unwanted inconvenience, expense, and perhaps publicity involved in judicial review. The suggestion, however, was not as welcome in judicial circles. The Massachusetts Supreme Judicial Court expressed outright disdain for the use of ethics committees in lieu of judicial review, but did acknowledge the potential usefulness of such a committee as an adjunct to judicial decision making:

> [T]he [trial] court judge may, at any step in these proceedings, avail himself or herself of the additional advice or knowledge of any person or group. . . . We believe it desirable for a judge to consider [the views of an ethics committee] wherever available and useful to the court. We do not believe, however, that this option should be transformed by us into a required procedure. We take a dim view of any attempt to shift the ultimate decisionmaking responsibility away from the duly established courts of proper jurisdiction to any committee, panel or group, ad hoc or permanent. Thus, we reject the approach adopted by *Quinlan*.(23)

Even the New Jersey Supreme Court, which first catapulted the idea of ethics committees into the public arena, seems to have backed off from its initial enthusiasm. In the *Conroy* case, decided almost a decade after *Quinlan,* the court decided not to rely upon ethics committees to make or review decisions about withdrawing life-sustaining treatment from patients in nursing homes, on the ground that "[f]ew nursing homes . . . have 'ethics' or 'prognosis' committees "(88). The same was even more true of hospitals a decade earlier, and yet that did not deter the New Jersey court from pronouncing their utility then. Recent surveys of hospitals estimate that between 66 percent and 70 percent of them have an in-hospital ethics committee (98,99). Hospitals that do not have an ethics committee may still have access to some type of ethics education or consultation outside the hospital. The Joint Commission on Accreditation of Health Care Organizations (JCAHO) now requires that hospitals have some mechanism for dealing with ethical issues (100), which usually takes the form of an institutional ethics committee. Additionally, two states mandate hospital ethics committees (101,102).

Discussion about establishing and using ethics committees for decisionmaking purposes continues and is largely positive, though there are occasional notes of caution and outright opposition. Most problematic is the fact that there do not seem to be any standards to which ethics committees are held. If they are to replace judicial review, there should be some regulation of their composition, process, and role (103), as well as a mechanism for evaluation of their consultation services (104,105). Ethics committees have been proposed to address questions about the determination of competence, the choice of a surrogate, and the appropriateness of honoring advance directives and current treatment decisions. In part, controversy over the use of ethics committees has been due to confusion about the range of their activities. Should they confirm a prognosis (basically a medical question), determine standards of decision making (basically a legal question), or resolve disputes when neither law nor medicine provides the answers (basically an ethical question)? It is only this latter category that is the proper domain of ethics consultation. The first issue arguably is not the province of an ethics committee at all, and the second relates to the educational role that ethics committees play.

Besides operating within the confines of a particular healthcare institution to review decisions about forgoing life-sustaining treatment, ethics committees often have several other functions, including education and policy making. Education takes place at several levels. The simplest is the self-education that committee members deliberately or necessarily undergo through committee service. Similarly, those who bring cases to committees for review—whether healthcare professionals or patients and families—are also educated in the process. The committee may also make conscious efforts to provide more formal educational programs for itself, health-care professionals, patients and families, or the community the hospital serves.

In their initial stages, ethics committees may deal with cases on an ad hoc basis. As their workload increases and their members become more sophisticated and knowledgeable, they will almost inevitably consider drafting policies for use in their healthcare institutions to provide guidance for the resolution of future cases, perhaps without resorting to the committee for advice. Such policies also serve an educational function and help to provide some consistency in how decisions are made within the hospital or nursing home. In jurisdictions where there is no law to provide guidance about forgoing life-sustaining treatment, or where the law fails to address other important issues, institutional policies may play an important role in the development of professional standards that, in the event of litigation, may aid in the resolution of the dispute (66)[5]

Conclusion

Decision making for incompetent patients poses great problems for all concerned. Physicians may be stymied by issues such as the standards and procedures to use in determining whether a patient is incompetent, identification of a surrogate to make decisions for incompetent patients, and determination of when to honor or override surrogate decisions. Decision making for incompetent patients may be complicated by conflicts among professional staff and the family members and friends of the patient. Finally, the fear of legal liability may subtly pervade the atmosphere in which treatment questions arise and make physicians inclined to err on what they believe to be the safe side by providing treatment when in doubt. In fact, the prospect of liability is extremely remote. Moreover, healthcare providers may be as much at risk of liability for providing unwanted treatment as for failing to provide medically indicated treatment.

Despite the large number of pitfalls that accompany caring for incompetent patients, reported judicial cases involving treatment of incompetent patients are relatively few compared with the large number of patient–physician contacts. When such cases do arise, more often than not they involve decisions to forgo

---

[5] More recently there has been a trend to consider the role of ethics committees in making decisions regarding organizational ethics. The Joint Commission on Accreditation of Health Care Organizations (JCAHO) 1997 standards require institutions to have a code of ethics that "addresses marketing, admission, transfer, discharge, and billing," as well as "the relationship of the hospital and its staff to . . . payers." Although the JCAHO standards do not specifically require the formation of an ethics committee, this is the usual mechanism for addressing clinical ethics issues in the hospital setting. Some authors have argued that the clinical ethics committee should address these organizational ethics issues (106, 107). There are likely to be some overlapping areas between clinical and organizational ethics, and thus having one committee to deal with both types of issues may be useful. On the other hand, there are also likely to be areas of conflict. Moreover, most committees as they are currently set up have no background in business or organizational ethics nor any basis for developing policy. While institutions would do well do develop mechanisms for dealing with organizational ethics issues, whether or not this mechanism should be the same as the one developed to address clinical ethics issues is unclear. With the increasing emphasis on healthcare organizational ethics this issue is likely to gain additional attention in the coming years.

life-sustaining treatment. As compared to other treatment decisions, such cases may be even more emotionally charged, and the fear of legal liability runs even higher. The present uncertainties regarding decisions to forgo life-sustaining treatment demand special sensitivity and diplomacy on the part of physicians and other healthcare personnel in dealing with dying patients and their families. Indeed, the complicated nature of decisions on behalf of incompetent patients requires that physicians and other health-care personnel develop special sensitivity and knowledge. Professionals must first be cognizant that a patient's incompetence relieves her physician of the usual requirement to obtain informed consent in only the most technical sense. Except in the case of emergency treatment, a patient's incompetence triggers the process of surrogate decision making. Thus, physicians must be knowledgeable about the requirements for such decisionmaking and should be sensitive to the special burdens that serving as a surrogate decision maker may place on already burdened family members or friends.

References

1. Feinberg, J. (1984) *Harm to Self.* New York: Oxford University Press.
2. Dresser, R. and Robertson, J. (1989) Quality of life and non-treatment decisions for incompetent patients: a critique of the orthodox approach. *Law, Medicine & Health Care,* 17:234–244.
3. Buchanan, A.E. and Brock, D.W. (1990) *Deciding for Others: The Ethics of Surrogate Decision Making.* Cambridge: Cambridge University Press.
4. Pratt v. Davis, 118 Ill. App. 161 (1905), *aff'd* 79 N.E. 562 (Ill. 1906).
5. Schloendorff v. Society of New York Hospital, 105 N.E. 92 (N.Y. 1914).
6. In re Long Island Jewish-Hillside Medical Center, 342 N.Y.S.2d 356, 358 (Sup. Ct. 1973).
7. Berg, J.W., Appelbaum, P.S., and Grisso, T. (1996) Constructing competence: formulating standards of legal competence to make medical decisions. *Rutgers Law Review,* 48:345–396.
8. U.S. v. Charters, 829 F.2d 479 (1987).
9. In re A.C., 573 A.2d 1235 (D.C. 1990).
10. Wilkins, L. (1975) Children's rights: removing the parental consent barrier to medical treatment of minors. *Arizona State Law Journal,* 31–92.
11. Wadlington, W. (1973) Minors and health care: the age of consent. *Osgoode Hall Law Journal,* 11:115–125.
12. Pilpel, H. (1972) Minors' rights to medical care. *Albany Law Review,* 36:462–487.
13. Rozovsky, F. (1990) *Consent to Treatment: A Practical Guide.* Boston: Little, Brown.
14. Grodin, M. and Alpert, J. (1983) Informed consent and pediatric care. In Melton, G., Koocher, G., Saks, M. (eds) *Children's Competence to Consent.* New York: Plenum.
15. Redding, R. (1993) Children's competence to provide informed consent for mental health treatment. *Washington and Lee Law Review,* 50:695–753.
16. Weithorn, L. and Campbell, S. (1982) The competency of children and adolescents to make informed treatment decisions. *Child Dev,* 53:1589–1598.

126   THE LEGAL THEORY OF INFORMED CONSENT

17. Ross, L.F. (1998) *Children, Families, and Health Care Decision-making*. New York: Oxford University Press.
18. American Academy of Pediatrics (1995) Informed consent, parental permission, and assent in pediatric practice. *Pediatrics*, 95:314–317.
19. Morrissy, J., Hofmann, A., and Thrope, J. (1986) *Consent and Confidentiality in the Health Care of Children and Adolescents*. New York: Free Press.
20. 21 C.F.R. 50.
21. Relf v. Weinberger, 372 F. Supp. 1196 (D.D.C. 1974).
22. Strunk v. Strunk, 445 S.W.2d 145 (Ky. 1969).
23. Superintendent of Belchertown State School v. Saikewicz, 370 N.E.2d 417 (Mass. 1977).
24. In re Weberlist, 360 N.Y.S.2d 783 (Sup. Ct. 1974).
25. Matter of Storar, 420 N.E.2d 64 (N.Y. 1981).
26. Moore v. Webb, 345 S.W.2d 239 (Mo. App. 1961).
27. Gravis v. Physicians and Surgeons Hosp., 427 S.W.2d 310 (Tex. 1968).
28. Demmers v. Gerety, 515 P.2d 645 (N.M. Ct. App. 1973).
29. Grannum v. Berard, 422 P.2d 812 (Wash. 1967).
30. Sugarman, J., McCrory, D., and Hubal, R. (1998) Getting meaningful informed consent from older adults: a structured literature review of empirical research. *JAGS*, 46:517–524.
31. In re W.S., 3M A.2d 969, 972 (N.J. Super. 1977).
32. Etchells, E., Shuchman, M., Workman, S., and Craven, J. (1997) Accuracy of clinical impressions and mini-mental state exam scores for assessing capacity to consent to major medical treatment: comparison with criterion-standard psychiatric assessments. *Psychosomatics*, 38:239–245.
33. Appelbaum, P.S. and Grisso, T. (1995) The MacArthur Treatment Competence Study. I: Mental illness and competence to consent to treatment. *Law Hum Behav*, 19:105–126.
34. Schreiber v. Physicians Insurance Company of Wisconsin, 588 N.W.2d 26 (Wisc. 1999).
35. Yahn v. Folse, 639 So.2d 261 (La. App. 1993).
36. Meisel, A., Roth, L., and Lidz, C. (1977) Toward a model of the legal doctrine of informed consent. *Am J Psychiatry*, 134:285–289.
37. Jones, C. (1990) Autonomy and informed consent in medical decisionmaking: toward a new self-fulfilling prophecy. *Washington and Lee Law Review*, 47:379–430.
38. Meisel, A. and Roth, L. (1983) Toward an informed dicussion of informed consent: a review and critique of the empirical studies. *Arizona Law Review*, 25:265–346.
39. Sulmasy, D.P, Lehmann, L.S., Levine, D.M., and Faden, R.R. (1994) Patients' perceptions of the quality of informed consent for common medical procedures. *J Clin Ethics*, 5:189–194.
40. Lane v. Candura, 376 N.E.2d 1232 (Mass. App. Ct. 1978).
41. Roth, L.H., Meisel, A., and Lidz, C.W. (1977) Tests of competence to consent to treatment. *Am J Psychiatry*, 134:279–284.
42. Drane, J. (1985) The many faces of competence. *Hastings Cent Rep*, 15:17–21.
43. Roth, L.H., Appelbaum, P.S., Sallee, R., et al. (1982) The dilemma of denial in the assessment of competence to consent to treatment. *Am J Psychiatry*, 139:910–913.
44. 42 U.S.C. §§ 405(j), 1383(a)(2).
45. Robertson, J. (1983) *The Rights of the Critically Ill*. New York: Bantam.
46. Baron, C. (1978) Assuring "detached but passionate investigation and decision":

the role of guardians ad litem in Saikewicz-type cases. *Am J Law Med*, 4:111–130.

47. President's Commission for the Study of Ethical Problems in Medicine and Biomedical and Behavioral Research (1983) *Deciding to Forego Life-Sustaining Treatment: Ethical, Medical and Legal Issues in Treatment Decisions.* Washington, D.C.: U.S. Government Printing Office.
48. Cruzan v. Director, Missouri Dep't of Health, 497 U.S. 261 (1990).
49. Capron, A.M. (1974) Informed consent in catastrophic disease research and treatment. *University of Pennsylvania Law Review*, 123:340–438.
50. Cohen, L., McCue, J., and Green, G. (1993) Do clinical and formal assessments of the capacity of patients in the intensive care unit to make decisions agree? *Arch Intern Med*, 153:2481–2485.
51. Gutheil, T.G. and Duckworth, K. (1992) The psychiatrist as informed consent technician: a problem for the professions. *Bull Menninger Clin*, 56:87–94.
52. Brakel, S.J., Perry, J., and Weiner, B. (1985) *The Mentally Disabled and the Law.* Chicago: American Bar Foundation.
53. Matter of Nemser, 273 N.Y.S.2d 624 (Sup. Ct. 1966).
54. President's Commission for the Study of Ethical Problems in Medicine and Biomedical and Behavioral Research (1982) *Making Health Care Decisions: The Ethical and Legal Implications of Informed Consent in the Patient-Practitioner Relationship.* Washington D.C.: U.S. Government Printing Office.
55. Sabatino, C. (1999) The legal and functional status of the medical proxy: Suggestions for statutory reform. *J Law Med Ethics*, 27:52–68.
56. 45 C.F.R. 46.
57. Ouslander, J., Tymchuk, A., and Rahbar, B. (1989) Health care decisions among elderly long-term care residents and their potential proxies. *Arch Intern Med*, 149:1367–1372.
58. Suhl, J., Simons, P., Reedy, T., and Garrick, T. (1994) Myth of substituted judgment: surrogate decision making regarding life support is unreliable. *Arch Intern Med*, 154:90–94.
59. Hardwig, J., Hentoff, N., Callahan, D., Cohen, F., Lynn, J., and Churchill, L.R. (2000) The problem of proxies with interests of their own: toward a better theory of proxy decisions. In Hardwig, J. (ed) *Is There a Duty to Die?* New York: Routledge.
60. Hafemeister, T.L. (1999) End-of-life decision making, therapeutic jurisprudence, and preventive law: hierarchical v. consensus-based decision-making model. *Arizona Law Review*, 41:329–373.
61. Berg, J.W. (1996) Legal and ethical complexities of consent with cognitively impaired research subjects: proposed guidelines. *J Law Med Ethics*, 24:18–35.
62. Hamann, A. (1993) Family surrogate laws: a necessary supplement to living wills and durable powers of attorney. *Villanova Law Review*, 38:103–177.
63. Sabatino, C. (1994) Legislative trends in health-care decisionmaking. *ABA Bioethics Bulletin*, 3:10–11.
64. Meisel, A., Grenvik, A., Pinkus, R., and Snyder, J. (1986) Hospital guidelines for deciding about life-sustaining treatment: dealing with health limbo. *Crit Care Med*, 14:239–246.
65. N.Y. Mental Hygiene Law sec. 80.01 (Supp. 1995).
66. Veatch, R.M. (1981) *A Theory of Medical Ethics.* New York: Basic Books.
67. Bartling v. Superior Court, 209 Cal. Rptr. 220 (Ct. App. 1984).
68. Severns v. Wilmington Medical Center, 421 A.2d 1334 (Del. 1980).

69. Matter of Eichner, 420 N.E.2d 64 (N.Y. 1981).
70. Leach v. Akron Medical Center, 426 N.E.2d 809 (Ohio Com. Pleas. 1980).
71. Tune v. Walter Read Army Medical Hosp., 602 F. Supp. 1452 (D.D.C.1985).
72. Kuczewski, M.G. (1999) Commentary: Narrative views of personal identity and sub-stituted judgment in surrogate decision making. *J Law Med Ethics*, 27:32–36.
73. Harmon, L. (1990) Falling off the vine: legal fictions and the doctrine of substituted judgment. *Yale Law Journal*, 100:1–71.
74. In re Martin, 538 N.W.2d 399 (MI 1995).
75. Malloy, S.E.W. (1998) Beyond misguided paternalism: resuscitating the right to re-fuse medical treatment. *Wake Forest Law Review*, 33: 1035–1091.
76. Terry, M. and Zweig, S. (1994) Prevalence of advance directives and do-not-resusci-tate orders in community nursing facilities. *Arch Fam Med*, 3:141.
77. U.S. General Accounting Office (1995) Patient Self-Determination Act: providers offer information on advance directives but effectiveness uncertain. Washington, D.C.: U.S. General Accounting Office, August 25.
78. Support Program Investigators (1995) A controlled trial to improve care for seriously ill hospitalized patients: the study to understand prognoses and preferences for out-comes and risks of treatments (SUPPORT). *JAMA*, 274:1591–1598.
79. In re Quackenbush, 383 A.2d 785 (N.J. Super. 1978).
80. Matter of Schiller, 372 A.2d. 360 (N.J. Super. 1977).
81. State Department of Human Resources v. Northern, 563 S.W.2d 197 (Tenn. Ct. App. 1978).
82. In re Sampson, 317 N.Y.S.2d 641 (Family Ct. 1970).
83. Custody of a Minor, 393 N.E.2d 836 (Mass. 1979).
84. Matter of Hoffbauer, 393 N.E.2d 1009 (N.Y. 1979).
85. Matter of Quinlan, 355 A.2d 647 (N.J. 1976).
86. Saunders v. State, 492 N.Y.S.2d 510 (Sup. Ct. 1985).
87. Gutheil, T. and Appelbaum, P.S. (1980) Substituted judgment and the physician's ethical dilemma: with special reference to the problem of the psychiatric patient. *J Clin Psychiatry*, 41:303–305.
88. Matter of Conroy, 486 A.2d 1209 (N.J. 1985).
89. Matter of Roe, 421 N.E.2d (Mass. 1980).
90. Rogers v. Commissioner, 458 N.E.2d 308 (Mass. 1983).
91. Matter of Spring, 4905 N.E.2d 115 (Mass. 1980).
92. John F. Kennedy Memorial Hospital v. Bludworth, 452 So.2d 921 (Fla. 1984).
93. Barber v. Superior Court, 195 Cal. Rptr. 484 (Ct. App. 1983).
94. Guardianship of Barry, 445 So. 2d 365 (Fla. Ct. App. 1984).
95. In re L.H.R., 321 S.E.2d 716 (Ga. 1984).
96. Pleak, R. and Appelbaum, P.S. (1985) The clinician's role in protecting patients' rights in guardianship proceedings. *Hosp Comm Psychiatry*, 36:77–79.
97. Teel, K. (1975) The physician's dilemma; a doctor's view: what the law should be. *Baylor Law Review*, 27:6–9.
98. Youngner, S.J., Jackson, D.L., Coulton, C, Juknialis, B.W., and Smith, E.M. (1993) A national survey of hospital ethics committees. *Crit Care Med*, 11:902–905.
99. Kelly, D. and Hoyt, J. (1996) Ethics consultation. *Crit Care Clin*, 12:49–70.
100. Joint Commission on Accreditation of Healthcare Organizations (1992) *Accredita-tion Manual for Hospitals*. Illinois: JCAHO.
101. Md. Health-Gen. Code Ann. §§ 19-370 to -374 (Supp. 1990).
102. N.J. Stat. Ann. § 2A:84A-22.10 (1990).

103. Wolf, S.M. (1991) Ethics committees and due process: nesting rights in a community of caring. *Maryland Law Review*, 50:798–858.
104. Symposium (1996) *J Clin Ethics*, Volume 7.
105. American Society of Bioethics and Humanities (1998) *Core Competencies for Health Care Ethics Consultation.*
106. Spencer, E.M. (1997) A new role for institutional ethics committees: organizational ethics. *J Clin Ethics*, 8:372–376.
107. Weber, L. (1997) Taking on organizational ethics. *Health Progress*, 20–23,32.

6

Legal Rules for Recovery

This chapter deals with the legal theory and procedural framework under which patients can obtain redress for their injuries resulting from treatment administered in the absence of informed consent. The evolution of the legal doctrine was driven by the demands of patients for redress for injuries, and more attention has been given by courts and legislatures to the questions of when and how compensation might be obtained than to providing guidance for clinicians. In some important respects, the distinction between the law as it applies to the physician engaged in medical decision making with a patient and the law as it applies to that same patient who later seeks compensation in the courts is an artificial one. Insofar as the spirit of informed consent is not embraced voluntarily by the medical profession, but is adhered to in large part to avoid the likely consequences of failure to observe the legal rules, physician behavior will be shaped not only by the rules themselves but also by the way they are enforced.

If, for example, the rules governing the means of redress were complex, time-consuming, and unlikely to yield the desired compensation, few injured patients would pursue a judicial remedy. As a result, physicians would eventually realize that adverse consequences were unlikely to follow from a failure to observe the relevant rules and, except to the extent that they had accepted the ethical theory of informed consent, their adherence to the doctrine would crumble. Some critics of the present system contend that this has already happened (see Chapter 7).

On the other hand, rules that make recovery easier and more certain would be likely to encourage compliance with the requirements for informed consent. Differential emphasis by the courts on particular kinds of lapses by clinicians might also shape their actions accordingly. For example, the courts' focus on risk information has led many physicians to tailor disclosure to emphasize risks. Thus, the issues addressed in this chapter, although framed in legal terminology, are important (some would argue crucial) determinants of the ultimate impact of informed consent.

Theory of Recovery

The law of informed consent represents the application of principles of tort law to medical practice and medical research. Tort law deals with private wrongs or injuries, in contrast to criminal law, which deals with public wrongs or crimes against society. The kinds of interests protected by tort law are varied, as are the particular legal theories behind that protection. So varied, in fact, are these interests that one legal scholar concluded that there is no such thing as a single law of torts, but only an unconnected set of pigeonholes into which the conduct of one who causes injury to another must be fit before the law will afford a remedy for that injury (1). Among the interests that tort law protects are individual interests in freedom from harm to person, to property, and to reputation. In addition, tort law serves broad social goals, such as the compensation of injured persons, the deterrence of harm-causing conduct, and the punishment of those who cause such conduct.[1] In the last four decades, an increasingly prominent goal of tort law has been the efficient allocation of economic resources. This goal has been accomplished by requiring harm-causing actors to internalize previously externally borne accident costs that arise from the conduct of those activities. In other words, the individual who can most easily bear the cost of changing his behavior should be responsible for paying for harms caused by his activity. Presumably this internalization will result in the cost bearer taking additional steps to ensure minimization of potential harms.

Since the middle of the nineteenth century, tort law has accomplished these goals through two predominant theories of liability: intentional tort and negligence. A third theory, strict liability, has gradually gained ascendance in some areas of conduct, including some areas related to medical practice, but the informed consent doctrine is traditionally associated with the first two theories. Strict liability doctrine holds the tortfeasor (the person who engages in the tortious action) liable for any and all foreseeable injuries arising from his conduct, even those that are unintentional or are not the result of negligence. Intentional

---

[1]In general, punishment objectives are achieved through criminal rather than civil law.

and negligent torts, by contrast, are designed to remedy injuries intentionally or negligently caused. Since physicians rarely intentionally cause harm to patients, the intentional tort theory might seem inapropos. Nonetheless, this theory is where the informed consent doctrine has its legal roots.

Battery

Assault, battery, and false imprisonment are the most common intentional torts. The one most relevant to informed consent cases is battery. A battery occurs when one person engages in conduct that is intended to, and does, cause harmful physical contact with another person, as when, for example, a person throws a punch in a barroom brawl or hits someone with a rock. Less obviously, a battery is also committed by contact, or *touching,* that is *offensive,* but not necessarily harmful, at least not in the sense of causing bodily injury (2, §18). Spitting can be a battery. Contact with another person is ordinarily considered offensive if it occurs without the consent of the person being touched. Thus, a physician who fails to obtain a patient's consent to a medical procedure that involves a touching of the patient commits the tort of battery even though the medical procedure may have helped rather than hurt the patient (3–6, but see 7). This is because the right of bodily integrity is the legally protected interest, and thus the patient can be wronged even if not physically harmed.

Perhaps because this reasoning is subtle, or perhaps because the common meaning of the words used in this analysis differs from their legal meaning, courts have long been reluctant to impose liability on physicians for intentional torts. Courts overcome this reluctance when the facts of a particular case make it clear that the physician intended to operate over a patient's express objection or (less likely) actually intended to harm, and not merely to have offensive nonconsensual contact with a patient.

Early cases involving a lack of consent to treatment were addressed under a battery theory. The same theory was generally applied in the precursor informed consent cases—that is, those cases in which the courts recognized that some legal wrong had been committed because of inaccurate or incomplete information delivered by the physician to the patient, but in which the courts' responses had not yet solidified into the present-day doctrine of informed consent. In these cases the courts concluded that a battery took place if consent was based on substantial misunderstanding of the nature of the procedure, or of its consequences for the patient, due to misinformation or lack of information (8).

Negligence

Negligence is the other major theory of tort law relevant to informed consent. The law of negligence imposes very broad and general requirements upon most persons to act (or to refrain from acting) in such a way that their behavior does not cause harm to other persons. In our various roles as pedestrians, vehicle operators, homeowners, business operators, employees, professionals, and others too numerous to mention, we are expected to comport ourselves in such a way as to avoid unintentional harm to others. Failure to use reasonable care in the conduct of such activities constitutes negligence. Any party causing harm through negligence is required to compensate the victim for injuries to person, property, and, increasingly, emotional well-being.

In order to recover under negligence theory, the plaintiff (the individual bringing the lawsuit) must establish four elements: (*1*) that the defendant (injurer or tortfeasor) had a *duty* to use reasonable care to prevent harm to the plaintiff; (*2*) that the defendant *breached* this duty; and (*3*) that the conduct that constituted the breach of duty was the *cause* of (*4*) *harm* (bodily injury, property damage, emotional harm, and/or economic loss) to the plaintiff.

Unintentional injuries to patients caused by physicians are remediable, if at all, under the theory of negligence. Such conduct is generally referred to as malpractice but is more properly called professional negligence. A physician is under a duty to possess and exercise the care, skill, and training of what the law terms a "reasonably prudent physician." If the physician fails in this duty and as a result a patient is injured, the physician has committed professional negligence. Examples include surgical errors like performing the wrong type of surgery or leaving surgical implements in the patient's body; error in prescribing dosage or kind of medication; and failure to take a thorough medical history, leading to an incorrect diagnosis and delay in instituting treatment.

In all cases, the mere fact that the physician makes what retrospectively can be characterized as a mistake, or that the patient suffers bad results (or fails to obtain good results) from the physician's care is not the critical feature; however, in the absence of harm, the patient has no right to obtain damages. The critical feature is whether the physician's conduct measures up to legally acceptable standards. These standards are almost always determined by reference to the prevailing custom and practice in the medical profession.

Originally, failure to obtain patient consent was treated as an intentional tort (battery) rather than as professional negligence. When the physician failed to give the patient adequate information about the potential consequences of the recommended procedure, the patient's permission to proceed did not amount to consent. Thus, the physician's contact with the patient was offensive, because no consent was given, and if any harm to the patient resulted, damages could be recovered not only for the offense but, under well-accepted rules, for any harm that occurred as well.

A few of the early informed consent cases, however, were brought as professional negligence cases. Unlike standard professional negligence (malpractice) cases in which the essence of a patient's complaint is that something the physician did (or failed to do) in the way of medical treatment caused harm, the basis of the complaint in an informed consent case is that the physician failed to provide the patient with adequate and/or accurate information.

Battery Versus Negligence

From the early 1960s to mid-1970s, a number of courts wrestled with the problem of whether an informed consent case ought to be treated as a battery or negligence. The difference between the two theories can be of substantial importance in terms of what a patient must prove, and whether or not damages are available at all. More fundamentally, the difference between the two theories reflects different underlying values that a legal doctrine of informed consent might seek to protect.

If lack of informed consent is remediable as a battery rather than as negligence, a patient has a right to recover damages for inadequate disclosure alone, even if not physically injured by the physician's treatment. The wrong to the patient is the failure to obtain consent or the deprivation of the right of personal choice (sometimes called a "dignitary" harm). In contrast, under negligence theory the right vindicated is the right to be free from bodily injury caused by substandard medical practice. If the negligence causes no bodily injury to the patient, no remediable wrong is considered to have occurred.

A further difference is that the focal inquiry under a battery theory is whether or not consent was given. As stated previously, in battery cases consent is not considered to have been given if the physician has failed to provide the patient with certain information (2). In the earlier battery cases, the only information that the physician needed to provide to assure that the patient's assent amounted to consent was an explanation of the nature of the procedure (8). By the mid-1950s, however, courts occasionally could be found to hold that it was necessary for the patient to be given a greater quantity of information in order for it to be said that consent had been given. Even so, the focus was still on the patient's consent or lack thereof. Under a negligence theory, in contrast, the issue of consent takes a decidedly secondary role to the duty of the physician to disclose information. The courts in negligence cases focus on the adequacy of the disclosure and judge adequacy using one of two legal standards described in Chapter 3: a lay standard that asks what a reasonable patient would want to know or a professional standard that asks what a reasonable practitioner would disclose. Under negligence, although a patient may have consented, if disclosure was inadequate the consent is not deemed "informed." The inquiry concerning the adequacy of the disclosure is made central rather than being subsumed under the aegis of the term "consent" as it is used in the context of battery theory.

Such matters have implications for proof at trial. Under a negligence theory, patients must demonstrate what constitutes adequate disclosure (duty) before they may attempt to show that there was inadequate disclosure (breach); that the inadequate disclosure resulted in a decision to undergo, or forgo, treatment (causation); and that the treatment, or failure to receive it, caused physical injuries (damages). They may need expert witnesses to establish some or all of these things. Under a battery theory, recovery is far simpler, since all that need be demonstrated is that an invalid consent was obtained. For this, expert witnesses need not be employed. Any ensuing harm will be deemed to be causally related to the battery; separate proof that provision of information would have altered the decision to undergo treatment is not required.

Finally, the choice of battery or negligence may affect whether a case gets to court and whether the physician's professional liability insurance coverage is available to reimburse injured patients. Statutes of limitation, which establish the interval within which a suit must be filed after a harm comes to light, differ for battery and negligence. In this respect, a negligence theory is more favorable to plaintiffs by allowing a longer time period between the action that caused the harm and the patient's decision to bring a lawsuit than would be allowed under a battery cause of action. Furthermore, malpractice insurance policies ordinarily do not provide coverage for intentional torts, so a patient suing under a battery theory would not have access to this potential pool of funds for compensation.

The dispute over whether a lawsuit alleging lack of informed consent ought to be treated as a battery or as professional negligence has slowly withered away. By the mid-1970s, almost all states that had considered the question had concluded that inadequate disclosure is actionable only as professional negligence, not battery. At present only one state, Pennsylvania, still uses a battery theory (9). At the same time, the administration of therapy without any consent at all, or outside the scope of the consent given, is still actionable as a battery in many states (10,11). Thus, for example, the decision to remove an organ during nonemergency exploratory abdominal surgery may be considered a battery in some states.

The predominance of negligence theory appears to have been based largely on judicial reluctance to stigmatize physicians with the label of having committed a battery, thereby lumping them into the same category as barroom brawlers, rather than on any clear analysis of the different effects of one option or the other. A battery theory of recovery for lack of consent has at least some basis, historically, in medical practice (see Chapter 3). A negligence theory based on a duty to disclose, on the other hand, has a more tenuous link to practice because, historically, disclosure was left to the discretion of medical professionals. Thus, in moving away from a battery theory, the courts moved informed consent law further away from customary medical practice.

Regardless of the legal theory used to bring a lawsuit for lack of informed consent, the fundamental legal duties imposed by the doctrine have the same general contours. A physician is still obligated to disclose information about treatment and to obtain the patient's consent. However, battery theory is generally viewed as more conducive to successful suits by patients. In fact, some commentators believe that the legal requirements of informed consent would be more carefully observed had the battery approach been widely adopted (see Chapter 7). On the other hand, a battery theory may be limited. In interpreting the application of informed consent under a battery theory, Pennsylvania courts have held that no battery can occur in the administration of medication since no "touching" occurs (12). Interestingly, this has even been extended to the provision of intravenous medication, an odd result at best (13).

The use of a negligence cause of action (theory of recovery) for informed consent also has its limitations (14). Negligence theories have more elements and are thus harder to prove. As a result, they are thought to restrict suits against physicians, thus encouraging physicians to be more controlling when medical decisions need to be made, and presumably to favor the value of health over the value of self-determination. Although the disclosure requirement of a negligence cause of action is not drawn from historical medical practice (see above), favoring health over self-determination is quite consonant with the traditional values of medicine. Substantially different consequences flow from the use of a battery versus a negligence theory. These consequences go to the heart of the interests served by the informed consent doctrine, the burdens it imposes on physicians, and the protections it affords to patients.

Causation

A lawsuit based on tort theory requires that the plaintiff must show both that he or she was injured and that the defendant *caused* the injury. In cases involving intentional torts such as battery, the requirements for establishing causation are simple (15). In fact, causation is rarely an issue under a battery theory, and few if any of the early simple consent cases even mention it. Once the patient demonstrates that no consent was given, all resulting injury is presumed to be caused by the physician's nonconsensual actions; for example, in Pennsylvania where a battery cause of action is still used, the plaintiff does not have to show proximate causation (see later under *Injury Causation*) to prevail (16).

Under negligence theory, causation can be far more problematic. There are actually two issues of causation, although few courts explicitly acknowledge them. One has received wide attention; it concerns the link between the physician's failure to disclose (or the disclosure of misinformation) and the patient's decision. The question is whether the disclosure or lack caused the patient to consent or to refuse. We refer to this as decision-causation. The other causation question, rarely acknowledged, involves the link between the physician's provision of treatment and the patient's injury. The question is whether the treatment caused the patient's injury (in contrast to an injury resulting from the underlying illness). We refer to this as injury-causation and will address it first.

Injury-Causation

When a patient is worse after treatment than before, it is not always clear whether the treatment was the cause of the worsened condition. It may be that the treatment was beneficial or neutral in effect and that the natural course of the illness was responsible for the deterioration. Injury-causation requires the plaintiff to show that the medical procedure performed by the defendant led to the deterioration. This requirement is merely a specific instance of the general one in negligence cases that the plaintiff prove *cause-in-fact*—that is, that the defendant's conduct was the actual cause of the plaintiff's injury (sometimes referred to as "but for" causation). Ordinarily, this requires plaintiffs to show that they would not have been injured if the defendants had exercised reasonable care, for example, had a correct diagnosis been made, or had medication side effects been monitored closely enough that the medication could have been stopped before they became irreversible.

Sometimes an injury is produced by more than one causal agent. Where that is the case, it is often impossible for plaintiffs to demonstrate that they would not have been injured if a particular defendant had not been negligent. For example, suppose a plaintiff had been simultaneously shot and killed by two careless hunters who thought they were shooting at a deer (17). If either bullet alone would have killed the plaintiff, both hunters could go free despite their negligence, because the plaintiff would have been killed even if one of the hunters had not been negligent. Each hunter could argue that her act alone was not a necessary cause of the harm.

To avoid blatantly unjust situations of this sort, when more than one causal agent is involved, a plaintiff must demonstrate only that the defendant's failure to use reasonable care was a *substantial* factor in bringing about the injury. In professional negligence cases the same rule is applied. If a patient's injury is caused in part by the underlying illness or injury and in part by the medical intervention, injury-causation is established by the medical intervention being found to have been a substantial factor in producing the injury.

Proof of injury-causation generally will require that the plaintiff produce expert testimony that it was the defendant's conduct, and not the plaintiff's original illness, that caused the plaintiff's injury (18). For example, an expert might testify that chloramphenicol has been shown to cause aplastic anemia, and that the patient who received this drug did in fact die as a result of aplastic anemia, not his underlying infection. In some cases the common experience of laypersons may be adequate to determine the cause of the injury, and expert testimony is not needed. The amputation of the wrong limb by a surgeon is a good example.

Courts and legislatures that have recognized the problem of injury-causation in informed consent cases have sometimes done so under the name of proximate causation—that is, a finding that the negligent act was sufficiently related to the injury to be a legal cause. Proximate causation refers to the primary cause of an injury and is sometimes called "legal" causation. This requirement, by whatever name, has been recognized explicitly in only a few jurisdictions, probably because it has been taken for granted as a necessary aspect of any action based on a negligence theory of liability (11). One court, for example, noted that lack of disclosure never "causes" physical harm; instead it is the provision of treatment based on inadequate disclosure that causes harm (19).

Decision-Causation

Decision-causation refers to the nexus between the physician's failure to disclose and the decision made by the patient. When it can be said that if the physician had made proper disclosure, the patient would have made a different choice, decision-causation exists. The question that has troubled courts and commentators is whether an objective or subjective test should be applied in determining the relationship between the physician's disclosure and the patient's decision. Under an objective test, for example, the plaintiff must prove that the undisclosed information would have led a reasonable person to decline the treatment in question; under a subjective test, the plaintiff must prove merely that he would have refused the treatment (20–22). A subjective test thus presents a lesser obstacle to recovery, since the patient need only present evidence regarding his decision.

Prior to *Canterbury v. Spence,* courts had given very little attention to causation in informed consent cases (23). While courts considering the problem both before and after *Canterbury* agreed that causation in negligence exists only when disclosure of risks (or conceivably other information, such as alternatives) would have resulted in a decision to forgo the treatment, the pre-*Canterbury* courts generally did not address the problem of whether causation is to be found by reference to an objective (reasonable person) or subjective (the particular patient) standard. Many commentators assumed that the subjective test should be applied (24–28). The courts, though seemingly unaware of the issue, concurred (29).

Because the doctrine of informed consent is premised on the right of persons to make decisions about what medical care they wish to undergo, regardless of the soundness of their reasons, the subjective test of decision-causation seems more consonant with the underlying rationale for informed consent than the objective test. By conditioning the availability of compensation on the congruence between the patient's own decision and what a so-called reasonable person would have decided, the objective test appears to undercut a patient's right of self-determination (30). However, under an objective test, plaintiffs still may testify as to what they actually would have done had they been properly informed. Although such testimony will not definitively settle the decision-causation issue, the jury is entitled to consider the plaintiff's views. Thus, the objective test does not completely undercut the patient's right of self-determination.

In fact, the majority of courts and legislatures that have addressed the issue have adopted an objective test (31,32). Even those few states that use a subjective disclosure standard (i.e., what the particular patient would have wanted to know) apply an objective causation requirement. It is not difficult to understand why the objective test has been favored. A subjective analysis calls for the jury to credit the plaintiff's answer to a hypothetical question— for example, "Mr. Smith, if Dr. Jones had told you that you might lose motion in your arm as a result of this procedure, would you have gone through with it?" Such a question "places the physician in jeopardy of the patient's hindsight and bitterness"(23). As *Canterbury* indicates, and as other cases have agreed, it is unlikely that medical accident victims would thwart their own chances to obtain compensation, no matter how much good faith we are willing to ascribe to them, by testifying that even had they been properly informed, they would still have consented. However, the fear of the courts may be overstated, if not misplaced. For the same reason that the *Canterbury* court was skeptical, it is reasonable to assume that most jurors will also be skeptical. Because it is the jury's function to evaluate all the evidence and to weigh the credibility of witnesses, there is ample opportunity for jurors to apply this natural skepticism.

To the best of our knowledge, no United States court has ever mentioned the possibility of applying any other type of test, nor have legislatures (33).[2] An attractive alternative is a material factor test, under which the jury would have to find only that the information withheld was material to the decisionmaking process. The use of a material factor test might pacify critics of both the objective and subjective tests. Patients would no longer be required to state that had disclosure been complete, they would have forgone treatment, and the jury would no longer be required to evaluate the credibility of that statement. If the jury simply found that the undisclosed information would have been important, even if not determinative, it could find the necessary causal connection to have been proved.

The insistence on a demonstration of decision-causation stems from the unwillingness of the United States courts to view inadequate disclosure alone as a harm to a patient. This constitutes the strongest judicial resistance to recognizing that a patient can be wronged by a physician's behavior—specifically inadequate

---

[2]The German courts have addressed the hindsight problem by requiring plaintiffs to give a plausible reason why they would have refused treatment when the reasons for refusing treatment are not apparent from the facts of the case. Thus, the issue is not whether a reasonable patient would have refused, but whether the particular patient can substantiate her claim that she would have refused. Basically this is a mixed test—subjective in that it looks at the particular patient, but objective in that it requires that the patient's rationale be "plausible."

disclosure— even when not physically harmed (30). This resistance conflicts with a fundamental purpose of informed consent: the protection of human dignity and promotion of autonomy.

Establishing Liability for Failure to Obtain Informed Consent

In a lawsuit based on a claim of lack of informed consent, the plaintiff-patient has the burden of producing evidence on each element of the *prima facie* case (i.e., the information set forth by the plaintiff that, barring any evidence from the defense, sets forth a case for recovery under a particular theory). As noted previously, there are four elements in any cause of action based on a negligence theory: duty, breach of duty, causation, and damages. To fulfill some of these elements, the plaintiff may need to produce expert witnesses.

First, the patient needs to establish that the defendant-physician owed the patient a legal duty. This question is ordinarily one of law, decided by the court rather than the jury. Duty is not often at issue in informed consent cases. It has been established as a matter of law in all United States jurisdictions that when a physician–patient relationship exists, the physician owes the patient duties of disclosure and obtaining consent before treatment may be commenced (34). Sometimes, however, there is a question about whether or not a physician–patient relationship existed or whether it was the kind of physician–patient relationship that required disclosure (35). This question can arise in a variety of ways (31). Often it occurs when one physician evaluates a patient and recommends a particular procedure but refers the patient to another physician for its performance. A referring physician, as opposed to a treating physician, is not required to explain a procedure to a patient. Or sometimes this issue arises when one physician inadequately informs a patient about a procedure but does not participate in its performance. In that case, it is again the treating physician who owes the patient a duty of reasonable disclosure (36).

Once duty is established, and usually there will be no dispute about this between the parties, the patient must introduce evidence of the second element of recovery, breach of duty. This element requires evidence about the standard of care; for informed consent, this would be the standard of disclosure. In a jurisdiction that adheres to a professional standard of disclosure, the plaintiff must call an expert witness to establish what information a reasonably prudent physician would have disclosed (37,38). Where no other expert is available or willing to testify, the plaintiff may attempt to use the defendant-physician as an expert witness (39), but for obvious reasons this method is decidedly less effective. To complete the proof of breach of duty, the patient is also required to prove that the defendant did in fact fail to disclose information that a reasonably prudent physician would have disclosed. This is one place where consent forms may come into play as evidence of what disclosure actually took place. (See Chapter 9 for a more complete discussion of consent forms.)

In a jurisdiction that adheres to a lay standard of disclosure, the plaintiff's task is simpler: the plaintiff need only prove that information was not disclosed. The jury will decide on its own whether the information is of a type that would be material to the decision of a reasonable patient or (in the jurisdictions using a subjective standard) the particular plaintiff. In either case the plaintiff is likely to need an expert witness to establish that the undisclosed risk is actually associated with the particular treatment provided, or that a particular therapeutic option that was not discussed actually is an alternative to the treatment that was performed (29).

The patient must then prove the third element, causation. To establish injury-causation, the plaintiff-patient may again need the services of an expert witness (29). In addition, the jury (or judge if jury trial is waived) must be able to find decision-causation. In most jurisdictions where an objective standard of causation applies, this will mean that the jury must find that reasonable persons would not have consented to treatment had they been told the information that the physician neglected to disclose. For this aspect of the patient's case, no expert witness will be needed. In those few jurisdictions where a subjective standard applies, patients may introduce evidence that they themselves would not have consented to treatment had the omitted information been provided. Evidence of this sort should also be admissible, though of less weight, in a jurisdiction applying an objective test of causation (8).

Finally, the plaintiff must prove the fourth element, damages. Damages in informed consent cases may include any added medical expenses, any other out-of-pocket expenses occasioned by the injury, physical pain and mental suffering, and lost wages, salary, or income. In general, recovery may not be obtained if the patient suffers no physical injury. Inadequate disclosure alone—that is, the deprivation of the right of informed choice—is not a legally protected interest under a negligence theory. In a case in which the omitted information concerned a risk of treatment, it must be this omitted risk that materialized and constituted the injury (40). If the physician neglected to inform the patient about an alternative treatment that the plaintiff claims she would have chosen had it been explained, the plaintiff may recover for injuries even if informed of the risk that materialized (41). This is so because the patient's argument is that she would not have chosen the given treatment over an alternative(s), had she been properly informed.

Some cases have allowed patient recovery based on a claim of emotional injury resulting from negligent non-disclosure of material information. In one case the issue was the physician's failure to disclose his HIV-positive status (42), another was the physician's failure to warn a pregnant woman about the dangers of an X-ray (43). In both cases the patients sustained no physical injury, only emotional harm. It remains to be seen whether these cases signal a trend toward the broadening of informed consent protections or are merely anomalous examples.

It is the plaintiff's responsibility to introduce evidence on all of the above matters. If the plaintiff does so, a *prima facie* case has been established. If the plaintiff cannot produce enough information on these matters to meet this production burden, then the case will be dismissed, before the defendant-physician is required to introduce any evidence at all.

If the plaintiff does establish a *prima facie* case and meets what is called the production burden, the defendant-physician has two general choices. He may introduce no evidence and let the case go to the jury solely on the plaintiff's evidence. If the plaintiff's case is exceedingly weak, or if it is likely that information damaging to the physician will come out if the physician chooses to present evidence, the physician may prefer this alternative.

More likely, it will be to the physician's advantage to introduce evidence designed to weaken the plaintiff's case. This may be done in a number of ways, but there are two general approaches. The first is to introduce evidence that weakens one, several, or all of the elements of the plaintiff's *prima facie* case. The simplest way is to deny the plaintiff's claim that there was incomplete disclosure. Testimony can be introduced—from the physician for example, or a nurse, or the patient's spouse (or other family member), if they were present when the doctor talked to the patient—that the patient was, in fact, informed of the information that the patient claims was not disclosed. Testimonial contests of this sort are a frequent occurrence in informed consent cases. Physicians are even permitted to testify in their own defense about their usual disclosure practices for the type of information at issue (44,45). In a jurisdiction adhering to a professional standard of disclosure, the defendant-physician may introduce the evidence of expert witnesses as to what is customarily told to patients about the procedure undergone by the patient.

Similarly, on the issue of injury-causation, the defendant may introduce evidence tending to show that the patient's injury was not caused by the treatment. Decision-causation is more difficult to counter, unless the patient indicated in some way that she would have undergone the procedure in question regardless of the risks involved. For example, if a patient has told the physician that she will consent no matter what the risks, or that she does not even want to know the risks, the physician will have a defense to an action charging lack of informed consent (31, p. 84).

The second general approach is to establish an affirmative defense. Rather than merely attempting to weaken the plaintiff's evidence, this method supposes, solely for the sake of argument, that the defendant breached the duty of disclosure or the duty to obtain consent (or perhaps even both), but asserts that the physician was legally entitled to do so. In other words, the defendant-physician claims that one of the exceptions to obtaining informed consent applies:

emergency, waiver, therapeutic privilege, or incompetence (see Chapters 4 and 5).

Some cases involve a claim of a patient's *contributory* negligence (46). Contributory negligence, allows a defendant to acknowledge his negligence but mitigates damages based upon the plaintiff's acts of negligence that contributed to the harm. In jurisdictions that allow claims of contributory negligence, the charge may serve to insulate the defendant from liability, or the court may apportion liability based on fault (e.g., if the plaintiff's actions contributed 30 percent to the harm, she may recover only 70 percent of the damages claimed from the defendant). Jurisdictions vary on whether they allow claims for contributory negligence at all and the effect of those claims on damage awards. The Wisconsin Supreme Court, in a case involving informed consent, held that although a patient could not be contributorily negligent by failing to ascertain the truth or completeness of the information disclosed, or in following a viable treatment option presented by the physician, she could be contributorily negligent by failing to provide a complete and accurate medical history, and thus remanded the case to the trial court to determine apportionment of damages (46).

For all affirmative defenses, the physician bears the burden of making out a *prima facie* case. That is, the physician must introduce sufficient evidence for the jury to find that the exception should apply (8). If the physician fails to do so, these matters of defense cannot be considered by the jury, and the plaintiff's case will stand on its own.

Conclusion

The legal rules for recovery developed out of cases brought by patients who were injured as a result of treatment (or lack of treatment). Physicians have sometimes, erroneously, viewed the resulting set of laws regarding how and when a patient may receive compensation as a step-by-step guide to obtaining informed consent. But although the legal rules for recovery can provide some aid in reducing exposure to liability, they cannot function as a primary guide for physicians engaged in medical decision making with a patient. Not only are the rules not designed to provide practical guidelines for clinicians, but there are also a number of criticisms of the legal doctrine as a whole. It is to these critiques that we next turn.

References

1. Keeton, W., Dobbs, D., Keeton, R. and Owen, D. (1984) *Prosser and Keeton on the Law of Torts.* St. Paul: West.

2. American Law Institute (1979) Restatement (Second) of the Law of Torts. St. Paul: ALI.
3. Lloyd v. Kull, 329 F.2d 168 (7th Cir. 1964).
4. Bailey v. Belinfante, 218 S.E.2d 289 (Ga. App. 1974).
5. Mohr v. Williams, 104 N.W. 12 (Minn. 1905).
6. Rolater v. Strain, 137 Pac. 96 (Okla. 1913).
7. Buzzell v. Libi, 340 N.W.2d 36 (N.D. 1983).
8. Meisel, A. (1977) The expansion of liability for medical accidents: from negligence to strict liability by way of informed consent. *Nebraska Law Review*, 56:51–152.
9. LeBlang, T. (1992) Informed consent. In *Medical Liability Issues for Lawyers, Physicians and Insurers: Current Trends and Future Directions.* Chicago: American Bar Association.
10. Cobbs v. Grant, 502 P.2d 1 (Cal. 1972).
11. Meisel, A. and Kabnick, L. (1980) Informed consent to medical treatment: an analysis of recent legislation. *University of Pittsburgh Law Review*, 41:407–564.
12. Dible v. Vagley, 612 A.2d 493 (Pa. Super Ct. 1992).
13. Wu v. Spence, 605 A.2d 395 (Pa. Super Ct. 1992).
14. Hudson, T. (1991) Informed consent problems becoming more complicated. *Hospitals*, 65:38–40.
15. Hodge v. UMC of Puerto Rico, 933 F. Supp. 145 (U.S. Dist. Ct. P.R. 1996).
16. Grouse v. Cassel, 615 A.2d 331 (Pa. 1992).
17. Thomson, J.J. (1984) Remarks on causation and liability. *Philosophy and Public Affairs*, 13:101.
18. Copeland v. Univ. Radiologists of Cleveland, Inc. 1993 Ohio App. LEXIS 2161.
19. Flores v. Flushing Hosp. & Med. Center, 109 A.2d 198, 490 N.Y.S.2d 770 (1986).
20. Arena v. Gingrich, 748 P2d 547 (Or. 1988).
21. Zalazar v. Vercimak, 633 N.E.2d 1223 (Ill. Ct. App. 1993).
22. Alaska Stat. § 9.55.556(a) (Cum. Supp. 1983).
23. Canterbury v. Spence, 464 F.2d 772 (D.C. Cir. 1972).
24. Waltz, J. and Scheuneman, T. (1970) Informed consent to therapy. *Northwestern University Law Review*, 64:628–650.
25. Plant, M. (1968) An analysis of "informed consent." *Fordham Law Review*, 36:639–706.
26. (1967) Informed consent in medical malpractice. *California Law Review*, 55:1396–1418.
27. (1970) Informed consent as a theory of medical liability. *Wisconsin Law Review*, 879–898.
28. (1962) Recent Cases: Physicians and Surgeons—Physician's duty to warn of possible adverse results of proposed treatment depends upon general practice followed by medical profession in the community. *Harvard Law Review*, 75:1445–1449.
29. Shetter v. Rochelle, 409 P.2d 74 (Ariz. App. 1965).
30. Goldstein, J. (1975) For Harold Lasswell: Some reflections on human dignity, entrapment, informed consent, and the plea bargain. *Yale Law Journal*, 84:683–703.
31. Rozovsky, F. (1990) *Consent to Treatment: A Practical Guide.* Boston: Little, Brown.
32. President's Commission for the Study of Ethical Problems in Medicine and Biomedical and Behavioral Research (1982) *Making Health Care Decisions: The Ethical and Legal Implications of Informed Consent in the Patient-Practitioner Relationship.* Washington, D.C.: U.S. Government Printing Office.

33. Giesen, D. (1993) The patient's right to know—a comparative law perspective. *Med Law*, 12:553–565.
34. Ga. Code Ann. § 31-9-6 (1996).
35. Nicholson v. Curtis, 452 N.E.2d 883 (Ill. App. 1983).
36. Hill v. Seward, 470 N.Y.S.2d 971 (Sup. Ct. 1983).
37. Bly v. Rhoads, 222 S.E.2d 783 (Va. 1976).
38. Gerrnan v. Nichopoulos, 577 S.W.2d 197 (Tenn. Ct. App. 1978).
39. Abbey v. Jackson, 483 A.2d 330 (D.C. Ct. App. 1984).
40. Cornfeldt v. Tongen, 262 N.W.2d 684 (Minn. 1977).
41. Logan v. Greenwich Hosp. Assoc., 465 A.2d 294 (Cann. 1983).
42. Faya v. Almaraz, 620 A.2d 327 (Md. Ct. App. 1993).
43. Jones v. Howard Univ., 589 A.2d 419 (D.C. App. 1991).
44. In re Swine Flu Immunization Products Liability Litigation, 533 F. Supp. 567 (D. Colo. 1980).
45. Sauro v. Shea, 390 A.2d 259 (Pa. Super. 1978).
46. Brown v. Dibbell, 595 N.W.2d 358 (Wis. 1999).

7

Critical Approaches to the Law of Informed Consent

A number of goals have been posited for the legal doctrine of informed consent. One author, for example, highlights four goals: "1) an ethical goal, in which the law promotes patient autonomy; 2) a decision making goal, in which the law promotes the ability of patients to make medical decisions; 3) a regulatory goal, in which the law attempts to control physicians' disclosure practices; and 4) a compensatory goal, in which the common law functions as a mechanism to provide monetary compensation for injuries" (1). Another author posits six goals: "1) promoting individual autonomy; 2) respecting human dignity; 3) encouraging professional self-scrutiny; 4) promoting rational decisionmaking; 5) avoiding deceit and coercion; and 6) educating the public" (2).

According to critics, the result has been a doctrine and a set of practices that compromise all values and satisfy none in their entirety (1). But commentators who have analyzed the law and practice of informed consent have each generally represented one point of view to the exclusion of others. The resulting debate over informed consent among healthcare practitioners, legal experts, and ethicists should come as no surprise. As long as one relies on a single perspective, it is remarkably easy to find critical things to say about informed consent. Those who would elevate any single value above all others, and steadfastly resist compromise, usually can offer a powerful, even devastating, analysis of the current state of affairs. In this chapter we focus on three critiques—a perspective concerned

146

with promoting individual autonomy, an approach that emphasizes the value of health, and a perspective that places primary emphasis on encouraging discourse and interaction between caregivers and patients—and assess their validity from a perspective that recognizes that the doctrine of informed consent must accommodate a number of competing interests and values.

The Autonomy-Oriented Critique

The most trenchant criticism of the state of informed consent law today focuses on the discrepancies between the goals highlighted by the ethical theories of informed consent—primarily, the enhancement of individual autonomy in making medical decisions—and the practical effects of the current system. Theorists of this school, most notably Jay Katz, are troubled by the failure of the current law to protect autonomy as fully as it might and by what they see as a consistent pattern of subordinating patient autonomy to the interests of the medical profession (3,4). Katz notes that "informed consent will remain a fairy tale as long as the idea of joint decisionmaking, based on a commitment to patient autonomy and self-determination, does not become an integral aspect of the ethos of medicine and the law of informed consent"(5, pp. 90–91). Ruth Faden and Tom Beauchamp, although they reject Katz's notion that the protection of autonomy requires shared decision making and argue instead for primacy of patient's autonomous authorization, also highlight the separation of the legal doctrine of informed consent from the ethical requirements (6). They refer to two senses of informed consent (ethical and legal) and argue that the legal requirements should promote conformance with the ethical standard. Thus, they would prefer a legal system that resulted in more informed consents (in the ethical sense) than one that results in fewer, but they leave room to accommodate practical concerns in the application of the doctrine.

One legal scholar tracing the evolution of informed consent questioned whether "autonomy . . . was put forward as the genuine rationale for the . . . doctrine of informed consent, or whether it was merely a convenient notion—an attractive philosophical and ethical symbol or benchmark at which to nod in passing"(7). He goes on to state that "it is arguable that informed consent was adopted not out of any sense that it would better promote autonomy, but because of essentially internal tort structure concerns" (7, p. 91). Another legal critic, Marjorie Shultz, notes that "autonomy has never been recognized as a legally protectable interest. It has been vindicated only as a byproduct of protection for two other interests—bodily security as protected by rules against unconsented contact, and bodily well-being as protected by rules governing professional competence"(8, p. 219).

Katz traces the problem with autonomy to the very cases that provided the foundation for the modern notion of informed consent. He points to the wording of the sentence in which the term informed consent was first applied to medical treatment, in the court's opinion in *Salgo v. Leland Stanford Jr. University Board of Trustees:* "[I]n discussing the element of risk a certain amount of discretion must be employed consistent with the full disclosure of facts necessary to an informed consent" (9). "Only in dreams or fairy tales," says Katz, "can 'discretion' to withhold crucial information so easily and magically be reconciled with 'full disclosure'" (3, p. 138).

For Katz, the courts' continual deference to medical paternalism, exemplified by their willingness to accept "a certain amount of [medical] discretion" (9), has served to restrict the impact of the law of informed consent. Katz sees the so-called discretion reserved to physicians in *Salgo* as the forerunner of courts' further obeisance to the medical profession, expressed in the use of a professional standard of disclosure and the acceptance of therapeutic privilege as an exception to the requirement of disclosure. Even those courts that have adopted a patient-oriented standard for disclosure have, in Katz's view, compromised the gain to patients' autonomy by choosing an objective (what a hypothetical reasonable patient would have found material), rather than a subjective (what the actual patient would have found material) standard. The same could be said in the area of causation (whether a patient would have been deterred from treatment had the information been disclosed), where the courts have again, by and large, accepted an objective rather than a subjective standard.

Katz's argument that the current law of informed consent is insufficient to compel physicians to share information with patients and thus enable autonomous decision making is supported by a number of empirical studies. Observational research has suggested that with the exception of decisions to employ surgical or other invasive procedures, physicians in hospital settings rarely provide any substantial information to patients about diagnostic and treatment decisions (10,11). Outpatients may receive somewhat more information, but this is often provided after the treatment decision is made and is geared more toward facilitating compliance than encouraging participation in decision making (10). Surveys show consistently that patients desire to have more information than physicians routinely provide (12–14).

Why are the courts, despite their rhetoric supporting patients' self-determination, so willing to contribute to the perpetuation of this state of affairs by continuing to bow to medical judgment? Largely, Katz believes, because they share the medical profession's low opinion of most patients' ability to understand the issues involved in medical treatment and to reach a reasonable decision. "Judges toyed briefly with the idea of patients' self-determination," he concludes, "and largely cast it aside" (3, p. 170).

As disturbing as Katz finds judicial deference to medical discretion, he is equally perturbed about the incorporation of informed consent into the law of negligence. Were the failure to obtain informed consent to lead to redress in an action for battery rather than negligence, Katz believes that plaintiffs would have a much easier time proving their cases, and the medical profession would be more punctilious in its observance of the consent requirements (see Chapter 6). In battery, plaintiffs would not be required to prove adverse effects of a failure to disclose in order to obtain a favorable verdict (although physical harms would certainly affect the size of any damages awarded). Nor would the law of battery necessarily require plaintiffs to demonstrate that their decisions about medical care would have been different had appropriate disclosure taken place. Thus the Supreme Court of Pennsylvania, the only state that still subscribes to a battery theory of informed consent, has held that when the patient proves inadequate disclosure, "[t]he sole issue remaining [is] a determination of damages" (15, p. 335). The failure to provide adequate information, under a battery theory, is viewed as the harm to the patient—that is, a *dignitary injury,* or insult to the personhood of the patient. This concept probably comes as close as any other to embodying Katz's view of the underlying rationale for informed consent.

Despite Katz's position as the most prominent theorist and critic of informed consent law, he has never formulated a comprehensive legal alternative to the current system. He would presumably favor addressing informed consent as a matter of battery law, and the adoption of subjective, patient-oriented standards. But he appears to recognize that this reorientation, which itself is unlikely to take place, would not necessarily improve matters all that much. Allowing patients to sue for dignitary harms, while theoretically appealing, is unlikely to increase significantly the number of legal suits filed. Such harms are likely to be compensated with only minimal damages, and few patients (not to mention attorneys) can be expected to pursue cases in which their time and effort will go largely unrewarded (3). This has proven to be the case, for example, in suits allowing nominal damages for emotional harm.

Proposed Changes in Legal Basis of Recovery

Particular attention has been given to Katz's autonomy-based critique of informed consent law because he has presented the most thorough analysis of the doctrine and its applications. Numerous other commentators, many of them probably influenced by him, have echoed and amplified his charges. Some have focused on individual elements of informed consent law, such as the acceptance by courts of the notion of therapeutic privilege (see Chapter 4). They have argued for the abolition of the privilege or for its limitation, for example, by excusing non-disclosure only of the information that itself is thought likely to cause the expected harm, but continuing to require otherwise complete disclosure (16,17).

Another favorite target of legal commentators is the professional standard of disclosure, seen by many as a major limitation on the right of patients to receive relevant information. Theodore Schneyer has offered probably the most interesting objection—namely, that the differing amounts of remuneration various procedures offer create such substantial conflicts of interest for physicians in informing their patients about the desirability of one treatment option over another that physicians cannot be trusted to establish the standards of disclosure (18). Schneyer believes that physicians, particularly surgeons, cannot separate their pecuniary interests from their fiduciary obligations to patients and will consistently recommend, and shape their disclosures to ensure that patients select, those procedures likely to yield the highest rates of compensation. His critique takes on added significance in light of the high degree of specialization of physicians. When the available options include procedures not performed by the physician with whom the patient is currently dealing, there is an economic disincentive for the physician to discuss those options, perhaps even an incentive not to see them as options at all. For example, it is often said that a patient will get a recommendation for surgery from a surgeon and for medical treatment from an internist. Prospective review by managed care organizations can substantially reduce this effect, but may involve other financial incentives (see Chapter 10). Although perhaps viewed skeptically when first proposed, Schneyer's analysis is likely to be given more credence now that the economic aspects of physicians' behavior are coming under extensive scrutiny (see Chapter 10).

Several commentators have offered more sweeping proposals for restructuring the law, in particular to allow recovery for the infliction of dignitary harms. One author calls for "the legislature . . . [to] fashion sanctions other than damages for injury, such as fines, probation, loss of license or other administrative penalties, which could be imposed on a sliding scale, depending on the gravity of the offense [of failing to disclose appropriate information]" (19). Another author calls for a system of non-insurable tort-fines that would have the desired punitive and deterrent effect on physicians (20). Marjorie Shultz suggests development of a new cause of action protecting patient autonomy that would be administered under either a tort or contract theory of recovery (8). Although she recognizes that damages in these cases may not be substantial, she notes that even awards of nominal damages would "dramatically strengthen protection of patient autonomy" (8, p. 291). The problem of encouraging patients to pursue these remedies in the absence of the prospect of substantial recovery of damages, however, has not yet been solved.

Leonard Riskin, whose concern "is based primarily on a commitment to human dignity as a value transcending even physical health," has offered two other suggestions (20). The first would, in essence, adopt a partial battery approach to informed consent cases by eliminating the current requirement for plaintiffs to prove the element of causation, that is, that their behavior would have been different had full disclosure been accomplished. Under this proposal, any undisclosed risk that materialized would warrant the assessment of damages. Alternatively, Riskin would reduce the standard of causation to require plaintiffs merely to show that they *might* not have consented had full, appropriate disclosure been made. Both suggestions would cut deeply against the negligence theory on which informed consent law has been based to date, and would approximate a system of strict liability for undisclosed risks that in fact occur (21).

Aaron Twerski and Neil Cohen also target the causation requirement (22). They criticize Shultz's autonomy cause of action, since it would allow only nominal damages when a procedure is successful. Instead, they base their model for recovery on the violation of a process right, specifically the right to participate in the process of decision making. As with other substantive process rights (e.g., election voting), they would allow recovery of substantial damages for violations of this right to participate. Compensation for a "bad result" would only be one part of the analysis; also included would be psychological harm from the sudden and unexpected manifestation of an undisclosed risk, harm from depriving the patient of the opportunity to choose and to accept the risks of a particular alternative, and harm from depriving the patient of choice among a range of benefits. They argue that if physicians "understood that the law encourages participation in decision making, rather than avoidance of bad results attributable to undisclosed risks, they would be more likely to foster that goal" (22, p. 665).

Proposed Changes in the Focus of the Doctrine

Rather than tinkering with the mechanisms for recovery, some critics would prefer to see a reorientation of the rules governing the informed consent process itself. Thus, Richard Simpson would substantially reconstruct the informed consent system to focus on patient understanding instead of physician disclosure. Simpson argues for a standard that evaluates whether patients actually understand what they have been told. He would require courts "to consider whether the physician has taken reasonable measures to ensure that the patient understands the information disclosed" (16). However, the difficulties with this approach are evident from his analysis. After a lengthy discussion of the importance of comprehension, Simpson backs away from suggesting a system that would require it. Fearful that patients who cannot comprehend the nature and risks of treatment, or who choose to remain ignorant, might thereby be deprived of medical care (a concern that appears to have motivated some of the courts that considered this issue as well), Simpson concludes merely with a detailed list of items physicians would be required to disclose. If the disclosure were made, and patients were encouraged to ask questions, he would presume comprehension.

Joseph Goldstein arrives at a similar solution from very different premises (23). In what might be termed an anti-Kantian mode of reasoning, he has argued that an emphasis on patients' comprehension would only serve to undercut their autonomy. If comprehension were to be the touchstone, he fears that uncomprehending patients would have their decisions made for them by others. Believing that even so-called irrational patients should have the right to determine their own medical care, Goldstein would focus entirely on the disclosure by the physician, shun any assessment of comprehension (or even competence), and allow patients to pursue compensation for dignitary harms.

The autonomy-based critics of informed consent command a wide following in legal and bioethical circles. The appeal of their arguments lies in their ability to identify substantial compromises of patient autonomy in current approaches to informed consent. However, they have had relatively little impact on the development of the law because they consistently have failed to deal effectively with their opponents' competing concerns— primarily, that too close an adherence to self-determination might encourage the harassment of physicians in the courts and lead patients to make decisions that would adversely affect their health. Katz comes closest to acknowledging the existence of these competing concerns but dismisses them as unsupported by empirical data. Most courts and legislatures, however, remain convinced that subjective standards and recovery for dignitary harms would encourage lawsuits and recoveries for plaintiffs in a manner that would be unfair to physicians. Moreover, they are generally willing to allow physicians some scope for paternalistic intervention, in the belief that patients sometimes require (and perhaps even desire) decisions to be made for, rather than with, them. Nevertheless, the autonomy-based critics have done a great deal to alert both the legal and medical professions to the danger that the spirit of informed consent might be lost in the process of creating legal rules to enforce it.

The Health-Oriented Critique

Most commentators who address the issue of informed consent believe that their approach, if adopted, will enhance the health of patients. We use the term health-oriented critique to refer to the position that favors the strengthening or relaxation of the current disclosure and consent requirements imposed on physicians on the basis of their probable effect on patients' health. This viewpoint is congruent with the "therapeutic jurisprudence" perpective— a method of analyzing law based on its potential therapeutic or antitherapeutic effects (24)—that has developed in the last decade. Although the majority of those who subscribe to the health-oriented critique focus on relaxing the current legal requirements, we address arguments of both those who favor strengthened rules and those who favor more lenient requirements.

Proponents of Strengthened Disclosure Requirements

Eleanor Swift Glass has suggested that therapeutic benefits would result from a rigorously defined requirement for informed consent (19). Arguing for patient-oriented standards of disclosure, administrative mechanisms for imposing sanctions on doctors who fail to provide adequate disclosure, and limitations on the therapeutic privilege, she maintains that these changes would improve the overall quality of health care. Informed consent was unnecessary, she claims, when doctors knew their patients for long periods of time and could, in making decisions for them, accurately reflect the patients' own value systems. Modern, technologically oriented medicine interferes with the development of such relationships by providing too many incentives for physicians to neglect the human aspects of their patients. As a result, physicians make poor decisions on behalf of patients they barely know, which leads to the improper choice of treatments and poor patient compliance. If physicians are compelled to discuss therapeutic options, risks, and benefits with patients, the result will be that additional relevant information will be elicited, personalized and joint decision making by doctor and patient will be encouraged, and a greater sense of teamwork and, therefore, compliance on the patient's part will ensue. Likewise, Robert Gatter, stresses the benefits that may result from better and more stringent disclosure rules. He focuses on the need for a tailored disclosure based on the patient's goals for treatment, and argues for a physician duty of reasonable inquiry regarding those goals (25). Enforcing such a duty, he argues, will result in (*1*) less unnecessary medical care, which will reduce costs, as well as avoid suboptimal care, (*2*) healthier outcomes because of greater patient involvement in decision making, and (*3*) fewer malpractice suits (25).

Empirical data in this area are problematic, but there are reasons to believe that the provision of appropriate information and collaborative decision making will enhance compliance with treatment (26). A complementary argument in favor of tighter informed consent requirements focuses on the benefits of reduced patient anxiety as a result of more complete disclosure (10), a suggestion supported by findings in classic studies of surgical patients (27). There have also been studies showing a general link between better physician–patient communication and improved health outcomes (28, 29).

The most cogent statement of the belief that increased patient participation in medical decision making will improve patients' health comes from the report on informed consent of the President's Commission for the Study of Ethical Problems in Medicine (30). The Commission emphasized that health, or well-being, must be defined broadly, and that the inability to make decisions congruent with one's values constitutes an impediment to the subjective, and probably objective, attainment of a state of well-being. In the commission's approach, well-being is seen as influenced by a combination of physical and psychological factors. A narrow focus on objective indicia of physical health, often characteristic of the medical profession's traditional approach, ignores the broader aspects of persons' satisfaction with their state of existence. Unfortunately, such a broad definition of benefit is difficult to measure. In fact, there are few data on the physical benefits of informed consent (14).

Proponents of Weakened Disclosure Requirements

Most health-oriented critics claim that informed consent is ineffective in achieving its primary goals. They generally make one of two points. First, patients do not understand or use the information they are given, and thus to require that physicians spend time disclosing information to patients constitutes a wasteful use of scarce health resources. Second, informed consent is actually deleterious to patients' health. Both arguments are rooted in a belief that patients are simply unable to deal with medical information in a manner that results in meaningful decisions.

Franz Ingelfinger, late editor of the *New England Journal of Medicine,* exemplified this approach in an editorial entitled "Informed (but Uneducated) Consent" (31). "The chances are remote," he noted, speaking in the research context, "that the subject really understands what he had consented to." Not only will the subject have difficulty comprehending the true import of discomforts and risks associated with any procedure, but "it is moreover quite unlikely that any patient-subject can see himself accurately within the broad context of the situation, to weigh the inconveniences and hazards that he will have to undergo against the improvements that the research project may bring to the management of his disease in general and to his own case in particular." Many research studies that purport to demonstrate poor patient understanding of relevant information are usually cited in support of such contentions.

One of the better early studies reported the results of testing fifty patients "within an hour of their admission to . . . [a clinical research] Center and their consent interview with the physician-investigator" (32). All subjects had just consented to a clinical research project and had presumably read and had signed a consent form (22 percent of the subjects failed to read the form in its entirety). Of the subjects, 52 percent were judged to be adequately knowledgeable, based on their responses to a nineteen-item questionnaire. Only a minority had what the investigators defined as sufficient knowledge of the procedures (34 percent), the purpose (22 percent), and the risks (20 percent) of the study. In assessing this poor performance, the authors found problems with the format and content of the consent forms, the manner of their presentation, and the circumstances in which the patient-subjects were situated.

This study suffered from the common defects of most investigations of patient or subject understanding. Oral disclosure was neither observed nor standardized, and the authors were forced to assume that the information whose comprehension they were measuring was actually conveyed, either in written form or in some unrecorded oral form. Furthermore, the ability to recall information, even a short time after a decision has been made, is not necessarily an indication of the understanding of the information at the time of the decision itself. Still, the authors in this study were more sophisticated than most in pointing to multifactorial causes of poor understanding and in suggesting improvements in consent practices rather than totally rejecting the idea of informed consent.

Data of this sort, produced repeatedly by different research groups (see references in 33), are often used to support the argument that understanding cannot be achieved. Such statements are easily refuted by reference to studies of situations in which reasonable comprehension actually has been achieved (34–36). A more sound interpretation of all these studies might be that patients and subjects can attain a good level of understanding in many cases, but that several factors—including the manner in which disclosure is made as well as patients' limitations—may get in the way (37–39).

A variation on the Ingelfinger argument relies not so much on patients' noncomprehension as on their proclivity to make decisions with little reference to the information they have. Carl Fellner and John Marshall, for example, studied decisions by kidney transplant donors (a most atypical population) and claimed that the decision to donate or not was always made before any information was provided, usually on grounds irrelevant to the medical issues at hand (40). In addition, a study of the effect of disclosure on contraceptive choice found that 93 percent of the patients reported having made up their minds before disclosure, and only 4 percent said the disclosure changed their decision (41). These results are difficult to generalize, however, since many patients may have considered transplant donation or contraceptive alternatives before speaking with a physician. In the majority of physician–patient encounters, the patient seeks consultation because of an as-yet-unidentified ailment or a condition for which the treatment options are not yet identified. Thus, the patient is unlikely to have seriously considered the choices beforehand.

Alternatively, it is argued that patients are so reliant on their physicians' advice that, regardless of the information they receive, they will passively place the decision in their physicians' hands. Even without such passive trust, some physicians have claimed that they can almost always get their patients to consent to any procedure they desire to perform, even in the research setting (42). If information is either not understood, or not considered in a patient's decision, the health-oriented critics maintain, it makes little sense to require physicians to provide it or to hold them liable for failure to do so. But evidence that patients will consent to whatever their physicians recommend does not necessarily support the notion that patients are not understanding or considering information. To the contrary, it is more likely to be a reflection of the congruence of physician recommendations and patient preferences. Moreover, two recent studies come to opposite conclusions about whether patients want physicians to make decisions for them, with one finding that patients preferred physicians to play the primary role in decision making (43), and the other that patients were reluctant to hand decisionmaking control over to their physician (44). Significantly, both studies found that patients wanted information in order to be involved in the decisionmaking process.

The second prong of the health-oriented critique concerns not only the waste of time and resources involved in an informed consent process but also the actual harm that might result from disclosure. Of course, the courts, beginning with *Salgo* (as Katz notes), have had similar concerns, which account for their deference to medical discretion, professional standards of disclosure, and the therapeutic privilege. A number of rather sensational case reports have purported to show instances when the disclosure of possible risks to patients led to untoward results, including cardiac problems, unjustified refusal of treatment, and death, either self-inflicted or as the result of the untreated disease (45–47). The conclusions drawn from these anecdotal accounts are that more patients are being harmed than helped by informed consent discussions. "I would propose," suggests one physician-author, "that we provide patients with reasonable explanations of what we feel is appropriate and not permit lawyers or administrators to set the rules" (46).

Few critics working from the health-oriented perspective make much more specific suggestions than this one as to what approach they would prefer to the current system. Implicit in many articles appears to be the wish that the legal requirements for informed consent would just go away, leaving physicians with the nearly total discretion they had in the days of "simple consent." In almost no case is any recognition given to the legitimate interest of patients in making their own decisions, participating in the decisionmaking process, or even knowingly ceding the right to make decisions to their medical caretakers. Insofar as the existence of competing interests and the impracticality of rolling back fifty years of case law and statutes are ignored, the health-oriented critique of informed consent has been a theoretical failure. Moreover, while this critique more than any other relies on empirical data to support its claims, the data relating to the harmful results of informed consent are generally so poor that few reliable conclusions can be drawn from them (33). The irony is, however, that even with weak empirical grounding and a monocular view of the world, this critique has had substantial influence on many of the courts and legislatures that have struggled to shape legal rules to govern informed consent. The discretion retained by physicians in current law, as Katz has noted, results largely from the lawmakers' fears of constructing a system that might actually cause harm to patients, even though such fears may be groundless.

The Interactionist Critique

The most original and provocative critique of informed consent rejects both autonomy and health as the ultimate goals. Robert Burt, in his book *Taking Care of Strangers,* has attempted to shift the focus of the debate away from the outcomes and toward the process (48). Burt's primary value in the doctor–patient interaction is respect for the humanity of each participant. In promoting this goal, Burt would reject both patients' and physician advocates' claims to dominance in the decisionmaking process. Dominance itself, in Burt's view, is incompatible with the kind of respect he is seeking to promote. His work is one of the only comprehensive efforts so far to rethink the rationale for informed consent and to offer a carefully worked out alternative. His analysis, despite some problems with the implications he draws from it, warrants careful examination.

Burt begins with a thoroughgoing skepticism about efforts to enhance patient autonomy through the process of disclosure and consent. Truly autonomous decision making, he believes, is an impossibility. Human beings operate within social frameworks, and any decision made within a dyadic relationship, such as that between doctor and patient, cannot help but be influenced by what both parties bring to the interaction. Moreover, both doctor and patient will change as they come to know and begin to share each other's values. This process is more emotional than rational. The intense feelings generated in a relationship in which life and death are often at stake will frequently have a more potent effect on the participants than any position they reach as the result of purely cognitive processes.

The resistance to recognizing the mutuality that must dominate the decisionmaking process, Burt would say, stems from fear: fear of acknowledging the dependency and impotence that both parties share in the face of often irreversible natural forces, fear of the inherent uncertainty of their situation, and fear of death. Doctors and patients alike attempt to master their fears by seeking complete control of the interpersonal scene. It is as if physician and patient are each saying to the other, "If I can master you and control this interaction in which we are engaged, then I can control anything. I will no longer be powerless and uncertain in the face of death."

If we are to humanize doctor–patient interactions, according to this view, we must transform this struggle for control into a collaborative effort to confront the participants' mutual fears. Doctor and patient could be encouraged or even compelled to talk with each other, in fact to negotiate with each other, respecting each other's independence and humanity. The law of informed consent can be a crucial tool in this process. Burt would compel such dialogue and negotiation by leaving all parties in doubt as to what the law requires of them. Since physicians could never be certain that anything they did effectively insulated them from suit, they would always be driven to ascertain patients' desires, work with them to shape a reasonable and mutually satisfactory plan of treatment, and in the process provide all the information patients want. Should a suit be brought after the fact, alleging that the physician had been negligent in the process, the case would be judged by a general standard of reasonableness, without predefined rules.

Burt's analysis has evoked considerable response, primarily from the legal profession. Most commentators have avoided criticizing his view of the emotional basis of the doctor–patient relationship and instead have targeted his proposed solution. Clearly, there would be immense legal difficulties in implementing Burt's scheme. Law works toward achieving certainty rather than uncertainty. A situation in which neither party could know with assurance the consequences of his behavior would strike many as unfair. In addition, it is difficult to imagine how that uncertainty might be maintained, that is, how one could prevent precedent from developing (e.g., in defining what constitutes a reasonable effort on the physician's part). It is almost impossible to envision how one might implement Burt's scheme.

Yet Burt's contribution, elements of which have been echoed by Jay Katz in his writings (4), should not be overlooked. Howard Brody, for example, has proposed a "transparency model" of informed consent that would focus physicians on conversation rather than legal standards (49). The idea is that informed consent "disclosure is adequate when the physician's basic thinking has been rendered transparent to the patient" (49, p. 7). Under this model, physicians would be required to share their thinking with patients, to allow patients time to ask questions, and finally to allow patients to participate in decision making to the extent that they chose. These actions are geared toward facilitating conversation, not avoiding liability.

Ezekiel and Linda Emanuel propose four models of the physician–patient relationship: paternalistic, informative, interpretive, and deliberative (50). They note that the legal doctrine of informed consent appears to promote the informative model. Although they state that different models may be appropriate in different cases, they generally advocate a deliberative model of informed consent whereby the "aim of the physician-patient interaction is to help the patient determine and choose the best health-related values that can be realized in the clinical situation" (50, p. 2222). Like Brody, they would shift focus away from the legal standards and toward helping physicians understand the values underlying informed consent.

Finally, Robert Veatch has proposed abandoning informed consent in favor of a model where the physician and patient are matched on the basis of what he refers to as "deep values" (51). These deep value pairings would reflect the "fundamental world views" of the physician and patient. He argues that traditional informed consent is outdated and that the goal should not be getting the patient to agree autonomously with the physician's offered options or recommendations, but to be an active participant in the choice among plausible alternatives. Although we agree with the ideal of promoting active participation by patients in medical decision making, we are unsure how such a value pairing would be achieved practically.

By emphasizing that the problem to be addressed is one of modifying interpersonal relationships, not formulating legal rules, the interactionist perspective tears us away from the arguments over legal standards of disclosure and causation. It refocuses our attention on the fact that the law is of dubious efficacy in regulating how people interact (14). Although the law can establish the prerequisites for interaction of the desired type (e.g., by requiring that a discussion about a patient's impending medical decision take place), it is quite helpless to affect the tone or goodwill of the interaction.

We know of only one suggestion for a legal system that would reflect the interactionist perspective, and that is to have "patients and doctors define jointly, based on their needs and expectation, what informed consent means to them" (52). Essentially the author advocates for private contractual agreements regarding the purpose of informed consent. Although an intriguing idea, it seems highly unlikely that the courts or legislatures will accept such a doctrine. Moreover, given the informational and time constraints of physicians, it is doubtful they will take the time to negotiate and establish a specific agreement with each patient. As Arnold Rosoff points out in his commentary on the proposal, it appears to be proposing a subjective professional standard—what a particular physician believes should be disclosed in a particular case (53). The result is less a collaborative process model, as the author claims, but instead a reversion to the old physician discretion standard of the past (53).

A Synthetic Approach

We find it difficult to question the validity of much of what critics on all sides of the informed consent controversy have had to say. Like the autonomy-oriented commentators, we believe firmly in the importance of patients having the opportunity to participate in making medical decisions. That conclusion appeals to us on deontologic grounds, since we take as fundamental the idea that patients should have the right to decide what happens to their bodies. On consequentialist grounds, our research, along with others', has suggested that patients are more likely to aid in their own care if they understand and have played a role in selecting the treatment they receive (10,54).

On the other hand, like the health-oriented critics, we recognize that whatever legal requirements are established to enforce the doctrine of informed consent, they should not so impede the delivery of medical care that, instead of improving patients' well-being, the doctrine actually causes patients harm. Thus, while we agree that steps need to be taken to encourage greater communication between physicians and patients, some proposals, including such punitive measures as a system of tort-fines that would be imposed whenever physicians are deficient in disclosing information, seem to us to have the potential for causing more harm than good. Physicians who are overly concerned about the possibility of being sued for what they say will say very little, at least spontaneously. The essential interactive nature of the physician–patient relationship will be lost, as physicians and patients glower at each other in suspicion. To save patient autonomy at the expense of destroying the very relationship that is essential for proper medical care is a Pyrrhic victory.

We part company with both autonomy and health-oriented critics—at least from the more extreme members of each group—in our belief that the law of informed consent cannot exclusively support either of these interests. To grant that the legal doctrine of informed consent compromises patient autonomy to some extent is not, as some would claim, to declare it worthless in that regard. There is little doubt that, however poorly the idea of informed consent has been implemented to date, its growing acceptance among doctors and patients has led to substantially greater communication of information than occurred in the past. If the legal requirements have not gone as far as they might in stimulating communication, a major obstacle has been the concern that patients' health might be harmed thereby—hardly a meretricious motivation.

Similarly, although the law of informed consent makes physicians' lives more difficult and permits some patients to make bad health decisions, this price is not an unreasonable one to pay for the support of a value as important as the right of individual choice. The argument that informed consent simply does not work because patients do not understand or utilize the information they receive also does not vitiate the value of the ideal of collaborative decision making. As noted previously, some studies suggest that the decisionmaking process, properly carried out, can result in patients having a good understanding of the information disclosed. Even if a fair number of patients fail to understand or decline to make use of the information they receive, informed consent still has value in that it offers all patients the opportunity to participate in their care. Patients do and should have the right to reject that opportunity, either implicitly by ignoring the information provided, or explicitly by waiver, and it is wrong to deny them the choice. Thus, the fact that informed consent is something less in practice than it is in theory in no way suggests that it should be abandoned, even if it has certain costs in terms of medical time and effort.

The compromises that have been struck between the values of autonomy and health, as detailed throughout this book, do not as a whole strike us as unreasonable ones. Although we might quarrel with one or another choice made by courts or legislatures, we do not share the apocalyptic visions of critics of both persuasions. In fact, the continuing attention paid to the nuances of the law of informed consent seems entirely misplaced. For the reasons so well described by the autonomy-oriented critics, and supported by empirical studies, the law has had surprisingly little impact on most doctor–patient interactions. It is unlikely that any legal rules can, by themselves, lead to very much additional alteration in physicians' practices without becoming so intrusive as to inhibit the effective provision of medical care.

How then can the idea of informed consent, with its vision of collaborative decision making between physicians and patients, be more nearly approximated in day-to-day medical care? We share the view of Katz and Burt that it certainly cannot be done without the cooperation of physicians (4,48). This cooperation in turn can only be garnered if the medical profession can be weaned from its view of informed consent as a pernicious, alien doctrine imposed by a hostile legal system. More stringent legal rules are not the answer, since they will only evoke increased resistance from physicians, who after all still remain largely in control of both the content and tone of doctor–patient interactions. Yet, the medical profession will not fully accept informed consent unless the belief that it is incompatible with good medical care can be dispelled.

We believe this goal is attainable. The development of the law of informed consent has been premised on a set of irreconcilable conflicts between autonomy and health, and the extent of those conflicts has been greatly exaggerated. Whatever the divergences in theory, when it comes to the clinical setting, the principles of good medical care and informed consent, properly conceived, are not in opposition. For physician behavior to change, physicians must be persuaded of two conclusions: that (*1*) patients should have the right to participate in decision making, and (*2*) appropriate implementation of informed consent actually reinforces the physician–patient dialogue that lies at the core of an effective therapeutic relationship, thus facilitating good medical care.

That many physicians now think otherwise is a function, in part, of their training about the relative rights and responsibilities of doctors and patients. (How physicians might come to accept the spirit of informed consent is considered in some detail in the concluding section of this book.) Physicians' views have also been shaped significantly by their experiences with a species of informed consent (what we call in the next chapter the "event model" of informed consent) that in paying obeisance to the legal requirements wholly ignores the realities of clinical care. We demonstrate in the following chapter that this need not be the case.

References

1. Merz, J.F. (1993) On a decision-making paradigm of medical informed consent. *J Leg Med*, 14:231–264.
2. 61 Fed. Reg. 51498, 51500 (October 2, 1996).
3. Katz, J. (1977) Informed consent—a fairy tale? *University of Pittsburgh Law Review*, 39:137–174.
4. Katz, J. (1984) *The Silent World of Doctor and Patient.* New York: Free Press.

5. Katz, J. (1994) Informed consent—must it remain a fairy tale? *J Contemp Health Law Policy*, 10:69–91.

6. Faden, R.R. and Beauchamp, T.L. (1986) *A History and Theory of Informed Consent.* New York: Oxford University Press.

7. Terry, N.P. (1993) Apologetic tort think: autonomy and information torts. *St. Louis University Law Journal*, 38:189–198.

8. Shultz, M. (1985) From informed consent to patient choice: a new protected interest. *Yale Law Journal*, 95:219–299.

9. Salgo v. Leland Stanford Jr. Univ. Bd. of Trustees, 317 P2d 170 (Cal. Ct. App. 1957).

10. Lidz, C.W. and Meisel, A. (1982) Informed consent and the structure of medical care. In President's Commission for the Study of Ethical Problems in Medicine and Biomedical and Behavioral Research, *Making Health Care Decisions: The Ethical and Legal Implications of Informed Consent in the Patient-Practitioner Relationship*, Volume 2, Appendices. Washington, D.C.: U.S. Government Printing Office.

11. Lidz, C.W., Meisel, A., Zerubavel, E., et al. (1984) *Informed Consent: A Study of Decisionmaking in Psychiatry.* New York: Guilford.

12. Harris, L., Boyle, J., and Brounstein, P. (1982) Views of informed consent and decisionmaking: parallel surveys of physicians and the public. In President's Commission for the Study of Ethical Problems in Medicine and Biomedical and Behavioral Research, *Empirical Studies of Informed Consent*, Volume 2, Appendices. Washington, D.C.: U.S. Government Printing Office.

13. Strull, W., Lo, B., and Charles, G. (1984) Do patients want to participate in medical decisionmaking? *JAMA*, 252:2990–2994.

14. Schuck, P. (1994) Rethinking Informed Consent. *Yale Law Journal*, 103:899–959.

15. Grouse v. Cassel, 615 A.2d 331 (Pa. 1992).

16. Simpson, R. (1981) Informed consent: from disclosure to patient participation in medical decisionmaking. *Northwestern University Law Review*, 76:172–207.

17. Rice, N. (1974) Informed consent: the illusion of patient choice. *Emory Law Journal*, 23:503–522.

18. Schneyer, T. (1976) Informed consent and the danger of bias in the formation of medical disclosure practices. *Wisconsin Law Review*, 124–170.

19. Glass, E. (1970) Restructuring informed consent: legal therapy for the doctor-patient relationship. *Yale Law Journal*, 179:1533–1576.

20. Riskin, L. (1975) Informed consent: looking for the action. *University of Illinois Law Forum*, 511–580.

21. Meisel, A. (1977) The expansion of liability for medical accidents: from negligence to strict liability by way of informed consent. *Nebraska Law Review*, 56:51–152.

22. Twerski, A. and Cohen, N. (1988) Informed decision making and the law of torts: the myth of justiciable causation. *University of Illinois Law Review*, 607–665.

23. Goldstein, J. (1975) For Harold Lasswell: some reflections on human dignity, entrapment, informed consent, and the plea bargain. *Yale Law Journal*, 84:683–703.

24. Wexler, D. (1990) *Therapeutic Jurisprudence: The Law as a Therapeutic Agent.* Durham: Carolina Academic Press.

25. Gatter, R. (2000) Informed consent law and the forgotten duty of physician inquiry. *Loyola University Chicago Law Journal*, 31:557–597.

26. DiMatteo, M. and DiNicola, D. (1982) *Achieving Patient Compliance: The Psychology of the Medical Practitioner's Role.* New York: Pergamon Press.

27. Janis, I. (1958) *Psychological Stress: Psychoanalytic and Behavioral Studies of Surgical Patients.* New York: Wiley.

28. Kreps, G.L. and O'Hair, D. (eds) (1995) *Communication and Health Outcomes.* Creskill, England: Hampton Press.
29. Stewart, M. (1995) Studies of health outcomes and patient-centered communication. In Stewart, M., Brown, J.B., Weston, W.W., McWhinney, I.R., McWilliam, C.L., Freeman, T.R. (eds) *Patient-Centered Medicine: Transforming Clinical Method.* Thousand Oaks: Sage Publications.
30. President's Commission for the Study of Ethical Problems in Medicine and Biomedical and Behavioral Research (1982) *Making Health Care Decisions: The Ethical and Legal Implications of Informed Consent in the Patient-Practitioner Relationship.* Washington, D.C.: U.S. Government Printing Office.
31. Ingelfinger, F. (1972) Informed (but uneducated) consent. *N Engl J Med,* 287:465–466.
32. Schultz, A., Pardee, G., and Ensinck, J. (1975) Are research subjects really informed? *West J Med,* 123:76–80.
33. Meisel, A. and Roth, L. (1983) Toward an informed dicussion of informed consent: a review and critique of the empirical studies. *Arizona Law Review,* 25:265–346.
34. Jensen, A.B., Madsen, B., Anderson, P., et al. (1993) Information for cancer patients entering a clinical trial—an evaluation of an information strategy. *Eur J Cancer,* 29A:2235–2238.
35. Quaid, K.A., Faden, R.R., Vining, E.P., et al. (1990) Informed consent for a prescription drug: impact of disclosed information on patient understanding and medical outcomes. *Patient Education and Counseling,* 15:249–259.
36. Wadey, V. and Frank, C. (1997) The effectiveness of patient verbalization on informed consent. *Can J Surg,* 40:124–128.
37. Lavelle-Jones, C., Byrne, D., Rice, P., et al. (1993) Factors affecting quality of informed consent. *Br Med J,* 306:885–890.
38. Mazur, D. and Merz, J. (1994) Patients' interpretations of verbal expressions of probability: implications for securing informed consent to medical interventions. *Behav Sci Law,* 12:417–426.
39. Silva, M. and Sorrell, J. (1988) Enhancing comprehension of information for informed consent: a review of empirical research. *IRB,* 10:1–5.
40. Fellner, C. and Marshall, J. (1970) Kidney donors—the myth of informed consent. *Am J Psychiatry,* 126:1245–1251.
41. Faden, R. and Beauchamp, T. (1980) Decisionmaking and informed consent: a study of the impact of disclosed information. *Social Indicators Research,* 7:314–336.
42. Beecher, H. (1966) Consent in clinical experimentation: myth and reality. *JAMA,* 195:124–125.
43. Bradley, J., Zia, M., and Hamilton, N. (1996) Patient preferences for control in medical decision making: a scenario-based approach. *Fam Med,* 28:496–501.
44. Deber, R., Kraetschmer, N., and Irvine, J. (1996) What role do patients wish to play in treatment decision making? *Arch Intern Med,* 156:1414–1420.
45. Kaplan, S., Greenwald, R., and Rogers, A. (1977) Neglected aspects of informed consent. *N Engl J Med,* 296:1127.
46. Katz, R. (1977) Informed consent—is it bad medicine? *West J Med,* 126:426–428.
47. Patten, B. and Stump, W. (1978) Death related to informed consent. *Tex Med,* 74:49–50.
48. Burt, R.A. (1979) *Taking Care of Strangers: The Rule of Law in Doctor-Patient Relations.* New York: Free Press.
49. Brody, H. (1989) Transparency: informed consent in primary care. *Hastings Cent Rep,* 19:5–9.

50. Emanuel, E.J. and Emanuel, L.L. (1992) Four models of the physician-patient relationship. *JAMA*, 267:2221–2226.
51. Veatch, R.M. (1995) Abandoning informed consent. *Hastings Cent Rep*, 25:5–12.
52. Piper, A. (1994) Truce on the battlefield: a proposal for a different approach to medical informed consent. *J Law Med Ethics*, 22:301–313.
53. Rosoff, A. (1994) Commentary: Truce on the battlefield: a proposal for a different approach to medical informed consent. *J Law Med Ethics*, 22:314–317.
54. Appelbaum, P. and Roth, L. (1982) Treatment refusal in medical hospitals. In President's Commission for the Study of Ethical Problems in Medicine and Biomedical and Behavioral Research, *Making Health Care Decisions: The Ethical and Legal Implications of Informed Consent in the Patient-Practitioner Relationship*. Washington, D.C.: U.S. Government Printing Office.

Part III

The Clinical Setting

8

The Role of Informed Consent in Medical Decision Making

How can informed consent be integrated into the physician–patient relationship in a manner that is respectful of both the idea of informed consent and the imperatives of clinical care? A realistic answer to that question could, we believe, remove much of the resistance of many healthcare professionals to the idea of informed consent. This chapter's goal is to offer a practical procedural framework within which clinicians can operate to facilitate patients' decision making in a manner that meets both these desiderata.

Decision Making and Informed Consent: Event vs. Process

The interactions of physicians and patients in making decisions about medical treatment can be conceptualized in two ways. Decision making can be approached as an event that occurs at a single point in time (an "event model"), or it can be viewed as a continuous element of the relationship between patients and their caregivers (a "process model"). The implications of these different ways of conceptualizing decisions about treatment are quite profound, rooted as they are in distinct visions of the relationship between physicians and patients.

Consent as an Event

The event model of informed consent is predicated on a relatively simple paradigm. A patient seeking medical care approaches a physician for assistance. After assessing the patient's condition, the physician reaches a diagnosis and formulates a recommended plan of treatment. The physician's conclusions and recommendations are presented to the patient, along with information concerning the risks and potential benefits of the proposed treatment, and possible alternatives and their risks and potential benefits. Weighing the available data, the patient reflects on the relative risks and benefits of each course of action and then selects the medically acceptable alternative that most closely fits the patient's particular values.

On the surface at least, the event model conforms well to the legal requirements for informed consent. The event model emphasizes the provision of full and accurate information to patients at the time of decision making. Consent forms are often used for this purpose; indeed, the consent form can be said to be the central symbol of the event model (see Chapter 9). Patients' understanding, although desirable in the abstract, is less crucial to this model than is the provision of information. Once information is provided, patients make clear-cut choices about treatment, offering physicians straightforward guidance as to whether legally effective consent has been obtained, and treatment can proceed.

In the event model, decision making is temporally circumscribed. Decision making begins when a physician offers a patient recommendations with accompanying information and ends with a patient's decision. Information that patients bring to this interaction, including previous communications from physicians, is considered outside the scope of the current decisionmaking event. Similarly, although patients are nominally free to change their minds about treatment, whatever occurs after the decision has been made is also irrelevant to the decision, unless one party or the other reopens the issue by initiating another decisionmaking event.

The event model offers several advantages (1), which help to explain the favor it finds in many medical settings, but also offers reason for pause. On the positive side of the ledger, the event model is clearly preferable to more physician-dominated modes of decision making, in which patients are offered little information and given no chance to participate in decision making. The event model, to its credit, provides patients with considerable information about their care and an opportunity to make choices.

Moreover, the event model fits well with the contemporary organization of hospital-, clinic-, and office-based medical care. Most modern health care facilities, whether a large medical center or a private office, now break down the care of patients into a series of discrete, smaller tasks. Each of these tasks may be the responsibility of a different member of a healthcare team. A receptionist obtains demographic and insurance information; a nurse elicits a chief complaint and measures some physiological parameters; a physician performs a physical examination and determines what additional data are needed; and a variety of technicians conduct tests that will provide these data. Even the responsibilities of physicians are subdivided by specialty and by time—patients may be assigned to the doctor "on call," rather than to "their" physician.

The growth of managed care, with its pressures to be efficient has reinforced the economic pressures on the informed consent process. Managed care has sought to control medical costs in a number of ways, including encouraging the most highly salaried members of the team to minimize the time spent with patients. Although comparisons with assembly-line procedures in factories are unfair in some regards, the underlying, efficiency-based rationale is similar. An event model of decision making meets the needs of this differentiated system. Decision making can be assigned to a particular place ("Will you please see Ms. Smith in Room 7 at the end of the hall"), person ("I am Ms. Smith, Dr. Jones's nurse; I will read you the consent form, answer your questions, and get your consent"), and time ("We need to have you read and sign this now"). In this model, obtaining the patient's consent need not be something to be concerned about before or after the assigned time, or by members of the team outside of whose responsibilities the task falls.

From the patient's point of view, too, the event model offers some advantages. There is little ambiguity about the roles of the members of the healthcare team; one person is assigned with whom the patient can interact. The time when a decision must be made is clearly demarcated. And, in the end, patients may have a good idea of just what they have consented to and when consent was obtained.

On the other hand, there are also substantial problems with the event model of consent. It presumes, for one thing, that medical care conforms strictly to the paradigm we outlined previously; that is, that medical care involves a single decision or a small number of decisions, which are made at discrete points in time when sufficient information is available. In contrast, observational research on the structure of decision making in medicine (2,3) suggests that it is rare for the care of a patient to involve only a single decision or for the needed information all to be available when a decision must be made. More commonly, treatment strategies evolve over time, as additional information becomes available, including data from diagnostic tests and the results of previous empirical therapy. This is particularly true for chronic illnesses but also applies to conditions of relatively recent onset, whose etiology is unclear.

A fever of unknown origin offers a good example here. When a patient with fever, but no localizing signs, is admitted to a hospital, a differential diagnosis will be constructed and a plan formulated to investigate each possibility. Although each test will yield some amount of information, as the tests become increasingly invasive and present greater risks of their own, more and more difficult decisions will have to be made about their value to the workup. In addition, indications may become stronger on empirical grounds for a trial of antibiotics, which itself entails risks related to potential side effects of the medication and to the possibility that the underlying cause of the fever will be obscured. There is no single decision to be made at a discrete point in time here, as is envisioned by the event model of decision making. Rather, multiple decisions must be made, often on a daily basis, as additional information becomes available. Adherence to the event model, with doctor and patient waiting for sufficient information to accumulate for a definitive decision to be made, will leave the patient out of decision making altogether while the physician conducts the workup. Yet, insofar as the evaluation may be difficult to separate from treatment (e.g., a trial of antibiotics is both a diagnostic and therapeutic procedure), and presents risks and benefits of its own, these are precisely the kind of decisions in which patient involvement is anticipated by the idea of informed consent.

In addition to situations involving a series of decisions, the event model may be problematic even in situations in which a single decision must be made, because of its assumption that the decision will be made at a discrete time. Evidence suggests that it is often extremely difficult to pinpoint the times at which medical decisions are made (4). Typically, information accumulates progressively, with each additional datum leading the doctor in the direction of recommending a particular treatment option. The cumulative effect of the information obtained over time may be to make the final "decision" appear to be preordained when the decisionmaking event finally arrives. At that point, neither doctor nor patient may feel as though there is a decision left to be made. If the patient has been excluded from the decisionmaking process until then, on the ground that the time for making a decision had not yet arrived, the goal of patient participation that underlies the idea of informed consent will be subverted.

Furthermore, the event model appears to be structured in the worst possible way as far as facilitating patients' informed participation is concerned. Educators have long known that provision of information repetitively, over a sustained period, results in better understanding and better retention than exposure at a single point. Information provided when patients are at relative ease is more effectively assimilated than information offered at times of stress. The event model encourages "one-shot" education of patients, with little opportunity for reflection and integration of the information obtained into the patients' underlying scheme of values, and at a time, given that a decision must be made imminently, when patients' anxiety is likely to be at a peak. Thus, the event model inhibits precisely the kind of understanding on which the idea of informed consent (although perhaps not the legal doctrine) is based. The numerous studies showing poor patient understanding and limited retention of information provided in physician disclosures and consent forms suggest, at least in part, the failure of the educational function of informed consent conducted according to an event model (see Chapter 9).

Even if patients were easily able to assimilate information on a one-time basis, a single discussion would still not be a good way of involving the patient in the decisionmaking process. Patients do not instantaneously consider all of the implications and all of the ways in which the information affects the things that they value. Indeed, many patients report that they only considered a particular aspect of a medical decision when discussing the matter with family or friends. For example, a cancer patient may object to receiving chemotherapy, only to change her mind when discussing with her husband the impact of her death on the family. Thus, the difficulties with patient participation in an event model are not only cognitive but social.

Many physicians sense these deficiencies in the event model, even as they employ it because it makes their lives easier in some respects. Their recognition that patients are not really participating in decision making, or are doing so with only limited understanding, contributes to their rejection of the idea of informed consent. It seems farcical to spend time talking with patients in detail about some of the least important decisions that need to be made—because the decision of the consent event has already been preordained by other events—when the earlier, more influential decisions have been made by physicians alone. It seems a waste of time to present patients with elaborate consent forms, when patients so rarely seem to understand the information critical to a decision. In short, the event model perpetuates a view of informed consent as something detached from the unique rhythm of the clinical setting—something imposed on medicine by an uncomprehending legal system.

These considerations suggest that a model of decision making is needed in medical encounters that recognizes both the temporal complexity of medical decisions and the complexity of patients' decisionmaking processes. Such an approach is found in the "process model" of decision making and consent.

Consent as a Process

In contrast to an event model, the process model of informed consent is based on the assumption that medical decision making is a continuous process, not a discrete event. The exchange of information, therefore, should take place throughout the course of the physician–patient relationship. We use the word "exchange," deliberately to imply a two-way transfer of information. To facilitate patient participation in decision making, physicians need to disclose information to patients about recommended and alternative diagnostic and therapeutic approaches, as it becomes available. In addition, patients need to discuss their concerns with their physicians, including their understanding of the choices that face them, questions that they may have, and values that they particularly want reflected in their medical care. The mechanics of the process model are explored in detail in the following section, but some of its general implications can be addressed here.

The process of information exchange, which we refer to as "mutual monitoring," because it permits each party to monitor the factors that are entering into the other's thinking at any given time, requires sensitivity on the part of both physicians and patients. Physicians need to offer information in an appropriate fashion that facilitates, rather than confuses, patient decision making. In no way does the process model call for stream-of-consciousness revelations by physicians of everything that is passing through their minds (5). Patients should not be greeted at the initial encounter, for example, with a terrifying list of potential diagnoses, including remote and usually fatal possibilities. Such disclosure is likely to immobilize rather than clarify their decision making. Instead, as information is developed that is relevant to the next stage of decision that has to be made, it should be offered to patients. Differentiation of disclosure according to the phase of the treatment relationship is implied by the process model, as will be described later.

Patients, too, have an active role to play in the process model, in comparison with the relatively passive part they play in the event model. Their role expands in three directions. First, it is anticipated that they will interact with their physicians as information is provided, asking questions, clarifying ambiguities, helping physicians understand the values they choose to promote. Second, the recognition that a number of decisions are involved in most medical care means that patients will be faced with an increased number of choices that must be made. Finally, since the selection of a course of treatment can usually be modified as interaction between the parties takes place, patients have a responsibility to provide feedback to physicians about the effectiveness of treatment in relation to the target symptoms and about the degree of satisfaction they experience with regard to their individual goals and values.

Of course, the patient retains the right to "waive" participation in the decision-making process (see Chapter 4). We are not advocating what Schneider has called "mandatory autonomy"(5). If the patient wishes to remain uninvolved, that is certainly a right that should not be infringed. Coerced participation is not autonomous and is unlikely to yield positive results for either patient or physician. We are, however, suggesting that it is in the best interests of good medical care, if nothing else, that physicians continue to encourage patients to participate in the decisionmaking process.

The advantages of a process model are substantial. The process model promotes the objectives of the underlying idea of informed consent and, at the same time, is equally in conformance with the requirements of the legal doctrine of informed consent as the event-oriented approach. Patients are brought actively into the decisionmaking process, in a manner that encourages their knowing participation. They receive information, over time, in a fashion that allows it to be contemplated, shared, and assimilated. Further, by participating in the stream of decisions as they are made, patients are not excluded from the "ultimate" decision, by virtue of being excluded from the many preliminary decisions that may, in effect, predetermine the outcome.

There are additional benefits from the enhanced alliance between physicians and patients envisioned by the process model. As patients perceive that treatment decisions are their own, not just their physicians', compliance may be improved. This can result both from the patient's greater identification with the decision and from an increased ability to understand what treatment entails (6). There is even significant evidence that patients do better when they are more engaged in treatment decision making (7–9). Further, patients who see themselves as intimately involved in medical decision making may be less likely to initiate suits alleging malpractice when a bad outcome ensues (10–13).

Finally, conceptualizing informed consent according to the process model, which better reflects the realities of medical care, should serve to make the idea of informed consent meaningful to physicians. No longer is the disclosure and decision-making process divorced from the real decisions that need to be made. To be sure, the process model will demand of physicians more substantial efforts to integrate patients' views into the decisions that need to be made, but in contrast to the event model, there will seem to be some point to the whole effort. Patients and doctors will be working together "where the action is."

As with all approaches to health care, however, there are also disadvantages to the process model. Although some medical school curricula have changed substantially in the past decade, most physicians are still not accustomed to discussing with patients their thoughts and the information on which they are based, except when an eventlike decision needs to be made. Substantial retraining might be required before most physicians could function comfortably in the process model. Similarly, patients who are accustomed, despite the frustration that results, to functioning passively in physician–patient relationships will have to be reeducated about their new role. Both these efforts will require time and money and may meet with resistance. The kind of interaction between physicians and patients envisioned here will also consume some additional amount of time, although perhaps not as much as many practitioners might fear. Hospital schedules and the organization of the average physician's day may have to be restructured to some extent to permit the mutual monitoring process to take place. The ratcheting down of physician and hospital payments that has occurred with managed care makes this evolution more difficult. Only a shift to a quality-oriented, rather than cost-driven, system will reward physicians and systems that take the time to engage patients in decisions about their care. Ranking health plans by patient satisfaction, among other measures, which is a process that has already begun in some venues, is an example of how this may occur.

Do the advantages of the process model outweigh its disadvantages? We believe they do. But many of the relative benefits and costs should be measurable in appropriately designed studies. Although there are significant a priori reasons to endorse a process model, they await empirical substantiation.

The Process Model and the Stages of Treatment

The basic principle of the process model of informed consent is that patients should be able to participate in decision making in every phase of patient care. Such participation is a continual facet of all interactions and ought to be woven into the very fabric of the doctor–patient relationship. How this principle works in practice may be envisioned most easily by examining its operation through the stages of patient care. These stages can be characterized by the primary tasks they address: establishment of a relationship, definition of the problem, ascertainment of the goals of treatment, selection of a therapeutic plan, and follow-up. Of course, the tasks will not always proceed in this order, and several may be addressed simultaneously. Each of these tasks requires physicians to provide patients with information relating to a key question, thereby enabling patients to make appropriate decisions.

Establishing the Relationship

The key question for patients at the point at which a relationship with a physician is first established is, "Do I want to entrust my care to this person?" This question is not always asked or answered definitively at the very beginning of a physician–patient relationship. If patient and physician first meet as the patient lies on a stretcher, writhing in pain, in an emergency room, treatment ordinarily will proceed with minimal attention by the patient to the question of whether this is the appropriate physician to handle the patient's care. Even in this setting, however, the physician must establish, to the patient's satisfaction, a basis for authority to treat. This may involve a statement as simple as, "I am Dr. Jones, the physician on call here tonight, and I have responsibility for all patients admitted." In an emergency setting, patients in need of care are likely to accept this information as sufficient to decide that the physician on call is precisely the person who should be in charge of their treatment. When patients are making decisions at greater leisure, of course, they may desire additional information about the physician before entrusting their care to that person. This may include data about the physician's specialty, particular interests and skills, and any unique aspects of the relationship (e.g., that the physician will nominally be in charge of the patient's care, but actual care will be rendered by a junior associate) (see Chapter 3).

Of course, the answer to the question "Do I want to entrust my care to this person?" is not resolved simply by factual information. Many patients will be much more interested in the "kind of person" that the physician is than in his or her credentials. There is ample evidence that patients choose physicians on the basis of other things rather than just their credentials (14,15). Nonetheless, providing an open, information-rich introduction is an important part of establishing a relationship. Although the substantive information may not be a central part of what many patients are looking for at this stage of the relationship, the willingness to provide it is likely to be seen in a positive light.

The establishment of a relationship, though rarely thought about explicitly by practitioners, is a constant element of medical care. In outpatient settings, where patients have a variety of options for health care, this process of evaluation of a physician often proceeds as a matter of course, with physicians providing the necessary information without even being aware that they are doing so. In hospital-based care, however, where patients are perceived as having limited choices as to who undertakes their treatment, physicians often neglect to provide the information that patients need to determine whether they want to be cared for by a given physician.

The problem here is compounded by the multiplicity of persons involved in inpatient care: attending physicians, house officers, consultants, physicians' assistants, technicians, nurses, social workers, and others. Patients are often least clear about who consultants are and why they should be allowed to participate in their care. Consultants are frequently senior physicians who are accustomed to being recognized in the hospital; they will often walk into a room, give their name, and begin an examination. Patients, who may previously never met these physicians, are understandably bewildered when this occurs, not knowing why such an examination is being conducted or who ordered it. They are unclear whether the consultant is someone who can present new information to them or who will make treatment decisions. The ambiguities in this situation are easy to clarify (as with a simple statement, "Your doctor, Dr. Jones, asked me to come in and take a look at your eyes because I am a specialist in ophthalmology; I will tell him what I find, and he can then decide whether further action is needed."). Yet, few consultants take the time to offer such an explanation.

How the doctor–patient relationship is established is crucial to all that follows in two ways. First, of course, if the patient declines to go any further with the relationship, no treatment will ensue. There is, however, a second and more subtle way in which the establishment of the relationship sets the tone for patient participation in all subsequent treatment decisions. If physicians communicate to patients that patients have little or no appropriate role in evaluating whether a particular physician should undertake their care, patients are likely to assume a fortiori that they have even less chance of influencing the treatment decisions that follow. On the other hand, physicians who set the tone by indicating to patients that patients have a right to know who the physician is and why the physician should be allowed to proceed with their care signal that patients' participation will be welcome in subsequent treatment decisions.

Defining the Problem

The second phase of the course of treatment involves defining the nature of the problem. The key question for patients here is, "What problem will be the focus of treatment?" Physicians often assume that this is a purely technical issue. In fact, some sociological theories of the professions distinguish professional groups from other workers by professionals' ability to reframe clients' complaints in terms that yield definitions of problems that differ from the clients' initial formulations (16). Researchers have demonstrated, however, that most medical problems are defined by a complex negotiation between physicians and patients (17,18). Physicians who ignore patients' definitions of their problems will often end up with patients who are dissatisfied with the interactions and resistant to medical recommendations. Conversely, to the degree that patients are committed to definitions of their problems and thus to particular treatment approaches, their inclinations to follow through with treatment are likely to be substantially greater (6).

An example of the importance of an interactive process of defining the nature of the problem was reported by a physician who was afflicted by a syndrome that resulted in progressive blindness (19). From the treating physicians' point of view the problem to be addressed was the underlying pathology, for which little could be done. The patient-physician, however, defined his problem more broadly as learning how to cope with his failing eyesight. Having never discussed the patient's formulation of his problem, his physicians felt they had little to offer and retreated in the face of the inexorable progression of his illness. This left the patient feeling embittered and abandoned. Ironically, although powerless to stop the advance of their patient's blindness, the treating physicians had a great deal to offer in terms of helping the patient adjust to his diminished sight. Their failure to grasp this fact vitiated their potential to help. Such is the unhappy consequence of the "ships passing in the night" phenomenon that occurs when patients and physicians have substantially different formulations of the problem to be treated.

Facilitating patients' participation at this point requires a rejection of what has been called the "high physician control" style of patient care (20–23). Typically, physicians employing this style of relating to patients begin by asking patients to describe their problems. Patients, perceiving difficulties in holding such physicians' attention, respond with brief accounts of their difficulties. Physicians then initiate a long series of questions dealing with current symptomatology and patients' medical histories. A physical examination will usually ensue, sometimes accompanied by blood, radiographic, or other tests. Finally, with the data all collected, physicians announce the nature of the problem to their patients and order appropriate treatment. Physicians may ask if patients have any questions, but patients, recognizing that the interaction is about to be ended, will either reply in the negative or ask a brief question, often focused on the details of the therapeutic regimen. Patients never have a chance to define the problem in their own terms. Although in some sense a caricature, this description is not markedly different from those that have been reported in several empirical studies (3).

In contrast, physicians operating under a process model of informed consent will encourage patients to participate actively in defining their problems. Since many patients have been socialized to passivity in doctor–patient relationships, this may require physicians to ask open-ended questions and to indicate explicitly their interest in complete responses. A recognition that patients are more likely to be disturbed by interferences with their daily lives than by underlying pathologic processes will help physicians to inquire appropriately. The ultimate, negotiated definition of the problem cannot ignore the need to address the pathology, but it must also take into account those results of the disease process that trouble patients the most.

The process of negotiating the nature of the problem does not end with the first few interactions. Indeed, physicians often discover, at what appears to be the end of treatment (either successful or unsuccessful), that the patient's definition of the problem has transformed into something related but different from what had been agreed upon previously. In part this may reflect the patient's changed circumstances. Thus, the successful treatment of a malignant tumor may result in the need to respond to the patient's sleep disorder related to anxiety about a recurrence. However, the change in the patient's definition of the problem may result from many other things including, for example, family discussions, occupational changes, and experiencing the side effects of the treatment.

Ascertaining the Goals of Treatment

Agreement between doctors and patients about the nature of the problem must be followed by consensus about the goals of treatment. Here the question for the patient is, "What are the reasonable goals of therapy for the problem we have defined?" Put somewhat differently, patients and physicians must collaborate at this point in defining the probable "health career" of the patient. As Timothy Quill and Howard Brody put it, "Focus first on general goals not technical options. Negotiating with the patient about the technical aspects of management without articulating the general goals of therapy often leads to the 'choosing' of treatments that are not in the patient's best interests" (24). Patients often have unrealistic expectations of what their future "careers" in the health system are likely to be, in part because many patients conceptualize medical treatment with models drawn from surgery or the treatment of acute infectious diseases. They may expect to be cured of their illnesses and may assume that treatment is a failure if that expectation is not achieved. Moreover, they may expect to be cured without much active effort on their part, which explains in part the documented difficulty in obtaining patient compliance with many forms of treatment, particularly those involving alteration of lifestyle (6).

One result of the prevalence of models of medical care drawn from the treatment of acute infectious diseases is that patients with chronic disorders often have particular difficulty understanding what constitutes reasonable goals (25). Patients with chronic cardiac disorders may conceptualize their problems as involving recurring attacks of a lingering illness. They may believe that if only the doctor could find the proper medication or dosage, their problems would be cured. Patients with severe congestive heart failure, for example, might expect to go back to blue-collar jobs as soon as they "get well."

Patients with unrealistic goals for the future cannot engage in a meaningful assessment of the risks and benefits of a proposed treatment. The risk of severe kidney damage with a 5 percent probability should be weighed quite differently by a patient for whom treatment offers the possibility of a complete restoration of function, than by a patient whose future will involve a continued struggle with a chronic disorder on a deteriorating course. Thus, physicians must ensure that patients have an accurate understanding of the reasonable goals of treatment. This involves monitoring patients' expectations and presenting sufficient information to correct distortions. Of course, this should be done sensitively, since it is always desirable to maintain some degree of hope, whether treatment involves a benign course of care or maximal efforts merely to alleviate pain. The physician should attempt to present the patient with a realistic goal(s) to be achieved in treatment but defer to the patient in his choice of whether to pursue the goal.

Physicians have not always made an effort to ensure the realism of patients' goals, particularly when that required disclosure of patients' diagnoses and prognoses. Katz pointed out that Hippocrates suggested that physicians

> perform [their duties] calmly and adroitly, concealing most things from the patient while you are attending him. Give necessary orders with cheerfulness and serenity, turning his attention away from what is being done to him. . . . revealing nothing of the patient's future or present condition. (26, p. 4)

The last few decades, however, have seen a strong movement in the direction of more open disclosure. A study for the President's Commission for the Study of Ethical Problems in Medicine found that substantial majorities of both physicians and patients favor disclosure of such information as a diagnosis of cancer (27). Attitudes of this sort have been supported by research findings showing that open disclosure to cancer patients leaves them with substantially less anxiety and depression (28).

In interviewing cancer patients about their relationships with their physicians, Lidz has found that patients had two major complaints: first, that they were not being told enough, and second, that they were given information in an insufficiently sensitive manner (unpublished data). Their angriest feelings were expressed toward the physicians who had told them, or other patients that they knew, that they would die in a specified period of time. By focusing on dying rather than on the fact that they might live for quite a while yet, the physician seemed to these patients to be removing any positive future. It is preferable, for example, to tell a patient who has had an auto accident that resulted in a damaged spinal cord, "With work, you will be able to get around in a wheelchair and do a lot for yourself," rather than "You will never walk again." Receiving bad news is different from being left without anything to live for.

In sum, patients' abilities to assess the reasonableness of what physicians recommend depend on the clarity of patients' vision of the future. Thus, it is important for physicians to reach an understanding with patients about the goals of treatment—especially when the goals are other than complete recovery.

Selecting an Approach to Treatment

Once the goals of treatment have been defined, patients and physicians must reach a decision on how to achieve those goals. For patients the key question is, "Which treatment will present the best possible balance of potential risks and likely benefits?" This is the aspect of the initiation of treatment that generally attracts the most attention, although as we have seen, effective participation by patients at this point is heavily dependent on what has already transpired between them and their physicians.

The disclosure required here is determined in part by the legal requirements for informed consent. That is, physicians must address the nature, purpose, risks and benefits of treatment, along with the alternatives and their risks, and benefits. Much of what should be included in the disclosure here is apparent from our earlier discussions, but additional points need to be made about disclosure of risks and alternatives and about the timing of the discussions.

The difficulty of specifying exactly which risks should be disclosed has been noted. Some sense of what information patients need to make truly knowledgeable decisions is probably the physician's best guide. But to encourage patients' reflections on what selection of a course of treatment is likely to mean to their lives, physicians may have to go beyond the narrow requirements of the law. The term "risks" of treatment may be somewhat limiting in its connotations here, since many of the negative aspects of a particular treatment are not risks, but certainties. Abdominal surgery, for example, always leaves patients with some degree of incisional pain, and in need of a period of bed rest, followed by a longer period of diminished activity. An adequate review of the expectable outcomes of surgery, including its negative aspects, should include disclosure of the particular discomforts patients are likely to endure. The law may not require this—since many jurisdictions exclude "commonly known risks" from the requirements for disclosure—but they may play a major role in patients' decisions. It is easy to see why a busy parent of young children might opt for a procedure that requires a shorter period of recuperation than for an alternative, whatever its other advantages, that involves prolonged bed rest.

Disclosure and discussion of alternatives raise important questions about the degree of neutrality that should be sought by physicians. This neutrality may be with respect to both values and opinions. Values describe physicians' deeply held beliefs, often grounded in religious and moral beliefs or in personal philosophies. There are some situations in which most people would agree that physicians' own values ought to play a minimal role in the decisionmaking process; for example, however strongly a physician may believe that elective abortions are immoral, that should not prevent patients from being informed that they have that option. (Of course, physicians who are opposed to abortion on religious or other grounds obviously have the right to refer a patient elsewhere rather than undertaking the procedure themselves.)

At the other end of the spectrum, there may be occasions when patients invite physicians to share their values with them; for example, a patient dying of cancer may ask, "Doc, if it were you, would you go through with another course of chemotherapy on the chance that you'd get three months to live?" These situations are often sensitive since patients may offer such invitations to acquire ammunition to use in disputes with family members, or being unable to make up their own minds, may at least find some comfort in accepting or rejecting physicians' advice. It is thus perfectly reasonable for the physician to say, "I don't know what I would do. I have never been in your situation." Nonetheless, with a proper appreciation for the delicacy of the clinical setting, physicians can legitimately make their values known, especially when invited to do so.

Values may play another role in the discussion of alternatives. In many medical decisionmaking situations, patients may lack clear ideas of how particular treatments may affect values they hold dear. Physicians, because they deal with certain situations routinely, have sometimes thought more extensively about the religious, moral, or emotional issues involved, or are familiar with the typical reactions of other patients. When it appears that patients have not recognized the implications of the choices they face, physicians might offer guidance by pointing out the values involved.

The difficulties that can arise when healthcare professionals attempt to be completely neutral were illustrated in observations of decisions in a psychiatric clinic (2). In the community in which the study was performed, the county mental health department had asked all hospitals treating psychiatric patients to provide it with certain types of personal information—including patients' names—in order better to track utilization of health facilities in the county. The administration of one psychiatric facility decided that automatic release of this information would be a violation of patients' right to privacy, and consequently that they would allow release only with patients' consent. Clinicians staffing the admissions unit were instructed that the decision was completely within patients' discretion.

In general, patients did whatever the clinician suggested, even though clinicians tried to keep from making patients' decision for them. Thus, if a clinician said, "The county likes us to send information about people who consent; do you mind?" patients readily agreed, and if a clinician suggested that it might be "unfair" to send such information, patients quickly denied permission to send the information. However, some clinicians followed their instructions to the letter. For example, consider this transcript:

CLINICIAN: Now one more thing. We send the county information about patients for statistics. If you don't want us to, you have the right to refuse to permit us to send any information about you. Write here [pointing] "OK" or not.

PATIENT: [didn't seem to understand]

CLINICIAN: If you don't want to, you can say no. It is up to you.

PATIENT: [hesitating] I don't see any reason why I wouldn't want the county to know.

CLINICIAN: If you don't want to, you can write that there.

PATIENT: I don't understand.

CLINICIAN: What don't you understand?

PATIENT: You want me to choose whether to send this information to the county?

CLINICIAN: Yes.

PATIENT: Will that benefit the hospital?

CLINICIAN: Don't worry about the hospital. I don't want to influence you. This is your decision. . . .

The patient eventually agreed to release the information but later told the interviewer: "Did you see me? I was so confused about the thing about the county. I thought: 'Now if I don't let them release the information, will they make me an involuntary patient or is it that if you want a job with them that they will have records on it?' I was so confused." Another patient wondered whether releasing the information would interfere with her getting a county job later, but her husband prevailed with the suggestion that the county might later hold it against her when she applied for a job that she had refused to release the information.

In general, these patients did not have the requisite background knowledge to assess what values were at stake. Part of this difficulty was a lack of purely factual information. Many poorer patients equated the county with its welfare component, and many working class patients knew it mostly as a source of jobs. The concept of a bureaucracy trying to control health costs and needing information to do so was alien to them. Likewise, however, the abstract value of a right to privacy—even when the release of the information could not be shown to do any direct harm—was difficult for them to comprehend. This is not to say, of course, that they had no feelings about these issues, but lacking an explanation about their relevance to the current decision, they were lost. One cannot take it for granted that patients will consider the issues fully unless they are explained. In some situations, part of an adequate informed consent process is a review with the patient of what values are at stake.

Physicians' opinions, in contrast to their values, relate to the conclusions they draw from medical facts, although it is impossible for a physician to form opinions without some influence from an underlying set of values. Some authors have concluded that the idea of informed consent, with its heavy emphasis on patient autonomy in decision making, obliges physicians to act solely as technical consultants (29). That is, physicians should provide information about the risks and benefits of alternative treatments, then retire from the scene to allow patients to decide. In this model, physicians function like the television weather reporter who provides an objective forecast and then allows the viewer to choose whether or not a 40 percent chance of rain creates sufficient risk to warrant cancellation of the July 4th picnic (30).

In the doctor–patient relationship, we believe this view is shortsighted. For the ostensible sake of promoting individual autonomy, patients are deprived of some of the most important information they may have in reaching conclusions about the appropriate choice of treatments. One of the most highly valued skills physicians have to offer is the ability to integrate a large body of information about risks and benefits to arrive at appropriate recommendations. Some patients may wish to accept a physician's recommendation with little further reflection (5,31). Other patients will consider physicians' suggestions as another piece of evidence—although not necessarily a decisive piece—to be taken into account as they arrive at their decision. Although recommendations from physicians that are too strongly stated may overwhelm some patients' independence in decision making, there is also a risk that patients will misinterpret physicians' silence as indicating that they believe that all treatment options are of equal desirability. Physicians must certainly be careful, except in extreme circumstances, not to throw so much weight behind a particular recommendation that patients' selection of an alternative would lead to rupture of the relationship. But patients deserve a judicious recommendation, especially when requested, as an important part of the decisionmaking process.

The final issue that needs to be considered is the temporal relationship between selection of a treatment approach and the actual initiation of treatment, particularly when therapy is focused on a single, major procedure, as in most surgery. By the time patients have prepared themselves psychologically for surgery, discussed it with family and friends, rearranged their schedules to accommodate the procedure, and checked into the hospital, they are clearly committed to having the operation. For such patients, the decision to have surgery has already been made definitively, at least from the patients' psychological perspective. Thus, they are hardly in a good position to make up their minds about whether or not to go through with a procedure to which they are already deeply committed. Consent obtained at this point is pro forma. Deferring serious discussion of treatment options to this time effectively deprives patients of a meaningful opportunity for decision making. On the other hand, physicians who have followed the process model and obtained patients' consent to a procedure prior to hospital admission offer little or no additional benefit to their patients by rehearsing the entire discussion again. The same is true in the case of patients for whom surgery was not definitively contemplated prior to admission, but who are kept apprised of relevant information about their course of treatment and about any diagnostic procedures throughout the course of hospitalization. In other words, patients who are kept well informed and included in the decisionmaking process as it unfolds prior to surgery being recommended do not need a stylized "consent procedure" at the eleventh hour. This certainly goes against current practice of routinely making disclosure (often accompanied by the signing of a consent form) just prior to surgery, invasive diagnostic tests, electroconvulsive therapy, and similar procedures. In fact, these discussions are often the only time that systematic disclosure takes place. Although a review of the experiences the patient will have and an offer to answer questions may be useful (32–34), serious consideration about whether or not to undertake surgery must take place at an earlier time.

Follow-up

Rarely, treatment will be a "one-shot" event, for example, the excision of a mole. However, usually once treatment is selected and implemented, the effectiveness of interventions must be evaluated and treatment modified accordingly. This is particularly true for the treatment of chronic illnesses, in which long-term doctor–patient relationships are the norm. Under the event model of decision making, the follow-up period is of little concern, unless a new event looms at some point in the future, when renewed interaction between physician and patient will be required. From the perspective of the process model, however, this position looks naive, since new information is continuously becoming available and decisions are always being made. The key question for patients at this stage is, "Where do I stand in relation to the decisions that were made when treatment was initiated?"

At follow-up sessions, physicians must naturally elicit from patients facts, relevant to their conditions and treatment, that have developed since the last interaction. This, however, is just one half of the process of mutual monitoring that must take place if patients are to remain involved in making decisions about their care. Physicians, too, must share information. They need to review the definition of the problem, the goals, and the treatment approaches that were decided upon previously in order to ensure that patients continue to share their understanding of these items. Patients' common reluctance to ask questions or admit to confusion means that physicians must take the initiative in exploring patients' understanding. As we noted earlier, change in patient (or physician) perceptions may require renegotiation of one or more issues. In addition, physicians should explain the existence and import of any new data and detail the relevance of those data for the agreements previously reached.

Empirical studies suggest that this process occurs infrequently. One study showed that less than 5 percent of a typical medical encounter (less than one minute out of twenty) was spent by physicians in providing information to patients (35). Physicians are often simply unaccustomed to explaining to patients the issues involved in making treatment decisions. Yet without this constant mutual monitoring process, there is good reason to believe that mutual understanding between physicians and patients will dissipate rapidly.

Even assuming that complete understanding by both parties is achieved during the initial encounter, patients' views of illness and treatment do not remain static. Patients continue to ruminate on what they know. Although this continuous reordering of knowledge is one of the human mind's strongest and most creative features, it is also the basis for a great deal of misunderstanding between physicians and patients. Each new event, such as the development of side effects from medication, and each new comment from physicians, family, or friends becomes an occasion to rethink and reconsider what patients already know. This tendency is increased by the structure of modern healthcare delivery. When a "team" of people (and sometimes three shifts of teams) engage in the delivery of clinic- and hospital-based care to a single patient, patients are likely to hear different and often conflicting information.

Moreover, new information is not a necessary stimulus to patients' reconceptualization of treatment. Patients use cognitive processes similar to what psychologists call "cognitive dissonance reduction" to reorganize and rethink their knowledge about treatment, even in the absence of new data. In reducing cognitive dissonance, patients try to build relatively simple cognitive fields that support the decisions that have already been made. Observational researchers found, for example, that patients had trouble understanding that a medication given to relieve the side effects of another drug might also have side effects of its own. Patients reduced the level of complexity of the information they were provided by reclassifying medications into those that caused side effects and those that relieved them. Thus, when they developed new side effects, they had trouble understanding why physicians might want to lower the dose of "the medication that relieves side effects" in response to their complaints (2).

It is evident that an adequate decisionmaking process must include an ability to monitor patients' understanding continually. Sometimes exploration of patients' views will reveal a need to renegotiate some previously agreed upon aspect of treatment. Sometimes, however, repetition or, in the light of new information, modification of the initial disclosure is what is required. Without repetition, the knowledge that was initially produced from disclosure can dissipate. However, if the repetition entails nothing more than the same words and phrases, it is unlikely that either patients or physicians will take them seriously. A good example of this type of disclosure is that which airplane flight attendants provide about the safety features of a plane. Because it has become an empty ritual to flight attendants and passengers alike, neither party pays much attention to the disclosure after the first few times it is made. The result is that no new learning and no reinforcement of what was learned previously occur, so learning quickly decays. (Hence, some flight attendants attempt to lighten their presentations with humor, and many airlines resort to catchy videos for the purpose.) Such a one-time only learning process is particularly problematic in medicine where the issues are continually changing, and the technical possibilities of medical interventions are evolving, sometimes gradually and sometimes dramatically. Therefore, what patients need to know may be somewhat different each time physicians and patients meet. Thus, physicians are continually challenged to remain flexible in their approaches to discussions with patients, to individualize disclosures to meet patients' particular needs and concerns, and to avoid sterile repetition.

Another issue arises in the follow-up of patients who have grown dependent on their caretakers, as most patients do to some degree. Now that they are recovering, they may harbor a sense of discomfort about their dependency. Seen from the perspective of the decisionmaking process, they may swing from an inability or unwillingness to participate in making decisions about their care to unwillingness to collaborate with anyone else in making decisions. They may therefore come to reject their physicians' advice as a means of reestablishing control. The issues involved in patients' rejection of treatment recommendations are discussed in detail in Chapter 11, but we should note here that the process model of consent can help patients to establish, maintain, or regain a sense of control without severing the therapeutic relationship. Physicians can help by providing information about the expected future course of the medical problem and by aiding patients in integrating that information with patients' understanding of their medical careers. Emphasis should be placed on patients' responsibility for management of their disorders, without giving the impression of abandonment by physicians. In this way, the continuing connection between physician and patient can be employed in the service of reestablishing patients' sense of autonomy.

Conclusion

The process model of medical decision making, as we have described it here, is in many ways an ideal. Few physicians and patients will be able to fulfill the aspirations of the model in its entirety. Sometimes this failure will be due to the intrusion of time or economic pressures, sometimes to the desire of one or both parties to play a dominant or a passive role in the relationship. But seen as an ideal, the process model provides a goal that concerned physicians and patients can strive to achieve. It is the concrete embodiment of the idea of informed consent and the logical extension of the ethical and legal theories from which that idea developed. Further, in providing a model of informed consent that conforms to the realities of clinical medicine, the process model replaces the artificialities of the event model—in which legal requirements are fit uneasily into clinical practice—with a meaningful and realistic alternative. Informed consent, using this approach, is no longer the intrusion, farce, or myth that its physician critics have accused it of being. It is an important and integral part of the doctor–patient relationship.

References

1. Wear, S. (1998) *Informed Consent: Patient Autonomy and Clinician Beneficence Within Health care*. Washington: Georgetown University Press.
2. Lidz, C.W., Meisel, A., Zerubavel, E., et al. (1983) *Informed Consent: A Study of Decisionmaking in Psychiatry*. New York: Guilford Press.
3. Lidz, C.W. and Meisel, A. (1982) Informed consent and the structure of medical care. In President's Commission for the Study of Ethical Problems in Medicine and Biomedical and Behavioral Research, *Making Health Care Decisions: The Ethical and Legal Implications of Informed Consent in the Patient-Practitioner Relationship*. Volume 2, Appendices. Washington, D.C.: U.S. Government Printing Office.
4. Brody, H. (1989) Transparency: informed consent in primary care. *Hastings Cent Rep*, 19:5–9.
5. Schneider, C.E. (1998) *The Practice of Autonomy: Patients, Doctors and Medical Decisions*. New York: Oxford University Press.
6. Meichenbaum, D. and Turk, D.C. (1987) *Facilitating Treatment Adherence: A Practitioner's Handbook*. New York: Plenum.
7. Ryan, R.M., Plant, R.W., and O'Malley, S. (1995) Initial motivations for alcohol treatment: relations with patient characteristics, treatment involvement and dropout. *Addict Behav*, 20:279–297.
8. Williams, C.G., Grow, V.M., Freedman, Z., Ryan, R.M., and Deci, E.L. (1996) Motivational predictors of weight loss and weight-loss maintenance. *J Pers Soc Psychol*, 70:115–126.
9. Kaplan, S.H., Greenfield, S., and Ware, J.E. Jr. (1989) Assessing the effects of physician-patient interactions on the outcomes of chronic disease. *Med Care*, 27(3 Suppl):110–127.
10. Cole, S.A. (1997) Reducing malpractice risk through more effective communication. *Am J Managed Care*, 3:649–653.
11. Levinson, W., Roter, D.L., Mullooly, J.P., Dull, V.T., and Frankel, R.M. (1997) Physician-patient communication: the relationship with malpractice claims among primary care physicians and surgeons. *JAMA*, 277:553–559.
12. Beckman, H.B., Markakis, K.M., Suchman, A.L., and Frankel, R.M. (1994) The doctor-patient relationship and malpractice: lessons from plaintiff depositions. *Arch Intern Med*, 154:1365–1370.

13. Lester, G.W. and Smith, S.G. (1993) Listening and talking to patients: a remedy for malpractice suits? *West J Med,* 158:268–272.
14. Haar, E., Halitsky, V., and Stricker, G. (1975) Factors related to the preference for a female gynecologist. *Med Care,* 13:782–786.
15. Roter, D., Lipkin, M. Jr., and Korsgaard, A. (1991) Sex differences in patients' and physicians' communication during primary care medical visits. *Med Care,* 29: 1083–1086.
16. Freidson, E. (1970) *The Profession of Medicine.* New York: Dodd, Mead.
17. Fisher, S. and Todd, A. (eds) (1983) *The Social Organization of Doctor-Patient Communication.* New York: Center for Applied Linguistics.
18. Eisenthal, S., Emery, R., Lazare, A., et al. (1979) "Adherence" and the negotiated approach to patienthood. *Arch Gen Psychiatry,* 36:393–398.
19. Stetten, D. (1981) Coping with blindness. *N Engl J Med,* 305:458–460.
20. Platt, F.W., and McMath, J.C. (1979) Clinical hypocompetence: the interview. *Ann Intern Med,* 91:898–902.
21. Laine, C. and Davidoff, F. (1996) Patient-centered medicine: a professional evolution. *JAMA,* 275:152–156.
22. Lang, F. Floyd, M.R., and Beine, K.L. (2000) Clues to patients' explanations and concerns about their illnesses: a call for active listening. *Arch Fam Med,* 9:222–227.
23. Frankel, R.M. (1983) Talking in interviews: a dispreference for patient-initiated questions in physician-patient encounters. In Psathas, G. (ed) *Interaction Competence.* New York: Irvington Publications Inc.
24. Quill, T.E. and Brody, H. (1996) Physician recommendations and patient autonomy: finding a balance between physician power and patient choice. *Ann Intern Med,* 125:763–769.
25. Lidz, C.W., Meisel, A., and Munetz, M. (1985) Chronic disease: the sick role and informed consent. *Cult Med Psychiatry,* 9:1–17.
26. Katz, J. (1984) *The Silent World of Doctor and Patient.* New York: Free Press.
27. Harris, L., et al. (1982) Views of informed consent and decisionmaking: parallel surveys of physicians and the public. In President's Commission for the Study of Ethical Problems in Medicine and Biomedical and Behavioral Research, *Making Health Care Decisions: The Ethical and Legal Implications of Informed Consent in the Patient-Practitioner Relationship.* Volume 2, Appendices. Washington, D.C.: U.S. Government Printing Office.
28. Gerle, B., Lundin, G., and Sandblom, P. (1960) The patient with inoperable cancer from the psychiatric and social standpoint. *Cancer,* 13:1206–1217.
29. Veatch, R. (1991) *The Physician-Patient Relation: Patient as Partner,* Part 2. Bloomington: University of Indiana Press.
30. Lidz, C.W. (1980) The weather report model of informed consent: problems in preserving patient voluntariness. *Bull Am Acad Psychiatry Law,* 8:152–160.
31. Ingelfinger, F.J. (1980) Arrogance. *N Engl J Med,* 303:1507–1511.
32. Langer, E.J., Janis, I.L., and Wolfer, J.A. (1975) Reduction of psychological stress in surgical patients. *J Exp Soc Psychol,* 11:155-165.
33. Vernon, D.T.A. (1971) Information seeking in a natural stress situation. *J Appl Psychol,* 55:359–363.
34. Stewart, M.A. (1995) Effective physician-patient communication and health outcomes: a review. *Can Med Assoc J,* 152:1423–1433.
35. Waitzkin, H. (1984) Doctor-patient communication: clinical implications of social scientific research. *JAMA,* 252:2441–2446.

9

Consent Forms: Documentation and Guidance

As suggested in Chapter 8, there are multiple reasons that obtaining informed consent is mistakenly considered to be a discrete event occurring at a particular moment in a patient's medical career, rather than a process that is (or should be) an integral part of the patient's healthcare experience. Perhaps the most common reason for this mistaken view is that the consent form has become the symbol of informed consent. Some physicians, in fact, equate informed consent with a patient's signature on the form. "Consenting the patient"[1] has become a too familiar shorthand for seeking the patient's authorization of treatment; behaviorally, "consenting the patient" often amounts merely to obtaining the patient's signature, rather than facilitating an informed, voluntary decision. One critic observes that "with informed consent having its roots in the law, it is not surprising that the idea was implemented through legalistic approaches" and that, therefore, the pursuit of patient autonomy has "achieved an ethics in practice that revolves around the signing and filing of pieces of paper" (1, pp. 179, 184).

Informed consent is a process, not a form—without the process, the form is just a piece of paper. In the absence of the elements of informed consent, a signed consent form is largely worthless. If appropriate disclosure was not made, if the

---

[1]The term is an indication of the problem, focusing on getting the patient's consent, in contrast to the perhaps more appropriate "informing the patient," which would shift the emphasis to disclosure.

form's signatory was not competent to understand the disclosure and make a decision, if the signatory signed the form but did not make a decision or understand what she signed, or if her signature was unduly pressured—the signed consent form will not serve any purpose. The continued focus on forms rather than the physician–patient interaction led one commentator to suggest that "instead of improving . . . consent forms, we should abolish consent forms—prohibit them by legal fiat as necessary" (2). Other commentators regard them as necessary evils (3).

We believe that both of these positions are, at least, exaggerations. Properly designed, appropriately employed consent forms might be more than necessary evils. They could actually modestly enhance the informed consent process and promote its goals. Before this can happen, "consenting the patient" must become less an empty ritual and more a meaningful social practice. Forms must be seen as tools that can facilitate the process of informed consent, rather than promoted as ends in themselves. Only then may forms become functional, not fetishistic.

In this chapter we discuss the multiple, and sometimes conflicting, purposes attributed to consent forms. Specifically, we acknowledge their use to document the informed consent process and discuss how they may be employed to facilitate patients' (and subjects') understanding and retention of information disclosed to them. We then suggest ways of making forms more useful and of minimizing their potential negative effects. Finally, we explain contexts in which the use of forms may be legally mandated, in clinical practice and research, as well as their status and role in legal actions, such as suits for failure to obtain informed consent.

The Purposes and Effects of Consent Forms

Consent forms are used for several purposes, which may be somewhat at odds with each other, if not outright contradictory. They are used, most often, to *document* that the informed consent process took place, as well as the particular authorization made by the patient (or research subject). As part of this documentation role, they may help to *protect* physicians (or researchers) from *liability* in some jurisdictions. Finally, with currently very limited success, they are also employed as *educational tools* in the informed consent process between physician and patient (or researcher and prospective participant), to help inform patients and prospective research subjects about a medical intervention or research protocol.

It would be simpler if we could discuss each of these purposes in turn, however, such a discussion would not reflect reality. Consent forms unavoidably serve these multiple purposes simultaneously. Yet these purposes may conflict. A form designed to fulfill one purpose may be inadequate for another, or at least not the best form that could be designed for that role. Most important, across these different purposes, there is a fundamental tension with respect to whose interests are being protected—those of the patient/subject or of the physician/researcher. We believe most strongly that, like the process of informed consent itself, the primary goal of consent forms should be to promote the interests of patients and subjects. Consent forms are used most appropriately as an adjunct to the dialogue between physician and patient (or researcher and potential subject) to facilitate and document the informed consent process. Only secondarily, and only insofar as they document actual informed consent, should they serve the interests of physicians, researchers, and institutions when questions of liability arise.

It would also be simpler if in this chapter we could focus solely on the use of consent forms outside of research, especially since Chapters 12 and 13 discuss informed consent to research in detail. For two reasons, however, we need at least to glance at their use in obtaining subjects' consent to research participation. First, participation in one or more research protocols is increasingly part of many patients' medical careers. Second, although the use of consent forms evolved somewhat differently in the research and clinical contexts, rules and requirements of research have influenced the norms of clinical practice with respect to documentation of the informed consent discussion.

In the research context there is evidence that consent forms were initially conceived to promote the goals of informed consent, rather than merely serve as documentation and thus liability protection. The Declaration of Helsinki first prominently introduced the idea of documenting consent to participate in research (see Chapters 12 and 13). It provides that after requisite disclosure to the prospective subject, "the physician should then obtain the subject's freely-given informed consent, preferably in writing" (4). Given the post–World War II historical context of the declaration, it is reasonable to understand this documentation requirement as being designed to increase researcher accountability and thereby enhance human subject protection. The more recent Department of Health, Education, and Welfare regulations, and then the Department of Health and Human Services Rules and Regulations governing human subject research mandated use of one of two types of forms for all federally funded research that is not specifically exempt from the documentation requirement. Exemption can occur either because the documentation itself would impose a sole and substantial risk to the privacy of subjects or, more frequently, because "the research presents no more than minimal risk and involves no procedures for which consent is normally required" (5). The Food and Drug Administration has imposed a similar requirement (6). A fair reading of these rules is that researchers may omit use of consent forms if their use might harm subjects' interests, or if their use is not viewed as necessary to safeguard subjects' interests. The implication is that the goal of consent forms is to promote subjects' interests, not merely to function as protection from liability.

Notwithstanding this evidence, in both medical practice and research there has been an unfortunate belief that consent forms should serve primarily to protect physicians (and researchers) from liability, rather than to promote patients' (and subjects') interests by facilitating the process of informed consent. Patients, too, do not understand that the information provided in a consent form is intended to benefit them rather than their doctors (7–9). One study of hospital consent forms found that:

> Aspects of many forms, such as the requirement of a witness countersignature, add to their legal appearance and further distance patients. Combined with concerns about legal jargon, these format issues help to explain why patients believe forms were created to protect hospitals or physicians. Anything that contributes to such appearances or perceptions is likely to hinder, if not counteract, the goals of informed consent. . . . Forms with a solely legalistic appearance may lead to either cursory or suspicious reading of forms, and therefore, an inadequate or distorted understanding. (10, p. 30)

These perceptions of the role of consent forms are problematic, because they undermine the process of shared decision making and hinder achievement of the goals of informed consent: the protection of patients' (and subjects') autonomy and well-being. The current format of consent forms not only may undermine patients' interests but also poorly serves physicians' interests in liability protection. The researchers in the previously cited study note that:

> Necessary legal statements—for instance, appraising [sic] patients of their rights and the hospital's obligations—might be better handled separately from the decision-making process such as in a general statement on the conditions of admission. A form that focuses instead on the promotion of information about the [medical] procedure might even lower the possibility of lawsuits, since shared decision making fosters a good patient-physician decision relationship, which may reduce litigation. (10, p. 30)

Signing a consent form could reinforce the goals of informed consent if signing the form documents, symbolizes, and thus reinforces the patient's understanding that he is authorizing the physician to act on his behalf and that he himself retains responsibility for the decision made. Being asked to sign a form may encourage patients to reflect seriously on the proposed intervention before consenting. Those who are deeply ambivalent about their treatment options may have an opportunity actively to resolve that ambivalence in the act of signing the form, or the prospect of being asked to do so may lead them to contemplation or further consultation with those whom they trust. To the extent that reflection and commitment to treatment are desirable ends, the use of consent forms may facilitate achieving them.

If signing the form takes place as part of a dialogical process of shared decision making, and if the form itself states what may be expected regarding treatment and the responsibilities of the parties (patient and physician) with respect to the treatment plan, the form may serve both to document important parts of that dialogue and to symbolize the collaborative, contractual nature of the treatment plan.

Of course, whether employing consent forms actually promotes subjects' interests is an empirical question. We are, in fact, very skeptical of their value in this regard, as they are currently employed. By virtue of being written in legalistic language or containing a laundry list of possible risks that, should they eventuate, might prompt subjects to sue, consent forms may sacrifice any actual usefulness in protecting subjects' interests. Forms may become so technical, formidably long, and frighteningly detailed that subjects fail to read them or cannot comprehend them. Moreover, they may omit information that subjects would find important in deciding whether to participate, for example information about inconveniences of participation, the omission of which is unlikely to give rise to lawsuits but could well affect subjects' lives.

Even the use of a well-crafted form may suffer from the aura that surrounds signing documents within American society. Signing the form is often taken by patients to mean that their role in decision making is over. This idea fits their experience with other signed contracts. In buying a house or car, the signature on the dotted line completes the transaction. Both buyer and seller are committed. In contrast, a patient's signature on a consent form does not constitute a legally binding contract to go through with the treatment described. Patients are always free to withdraw their consent. Forms for consent to research generally state this explicitly, but it is true whether contained on the form or not. Nonetheless, whatever the legal implications, psychologically a signed consent form represents a commitment on the part of the patient. Research has shown that the major factor inhibiting subject participation in survey research was the requirement that they sign consent forms (11,12). In short, the formal documentation of informed consent is not a psychologically neutral factor in the patient's (or subject's) decision making.

As the process model detailed in Chapter 8 noted, in the ideal situation patients continuously gather information relevant to their treatment not only before deciding which treatment plan to pursue but during and after that decisionmaking process. However, most people have learned in childhood that signing a document commits them to what is on the paper. There is usually no turning back, and there is little incentive to continue to mull over the benefits and risks of the situation, as is desirable to do in the healthcare context. In fact, the understandable human tendency is to persuade oneself that the best decision has been made and to put the issue out of one's mind. There is thus a tendency to see the signing of the consent form as a time to relinquish one's concerns about medical treatment, rather than as one phase of a continuing process of education about treatment and one decision among many to be made. For these reasons, it is important to stress that signing the consent form is neither a trivial legal formality, nor a final act. Physicians should make extra efforts to ensure that patients understand both that the physician expects and welcomes their continuous participation in decisions and that they are not signing their bodies over to the medical system. If information continues to be provided, if practitioners continue to inquire about patients' desires, and if patients' efforts to participate in decision making are not treated dismissively, patients may come to see the act of signing a consent form in its proper light.

Because of the potential difficulties of employing consent forms it might seem that it would be advisable simply to abandon their use whenever possible. For example, the American Psychiatric Association recommends that documentation of the patient's consent or refusal be accomplished by an explanatory note in the patient's chart about what has been told and what the patient understood, rather than through consent forms (13). From the clinician's perspective, entering notes in patients' charts at the time consent is obtained may offer as much legal protection as a consent form, without the clinical complications that consent forms may entail. Fay Rosovsky emphasizes that "notes in the patient's health record . . . that outline the nature, risks, and benefits of the proposed treatment, the reasonable alternatives to it, and the consequences of foregoing all care . . . [as well as] any questions the patient had on the matter and the answers given . . . may prove very useful for the defense" (14, p. 89). Clinicians could formulate a core disclosure for a particular intervention—items likely to be of importance to all patients for whom the treatment or procedure is recommended. This core disclosure could be modified by deleting some items or adding others, as the mutual monitoring process occurs (described in Chapter 8). The physician's note, written just after the disclosure and subsequent dialogue, could simply record that the core disclosure took place and note any modifications made to it to meet the interests of the particular patient. Since disclosure and discussion of the treatment plan is likely to be an ongoing process, follow-up notes could record patients' later questions and the responses and additional information provided.

As attractive as this approach might be, in some circumstances it is not feasible or is simply less desirable than employing consent forms. Some states, many institutions, and most research projects require the use of consent forms. Hospitals typically require them for invasive procedures, whether therapeutic or diagnostic, though generally not for treatment with medication per se. Some clinicians want to take advantage of whatever legal protection consent forms may afford (see later under *The Legal Status of Consent Forms*), and others may wish to incorporate consent forms into the informed consent process because of their potential for enhancing patient comprehension and retention of information about their health care. The use of consent forms places in the hands of patients information on which to base their decision and to which they may later refer. It also involves patients in the documentation of their decision. Therefore, addressing the practical challenges of designing readable consent forms and of implementing them effectively in clinical and research settings is of critical importance.

Challenges in Design and Use

Having established that the appropriate goal of using consent forms is the protection of patients' and subjects' interests, two sets of challenges remain if forms are to be beneficial as appropriate documentation and educational tools in the informed consent process. These challenges arise first in the construction of the forms themselves with respect to their style and content. The second set of challenges arises in their use, with questions centering on who should administer and retain them, and when in the course of a patient's medical career (or subject's research career) they should be presented for consideration.

Content

In clinical practice, there is no unified set of guidelines specifying the contents of forms for consent to treatment.[2] It should by now be obvious, however, that if the form is to serve as an aid to and record of oral disclosure and subsequent discussion, it must contain the same essential information as the oral disclosure. At the very least, the form and oral disclosure must not provide contradictory information. The oral disclosure and subsequent discussion with the patient should explain the informational elements provided in the consent form. Federal regulations specify the elements to be disclosed in obtaining informed consent to research participation (16), and the "long" version of the two types of forms that may be used to document consent should itself contain these elements (see Chapter 12).

A form for consent to treatment might begin by stating that the patient is being asked to make a choice about treatment and to authorize a physician to implement that decision, and also that information is being presented to aid in the patient's decision making. The form should then contain a description of the proposed intervention and the major risks and potential benefits associated with the intervention that reasonable patients would find relevant to their decision making, as well as a description of alternatives to the proposed intervention and their risks and potential benefits. A statement might be included that notes, for example, "These are the major risks of (or alternatives to) this intervention. There are other problems that occur less frequently or are less severe. If you would like to know more about them, your doctor will be happy to discuss them with you." Care must be taken in assuring that forms are used to encourage rather than fore-

[2]Some states provide model consent forms for particular treatments (15).

close discussion and also to prevent the oral disclosure from becoming rote or unresponsive to the explicit questions and implicit informational needs of patients. When in the course of discussion with the patient the physician supplies additional information that is material to the patient's decision, the consent form—often a preprinted form—should be modified to reflect that additional disclosure. This modification is important if the consent form is to document the discussion that actually took place and to provide patients with a written aid to help them remember what was discussed.

In both research and clinical practice, it is advisable to omit unnecessary, irrelevant, and potentially misleading information from the consent form, insofar as such omission is permitted by pertinent laws, regulations, or institutional policies. (In cases where such policies result in the frequent routine inclusion of standardized information that tends to mislead or confuse patients and subjects, it may be a good idea to reexamine such policies.) It is confusing, for example, for an Institutional Review Board (IRB) to require inclusion of standard language stating that "no compensation will be paid for physical injuries incurred as a result of participation" in a consent form for research in which subjects only complete a survey (17). This suggestion to omit some information should not be construed as providing an excuse to omit information that patients (or subjects) would find relevant if only it were presented in a manner that they could comprehend. Rather, we are suggesting that it is misleading to include irrelevant information simply because it is easier for those constructing and reviewing consent forms to include the standard "boiler plate" points, rather than tailor the form to the particular intervention (or type of project). In most cases, the information that needs to be disclosed is of sufficient magnitude and complexity that adding irrelevant information can only increase the risk of "information overload."

Evidence exists that patient understanding of information on consent forms is inversely related to their length (18). Overly inclusive consent forms may have the paradoxical effect of decreasing the level of patient understanding, perhaps even increasing the chance that a patient will feel misled, aggrieved, and inclined to sue. Despite this fact, one study of the use of consent forms for research within a Veterans Administration medical center found that the mean number of lines in information sheets almost doubled between 1975 and 1982 (19). Since the 1980s, much attention has been paid to enhancing the readability of consent forms, but little has been done to limit the sheer amount of information that patients and subjects must process in order to authorize treatment or participate in research. To be sure, in condensing there is some risk of deleting just that information that might have been crucial to the patient's decision; forms may be too short as well as too long. However, if forms are conceptualized as adjuncts to direct physician–patient discussion, there is little need for them to be comprehensive. It is preferable to err on the side of brevity, since encyclopedic forms that overwhelm patients do no one any good.

Another approach that retains the documentary value of consent forms, but avoids the dilemmas associated with trying to encapsulate complex disclosures on paper, involves the use of a different kind of consent form. This form, which can be used for all treatments and procedures in a facility that has requirements for written consent, is built around a notice to patients that their physicians will be disclosing certain categories of information to them about the proposed intervention: nature, purpose, risks, benefits, and alternatives. Space is available for physicians to include additional information that might not be part of their routine disclosure for the procedure, for example, the heightened risk in a particular case because of the patient's debilitated physical condition. Physicians are asked to attest by their signature that they have provided the information, and patients by their signature that they have received the disclosure and have been given an opportunity to ask questions. This may be a reasonable alternative for physicians and facilities concerned that extensive presentation of written information may detract from the focus on the physician–patient interaction.

Readability and Style

Patient comprehension and the comprehensibility of consent forms are the most thoroughly studied aspects of the forms themselves. It is important to note that studying the comprehensibility of forms—for example, the reading level at which they are written—is not the same as studying how much patients actually understand the content of the forms they read. Both are important, and writing comprehensible forms is certainly a prerequisite for enabling patients to understand the information they contain.

Complex and technical language presents a major challenge to constructing forms that most patients can understand. It is clearly more precise to write, "Research has shown that there is a statistically significant chance of a reduction in the circumference of a malignant sarcoma with this treatment," than to say, "This treatment is likely to increase the chance that there will be some improvement in your condition, but it will not do away with your cancer altogether." Most physicians, accustomed to communicating with colleagues and writing for professional audiences, automatically gravitate toward the polysyllabic words that make for greater precision. There is no doubt, however, that most patients would understand the second version more clearly than the first.

Several studies have examined the reading level at which forms for both research and clinical use are written (20–22). Studies published in the late 1970s and 1980s found that many forms are written with a complexity requiring at least college level, and often postgraduate, reading skills (7,23,24), despite the fact that, during the same years, 20 percent of Americans were reported to have reading skills at the fifth grade level or below (25,26). More recent studies suggest that consent forms continue to be written "at a higher reading level than is appropriate for the intended population" (27) or that "the majority of the U.S. adult population would be unable to comprehend" the forms studied (28). One study reported that of the seventy-six forms evaluated, 96 percent had readability levels higher than the target level of eighth grade (29), while in another study less than 10 percent of the 284 forms examined were written at the tenth grade level or below (30). Most studies focus on forms used for clinical research. Although it is possible to imagine that in comparison to consent forms for standard treatment, research protocols require more complex technical language for their explanations, it is also the case that many IRBs review research consent forms for their readability. If these are the products of even careful oversight, there is ample reason for concern about the less regulated, typically less scrutinized forms used in clinical practice.

Some researchers of form readability advocate striving for approximately a tenth grade reading level as an appropriate target for research consent forms (3,31), or more recently, an eighth or sixth grade level (32,27). In 1988, for example, Minnesota enacted legislation requiring that documents such as consent forms be written at the 7.5 grade level (33). Yet, despite development and advocacy of tools to test and rewrite consent forms, the reading level of many, perhaps most, consent forms continues to exceed these targets.

When interest in improving the readability of consent forms first emerged, two scales used by educational researchers were typically employed. The Fry Readability Scale counts the number of words per sentence, and the Flesch Formula counts the number of syllables per 100 words. Stuart Grossman and colleagues observed that in the 1970s determining the reading level of consent forms was cumbersome, but that today there are numerous software programs to aid in this task, including some routinely incorporated into personal computer software packages (25). As with the Fry and Flesch instruments, these common tools can indicate when words or sentences are too long (e.g., over 3 syllables or 30 words). The writer can then respond by splitting long sentences and using simpler synonyms. Tom Grundner suggests that a consent form should not have fewer than 4.5 sentences per 100 words and not more than 150 syllables per 100 words. Such formulas are not infallible, however. Robert Levine has pointed out that the following sort of statement may be helpful: "In the preparation of this consent form it was necessary to use several technical words; please ask for an explanation of any you do not understand" (3, p. 138). He then notes, parenthetically, that this sentence itself scores in the upper college reading level on the Fry Scale, and measures in the scholarly range using the Flesch Formula. Both scales would rate the following revised version as more readable: "Some arcane words are on this page. I will construe them as you wish." However, despite a better readability rating, subjects are less likely to understand this second version.

A peculiar irony arises in the simplification of language on consent forms. Given that polysyllabic medical jargon is often shorthand for longer descriptions using simpler words, efforts to reduce the complexity of consent forms almost inevitably increase their length. To simplify the sentence, "We are conducting an investigation of the pathogenesis and pathophysiology of hyperlipidemia," which consists of twelve words, we would have to resort to something like: "We are trying to find out more about persons who have unusually high levels of fats in their blood. In particular, we are studying what leads to the development of this condition and related changes in the way the body works." Although eminently clear, the more colloquial version more than triples the number of words used in the more technical version. Moreover, sometimes medical jargon becomes better understood by the public than "simpler" explanations would be. There is, for example, an "urban legend" that recounts how one group of AIDS researchers, who were required by their IRB to avoid using medical jargon and abbreviations in their consent forms, deleted "AIDS" and inserted "acquired immune deficiency syndrome" in their consent forms, thereby reducing the actual comprehensibility of the forms by their study population. These examples illustrate two points. First, guidelines for enhancing readability must be applied flexibly. Second, some compromise between simplicity and length must be struck.

Finally, various alternatives to conventional consent forms might avoid some of these problems and serve to educate patients and subjects more thoroughly and efficiently. Clinicians and investigators have experimented with using video or audio tapes to supplement oral disclosure (34–36). Given that a large segment of the population has difficulty reading at the high school level or even the fifth grade level, and that many patients may have impaired eyesight, there may be real advantages to these alternatives. Their use warrants additional study, especially as there is some indication that although providing patients with audiotapes of their discussions with their physician increased patient satisfaction, it did not enhance patients' retention of the information they discussed (36).

Another alternative to the conventional consent form is use of a two-part form (31). The first part consists of the usual written disclosure. After oral disclosure and discussion, the second part, consisting of a simple questionnaire, is given to patients to assess their comprehension of the essential features of their situation and decision. Although it is crucial to monitor patients' understanding of what they are authorizing, the use of a questionnaire may embarrass those who feel they are being "tested" and could miss barriers to understanding that are not included on the form's second part. In like manner, patients who "pass the test" may feel falsely reassured of their understanding and be reluctant to raise additional questions. The monitoring of patients' understanding might better be conducted in discussion between physician and patient. At the same time, physicians' roles in this discussion might be more effective if they were to begin with some ideas about areas of likely misunderstanding. A thought process similar to that involved in constructing the two-part form could stimulate such awareness on their part.

Constructing readable forms does not guarantee the success of the informed consent process, but may aid it. Clear, well-organized oral disclosure and unhurried discussion of the patient's questions are more important contributors to patient understanding than consent forms. And while a good consent form may serve to remind patients of what was discussed, rates of retention among patients (and research subjects) are alarmingly low (9,17).

Timing of Presentation

If the consent form is being used after oral disclosure, the physician—after discussing the nature, purpose, risks, and benefits of a recommended intervention, and describing alternative options—might say something like, "I use this form to remind myself and my patients that I am trying to provide the treatment that they want. This form is a written version of what I think we have agreed on as the appropriate treatment. Read it and tell me if that is what we have agreed on. If it isn't, then we need to continue talking, because I haven't understood what you want."

Alternatively, some physicians may prefer to provide patients with consent forms *before* the major part of the oral disclosure and subsequent discussion, to enable patients to study the material on their own, at their own pace, and to formulate questions for discussion. Some research has suggested that overall patient comprehension can be improved with the use of this technique (37). Patients who receive consent forms prior to the formal stage of decision making can review them with friends, relatives, or other trusted individuals who may help them understand the information and better appreciate the consequences of a decision. Used in either of these ways, consent forms serve both as adjuncts to patient education and symbols of the agreement reached between physician and patient. What has no educational benefit is the all-too-frequent "eleventh hour" presentation of the consent form accompanied by hurried oral disclosure. Moreover, as Chapter 8 argues, a patient who is kept well informed by the mutual monitoring process throughout his medical "career" will have no need for such last-minute decision making.

Manner and Means of Presentation

In addition to the timing of the presentation of consent forms, the manner of their presentation is of some importance. If the patient's signature were sought merely as a legal formality, it would matter little who was present. However, if consent forms are to be integrated into the decisionmaking process, these matters assume a larger meaning. As noted previously, consent forms have an effect of their own in this regard. Thus, how consent forms are presented and by whom may influence the decisionmaking process.

Even among clinicians who are committed to the goals of informed consent, the temptation is strong to use the forms, once they are constructed, as a time-saving device, to thrust them into the hands of patients, to allow them a few minutes to read them over, and then to ask if there are any questions. Among busy physicians, this temptation may subvert the clinical instinct and lead them to substitute the signing of a form for a meaningful disclosure and discussion. Managed care structures with their increased time pressures, as well as the general trend toward standardization of clinical practice, reinforce the temptation to rely on the form either as a substitute, or fairly rigid guideline, for the oral disclosure. Clinicians are not the only ones worn down by "the system." Franz Ingelfinger remarked, two decades before managed care appeared on the scene, about the

> . . . dilution and deprecation of the important by a proliferation of the trivial. The patient, asked to sign countless releases or consents, may respond with a blanket refusal or with a pro forma signature. The physician, immersed in a profusion of unimportant detail, will lose sight of, and respect for the important issues. Perhaps he will feel compelled to practice defensive ethics—no more honorable than defensive medicine. For medical ethics, in short, trivialization is self-defeating. (38, quoted in 2, p. 143)

In myriad ways, the environment of health care itself, as well as physicians, nurses, and other clinicians may convey the impression that signing consent forms, and even giving informed consent, are extraneous to the treatment process. Despite the fact that many of today's clinicians (and researchers) began their careers after informed consent became a cornerstone doctrine in health law and bioethics and sincerely believe in its patient empowering goals, consent forms are still frequently introduced with the phrase, "I have to ask you to sign this," or "We are required to tell you" (39, pp. 93-94). Despite clinicians' best intentions and—in principle—support of the goals of informed consent, in daily clinical practice consent forms and consent are seen as just one more bureaucratic process imposed on physician and patient (or researcher and subject) from the outside. Because actual healthcare decision making is an iterative, ongoing process, not a one-time event, signing consent forms continues to feel somewhat interruptive of the flow of continuous decision making. Pursuing the process model of informed consent, and incorporating consent forms into that process, is the best antidote to this perception that informed consent and consent forms are unrelated to medical decision making and patient care.

The question of who obtains the patient's signature on the consent form raises complicated issues. It is common practice in many institutions for a nurse or someone other than the treating physician actually to obtain the patient's signature. If legal protection were all that is at stake, this might be acceptable, so long as adequate provision was made to address patients' questions at some other time. If use of the consent form is to be integrated into physician–patient decision making and is maximally to serve an educational function, then it is desirable for the physician to be involved in its use. It can be argued, with some justification, that patients might be less intimidated about asking questions of a non-physician or that some non-physicians receive more extensive training in methods of patient education (3). Although such a non-physician might be less able to answer patients' questions, these could then be referred to the physician or the answers discovered and conveyed to the patient. Thus, perhaps the most important reason for physicians to be involved in the discussion surrounding signing of the consent form is that only in this way will they be able to learn of their patients' concerns firsthand. Physicians have the opportunity to be certain that they understand their patients' level of understanding and authorization of treatment. By gaining this insight into patients' concerns and informational needs, physicians may be better able to address them in future disclosures. Moreover, in situations in which physicians must make decisions on behalf of their patients, as in emergencies or when patients waive informed consent, their decisions may be guided by an enriched patient–oriented perspective, as well as their medical experience. Furthermore, because of the social authority accorded physicians, the participation of physicians in discussions surrounding the signing of consent forms symbolizes and reinforces the importance of the patient's authorizing the physician's medical intervention on her behalf.

Retention and Storage of Consent Documents

In research, it is required that subjects be given a copy of the consent form they sign. In some cases, the IRB that approves the form's content will specify that particular information be included in the consent form for the patient's future reference, such as how to contact the project's principal investigator or the head of the IRB. Forms used to document consent to research typically also include information to which subjects may wish to refer, such as likely physical effects of the intervention or the right to withdraw from the study without prejudice. In addition, the IRB itself is required by federal regulations to retain sample copies of the consent form, as well as other documentation of the research project. Many institutions have policies governing how long researchers should retain their collected research data, and signed consent forms should be retained at least as long and also "should be retained for a sufficient period longer than the statute of limitations as usually advised for physicians who are concerned with potential malpractice litigation," which may range from six months to forever (3, p. 139). Some institutions will require that the signed consent forms, like research data, become the property of the institution. How signed consent forms are stored may be of interest to subjects, because consent forms are one means (and in some studies the only means) of identifying study participants. Forms must be stored securely to protect subjects' privacy and confidentiality.

Documentation of consent to treatment in clinical practice may be handled somewhat less formally; however, privacy protection is no less important here than in research. Laws, regulations, and institutional policies regarding confidentiality apply both to the physician's note in the patient's chart, and to a copy of a signed consent form retained as part of the patient's medical record (40). If a consent form is employed, patients should be given a copy of the form so that they may refer to it during the course of their treatment. Giving patients a copy of the form is one—but as discussed earlier, need not be the only—means of supplying patients with written educational material about a medical intervention. One commentary suggests that the managed care–induced trend away from inpatient treatment to outpatient procedures may increase patients' reliance on consent forms when questions arise and their primary healthcare providers are unavailable (25).

From the perspective of patients (and subjects), retaining a copy of their consent form has an educational function. Possessing a copy while making their decision can, in some circumstances, help inform that decision and prompt them to inquire about what they do not comprehend. Retaining a copy of the signed form may help patients retain information disclosed to them or help them formulate questions about what they forgot.

The Legal Status of Consent Forms

Even if the primary and intended purpose of consent forms is to help guide and document informed consent and educate patients, consent forms will continue to play a role in legal proceedings. Therefore, in this final section, we consider the legal status of consent forms and their potential to provide protection from liability. The use of consent forms can indeed serve the interests of physicians, researchers, and institutions; however, their primary purpose is to protect the interests of patients and subjects.

Although the history of the use of consent forms is unclear, what we now call a consent form probably evolved from the simple release of liability, a common legal document in hospital treatment, in which patients acknowledged that they agreed to the proposed medical procedures and would not hold physicians liable for any resulting ill effects. Indeed, some simple consent forms are still entitled "Release of Liability" or "Release." The modern consent form (often called somewhat optimistically an "informed consent form"), which provides some information about the contemplated treatment, probably evolved from simple consent forms more or less contemporaneously with the early court cases requiring disclosure (see Chapter 3).

There is no common-law requirement that consent forms be used, and a number of courts have specifically stated that they are not necessary (41). But the Medicare Conditions of Participation (42) and the Joint Commission on Accredi-

tation of Healthcare Organizations (JCAHO) (43) both have explicit requirements for informed consent that are often interpreted to require consent forms. In
the absence of any statutory provision governing the effect of a consent form
signed by a patient, it has been held that the consent form "is simply one additional piece of evidence for the jury to consider. . . . [U]nless a person has been
adequately apprised of the material risks and therapeutic alternatives incident to a
proposed treatment, any consent given, be it oral or written, is necessarily inef-
fectual" (44). Thus, in many states, the presence or absence of a consent form
serves merely as some evidence of consent, but is not conclusive (14,44–48). As
one court stressed, "[a] form signed by the patient does not always indicate that
the patient's consent was in fact informed consent" (49).

A few states, however, have statutes that appear to encourage consent forms by
according those that comply with the statutory requirements a "presumption of
validity." These statutes require a written consent form to be signed by the patient
as part of the informed consent process. But although the absence of a consent
form may be evidence of the lack of informed consent, it does not preclude the
admission of other information (or documentation) that the patient was informed
and did indeed consent to the treatment. However, the weight given to an official
consent form in subsequent litigation in these jurisdictions will be substantial.
For example, in some of these states a signed consent document may be viewed
as a conclusive presumption that valid informed consent was obtained (50–57).
The plaintiff-patient may overcome this presumption only by showing that informed consent was not in fact valid because of misrepresentations, omission of
material information (58), failure to meet statutory requirements (59,60) or mal-
ice (61) on the part of the physician (14). In addition, the patient may show lack
of understanding on her own part (62)—for example, due to language barriers
(63), or sensory (hearing or visual) or cognitive impairments (64)—or that she
was unduly pressured into signing the form (62). In a 1996 Florida case, for example, plaintiffs (the class of pregnant women enrolled in a study) sought damages due to lack of informed consent, claiming both that the forms were written
in language too technical for the women to understand and that the subjects were
coerced into signing the forms (65,66).

Although these statutes were enacted specifically to protect physicians from
lawsuits, their meaning and effect are ambiguous at best. Some statutes refer to
"conclusive" presumptions, while others refer to a presumption of "valid" consent or simply a presumption of informed consent (67). The implications of all
these statutes are unclear in ways that should not be reassuring to a physician
who wishes to rely on them. The precise kind of presumption a statute creates
could be extremely important to the litigants in an informed consent case; the
consequences of a signed consent form could range from decisive to irrelevant.
But although it would seem that a consent form creating a conclusive presumption that the patient both was adequately informed and gave consent could put a

stop to a lawsuit almost immediately, most of these statutes have not actually been construed in this manner by the courts. Rather, the statutes have been held to create a presumption of consent, but not to speak to the adequacy of disclosure. As one court stated, the consent form in question did "not reveal the specific information disclosed and whether the information was adequate; however, the documents constitute some evidence supporting [the] claim that informed consent was indeed obtained" (68).

If the consent form is conclusive merely as to the issue of consent and not the adequacy of disclosure, a signed form serves as a defense only to a charge of unauthorized treatment (i.e., battery) and not to a claim of inadequate disclosure (i.e., negligence) (69). Moreover, as noted earlier, most states with consent form statutes do not create conclusive presumption even with respect to consent, but merely a rebuttable presumption—one that can be challenged by the plaintiff-patient on a variety of grounds. Thus, at most, the consent form assists the defendant-physician by establishing a *prima facie* case of adequate disclosure and consent, which may be overcome by the patient's evidence of fraud, misrepresentation, duress, or mistake. Statutes that create such a *prima facie* presumption work no change in existing law. It has always been the plaintiff-patient's responsibility to plead and prove inadequate disclosure and lack of consent (see Chapter 6), regardless of any statutory presumptions to that effect. Thus, there is no apparent benefit from the existence of many statutes that encourage consent forms.

In summary, then, a signed consent form's main legal use is as evidence that the patient at least had an opportunity to read the information on it. This is the case in most jurisdictions having statutes and the vast majority of jurisdictions without them. If the information presented in the consent form contains a description of the risk that actually came to pass and other information adequate for a reasonable person to make a decision, it will probably be helpful to a physician in the defense of a lawsuit. However, the same information documented in another way (e.g., recorded in the medical record) may serve a similar purpose.

Moreover, if the form presents inadequate or overly complex information, this evidence may support the plaintiff-patient's case. If the form merely acknowledges that disclosure was made but fails to contain the content of what should have been disclosed, it is unlikely to provide the physician with any added advantage with respect to the main issue of litigation: what was disclosed and whether it was adequate (68). Often a consent form of any sort merely provides the opposing lawyer with a good target to attack. Consent forms may provide a false sense of security to physicians and hospital administrators, leading them to believe that a signed consent form constitutes informed consent. James Vaccarino has concisely summarized the dangers of consent forms in this respect:

> By failing to distinguish between informed consent and its documentation, the legal profession has precipitated the most egregious misconception by physicians con-

cerning informed consent, namely that if a consent form is signed, informed consent has been obtained. At the outset, the consent form must be recognized for what it is: nothing more than [one piece of] evidence that informed consent has been obtained (70).

References

1. Smith, D.H. (1996) Ethics in the doctor-patient relationship. *Crit Care Clin,* 12(1):179–197.
2. Meisel, A. (1982) Commentary on Grundner. *IRB: Rev Human Subjects Res* 4(1):9.
3. Levine, R.J. (1988) *Ethics and Regulation of Clinical Research,* 2nd ed., New Haven: Yale University Press.
4. World Medical Association (1964) *Declaration of Helsinki.* http://www.bioscience. org/guides/declhels.htm (accessed October 11, 2000).
5. 45 C.F.R. 46.117.
6. 21 C.F.R. 50.
7. Cassileth, B.R., Zupkis, R.V., Sutton-Smith, K., et al. (1986) Informed consent—why are its goals imperfectly realized? *N Engl J Med,* 302:896–900.
8. Olver, I.N., Buchanan, L., Laidlaw, C., and Poulton, G. (1995) The adequacy of consent forms for informing patients entering oncological clinical trials. *Ann of Oncol,* 6(9):867–870.
9. Olver, I.N., Turrell, S.J., Olszewski, N.A., and Willson, K.J. (1995) Impact of an information and consent form on patients having chemotherapy. *Med J Aust,* 162(2):82–83.
10. Botrell, M.M., Alpert, H., Fischbach, R.L., and Emanuel, L.L. (2000) Hospital informed consent for procedure forms: facilitating quality patient-physician interaction. *Arch Surg,* 134:26–33.
11. Singer, E. (1978) Informed consent: consequences for response rate and response quality in social surveys. *American Sociological Review,* 43:144–162.
12. Singer, E. (1980) More on the limits of consent forms. *IRB: Rev Human Subjects Res,* 2(3):7.
13. American Psychiatric Association (1992) *Task Force on Tardive Dyskinesia.* Washington, D.C.: APA.
14. Rozovsky, F. (1999 Supp.) *Consent to Treatment: A Practical Guide.* Boston: Little, Brown.
15. Louisiana Rev. Stat. Ann. 40:1299.40 (LEXIS 2000).
16. 45 C.F.R. 46.116
17. Rogers, C.G., Tyson, J.E., Kennedy, K.A., Broyles, R.S., and Hickman, J.F. (1998) Conventional consent with opting in versus simplified consent with opting out: an exploratory trial for studies that do not increase patient risk. *J Pediat,* 132:606–611.
18. Epstein, L.C. and Lasagna, L. (1969) Obtaining informed consent—form or substance? *Arch Intern Med,* 123:682–688.
19. Baker, M.T. and Taub, H.A. (1983) Readability of informed consent forms for research in a Veterans Administration Medical Center. *JAMA,* 250(19):2646–2648.
20. Handelsman, M.M., Kemper, M.B., Kesson-Craig, P., McLain, J., and Johnsrud, C. (1986) Use, content, and readability of written informed consent forms for treatment. *Professional Psychology—Research & Practice,* 17(6):514–518.

21. Murgatroyd, R.J. and Cooper, R.M. (1991) Readability of informed consent forms. *Am J Hosp Pharm,* 48(12):2651–2652.
22. Tarnowski, K.J., Allen, D.M., Mayhall, C., and Kelly, P. (1990) Readability of pediatric biomedical research informed consent forms. *Pediatrics,* 85(1):58–62.
23. Grundner, T.M. (1980) On the readability of surgical consent forms. *N Engl J Med,* 302:900–902.
24. Gray, B.H., Cook, R.A., and Tannenbaum, A.S. (1978) Research involving human subjects. *Science,* 201:1094–1101.
25. Grossman, S.A., Piantadosi, S., and Covahey, C. (1994) Are informed consent forms that describe clinical oncology research protocols readable by most patients and their families? *J Clin Oncol,* 12(10):2211–2215.
26. U.S. Department of Education Office of Educational Research and Improvement (1986) *Digest of Education Statistics 1985–1986.* Washington, D.C.: U.S. Department of Education Center for Statistics.
27. Ogloff, J.R.P. and Otto, R.K. (1991) Are research participants truly informed? Readability of informed consent forms. *Ethics Behav,* 1(4):239–252.
28. White, L.J., Jones, J.S., Felton, C.W., and Pool, L.C. (1996) Informed consent for medical research: common discrepancies and readability. *Acad Emerg Med,* 3(8):745–750.
29. Philipson, S.J., Doyle, M.A., Gabram, S.G.A., Nightingale, C., and Philipson, E.H. (1997) Informed consent for research: a study to evaluate readability and processability to effect change. *J Invest Med,* 43(5):459–567.
30. Goldstein, A.O., Frasier, P., Curtis, P., Reid, A., and Krecher, N.E. (1996) Consent form readability in university-sponsored research. *J Fam Pract,* 42(6):606–611.
31. Miller, R. and Wilner, H.S. (1974) The two-part consent form: a suggestion for promoting free and informed consent. *N Engl J Med,* 290:964–966.
32. Young, D.R., Hooker, D.T., and Freeberg, F.E. (1990) Informed consent documents: increasing comprehension by reducing reading level. *IRB: A Review of Human Subjects Research,* 12:1–5.
33. Minn. Stat. §689.2:123 (1988).
34. Reynolds, P.M., Sanson-Fisher, R.W., Poole, A.D., et al. (1981) Cancer and communication: information-giving in an oncology clinic. *Br Med J,* 282:1449–1451.
35. Malone, M.L. (1983) Informed consent and hospital consent forms: paper chasing in a video world. *Journal of Urban Law,* 61:105–125.
36. Dunn, S.M., Butow, P.N., Tattesall, M.H.N., et al. (1993) General information tapes inhibit recall of the cancer consultation. *J Clin Oncol,* 11:2279–2285.
37. Morrow, G., Gootnick, J., and Schmale, A. (1978) A simple technique for increasing cancer patients' knowledge of informed consent to treatment. *Cancer,* 42:793–799.
38. Ingelfinger, F.J. (1975) The unethical in medical ethics. *Ann Intern Med,* 83:264–269.
39. Lidz, C.W., Meisel, A., Zerubavel, E., et al. (1984) *Informed Consent: A Study of Decisionmaking in Psychiatry.* New York: Guilford Press.
40. Roach, W.H., Garwood, J.C., Conner, C., Cartwright, K.K., Kole, S., and Forsyth, J. (1998) *Medical Records and the Law.* Gaithersburg: Aspen Publishers.
41. Foreman v. WI, 1998 Ohio App. LEXIS 4625.
42. 42 C.F.R. §482.24(c).
43. Joint Commission (1998) *Comprehensive Accreditation Manual for Hospitals.* Oak Brook: JCAHO.
44. Sard v. Hardy, 379 A.2d 1014 (Md. App. 1977).
45. Gassman v. United States, 589 F. Supp. 1534 (M.D. Fla. 1984)

46. Gordon v. Neviaser, 478 A.2d 292 (D.C. 1984)
47. Keane v. Sloan-Kettering Institute for Cancer Research, 464 N.Y.S.2d 548 (App. Div. 1983).
48. Desgravise v. St. Vincent Charity Hosp., 580 N.E.2d 818 (Ohio Ct. App. 1989).
49. Barner v. Gorman, 605 So.2d 805 (Miss. 1992).
50. Tex. Rev. Civ. Stat. Ann. art. 4590i (2000 Lexis).
51. Utah Code Ann. §78–14–5 (2000 Lexis).
52. Rev. Code Wash. §7.70.060 (2000 Lexis).
53. Iowa Code § 147.137 (1999 Lexis).
54. Cardio TVP Surgical Assocs. v. Gillis, 272 Ga. 404, 528 S.E.2d 785, 787 (Ga. 2000).
55. Shabinaw v. Brown, 131 Idaho 747, 963 P.2d 1184, 1188 (Idaho 1998).
56. Earl v. Ratliff, 998 S.W.2d 882, 891 (Tex. 1999).
57. Church v. Perales, 2000 Tenn. App. LEXIS 567.
58. Schaefer v. Miller, 587 A.2d 491 (Md. 1991).
59. Allan v. Levy, 816 P.2d 274 (Nev. 1993).
60. Distefano v. Bell, 544 So.2d 567 (La.Ct. App. 1989).
61. Idaho Code §39–4305 (1975)
62. American Law Institute, *Restatement of Torts (Second)* §892[B][2].
63. Ohio Rev. Code Ann. §2317.54 (Baldwin 1977).
64. Greynolds v. Kurman, 632 N.E.2d 946 (1993).
65. Hudson, T. (1991) Informed consent problems become more complicated. *Hospitals,* 65(6):38–40.
66. Diaz v. Hillsborough County Hospital Authority, 165 F.R.D.689 (M.D. Fl 1996) (granting class certification).
67. Hondroulis v. Schuhmacher, 553 So.2d 398 (La. 1989).
68. Palmer v. Bilozi, 564 So.2d 1346 (Miss. 1990).
69. Hartsell v. Fort Sanders Reg'l Med. Ctr., 905 S.W.2d 944, 947 (Tenn. Ct. App. 1995).
70. Vaccarino, J.M. (1977) Malpractice: the problem in perspective. *JAMA,* 238: 861–863.

10

Managed Care and Informed Consent

In the last decade, American medicine has been transformed by a series of changes in the economic arrangements governing clinical practice that have come to be known generically as "managed care." Since the nature of these changes is complex and the process of evolution incomplete, managed care evades efforts at easy definition. However, it is probably fair to say, as Iglehart has, that "[a]ll forms of managed care represent attempts to control costs by modifying the behavior of doctors, although they do so in different ways" (1, p. 1167).

Managed care's alteration of some of the basic premises of the physician–patient relationship, has raised serious questions about its effect on the doctrine of informed consent. To take but one example, if the physician is now subject to incentives from a managed care organization to decrease the amount and cost of care provided, would this information be material to the decision making of a reasonable patient? Should the law therefore require that such information be disclosed? If so, who should disclose this information, and when should the disclosure be made? At this stage, most of the questions that can be framed are, like this one, not susceptible to definitive answers from a legal or ethical perspective. But the potential impact of these new means of authorizing and paying for medical treatment is so substantial that there is value in laying out the issues to which jurists and legislators will have to respond, and in providing some initial guidance to clinicians and administrators. These are the goals of this chapter.

What Is Managed Care?

To understand the changes wrought by managed care in the practice of medicine—and their possible relevance for informed consent law—one needs to begin by recalling the economic framework of medical care during the development of the doctrine of informed consent. With the growth of employer-provided health insurance following World War II, most middle-class Americans and their families were freed of the spectre of bankruptcy attending serious medical illness (2). Indeed, with health insurers covering the charges for medically necessary care, neither these patients nor their physicians were compelled to pay attention to the costs of treatment or to feel obliged to limit interventions for financial reasons. The introduction of Medicare for the elderly and disabled and the joint federal-state Medicaid program for the indigent, in 1965, extended this model to additional large segments of the population (2).

Informed consent as we know it was born in this milieu. The implicit assumption in *Natanson* (3), *Canterbury* (4), and the other formative cases discussed in Chapter 3 was that the provision of information to patients about the options for their care would lead them to make autonomous choices of preferred treatments unconstrained by economic considerations. Money—that powerful determinant of most worldly decisions—went conspicuously unmentioned and apparently unnoticed by those who framed the doctrine. They appear to have presumed that whichever treatment options patients selected would be provided regardless of expense. Thus, the crucial list of information to be disclosed to patients about their options omits any reference to such matters as the relative costs of care. With the insurance company footing the bill, it simply was unclear why the average patient would find such details to be material to a decision. It is worth noting that, for this reason, the doctrine better served the interests of more affluent patients or those with adequate health insurance coverage than those patients who lacked financial resources.

The mechanism of physician compensation is another contextual aspect of medical decision making that was so taken for granted as not to warrant explicit mention in the early common law of informed consent. Physicians were paid for providing care. Their income might vary as a function of the amount and type of care provided (e.g., surgical intervention might be more lucrative than "watchful waiting"), but the early informed consent cases gave no direct attention to the incentive for physicians to increase their provision of care so as to augment their income. Insofar as this possibility may have entered the minds of the judges who were shaping informed consent law, one suspects that the concern was assuaged by the fact that the "incentive structure was fairly transparent; patients understood that if their doctor did more, the bill would rise" (5). Well-informed patients could protect their interests by selecting the intensity and type of treatment that best reflected their preferences, perhaps to the financial detriment of their treating physicians.

This "purity" of the insurance-based medical care system—free of concern about financial issues—was, of course, illusory. Someone, usually the patient's employer or the government, was paying the bill, and over time the bill grew steadily. By the late 1980s, pushed by the growth of medical technology, employers' healthcare costs were increasing at annual rates approaching 20 percent. In 1989, "employers' health insurance expenditures represented 8.9 percent of wages and salaries, up from 2.2 percent in 1965" (6, p. 1004). Pressure mounted to identify mechanisms to reverse or at least to restrain spiraling costs. Employers turned to health maintenance organizations (HMOs), initially designed to improve the comprehensiveness and efficiency of care. These entities assumed the responsibility of covering workers' healthcare benefits for a fixed fee, always less than would be charged by traditional indemnity insurers for comparable coverage, and then aggressively managed the utilization of services to hold down overall costs. HMO development had been encouraged by the federal HMO Act of 1973, which required employers of more than twenty-five workers to offer an HMO option if it was available in their area. But the real growth of HMOs and related managed care organizations awaited the explosive increase in healthcare costs in the late 1980s (6).

By the end of the 1990s, approximately 75 percent of employees in the United States received their healthcare insurance coverage through some form of managed care (7). This number included millions of Medicare and Medicaid recipients, as state and federal governments, no less desirous than private-sector employers of reducing healthcare expenditures, though somewhat slower to act, turned to managed care organizations for this purpose (8–9). The structure of the managed care entities that oversee this care and the mechanisms they use to hold down the costs of care vary greatly. In general, though, three forms of managed care can be discerned:

- Modified fee for service. Resembling the traditional indemnity or "fee for service" model, this approach continues to pay physicians and other caregivers based on the units of service they deliver. More visits, consultations, or procedures mean more dollars going to the providers of care. But managed care organizations typically negotiate a reduced fee schedule with physicians and healthcare facilities (compared with indemnity insurers), using as leverage to drive down reimbursements their control of a substantial portion of the doctor's potential patients. Patients covered by these plans are generally limited to using physicians in a predefined network or paying extra for the privilege of obtaining "out-of-network" care. In addition to negotiating lower fees, these managed care entities (which may call themselves HMOs, preferred providers organizations [PPOs], or simply health insurers) control utilization by requiring preapproval of many kinds of non-emergent care, for example, elective surgery, consultations with specialists, and many psychiatric services. They will often conduct concurrent utilization review of ongoing care for more persistent conditions to determine if further coverage is warranted. In this model, managed care entities are closely involved in monitoring proposed care, and they restrain costs primarily by declining to cover care that they consider not to be medically necessary.

- Risk sharing. When insurers accept a fixed premium in exchange for covering all needed medical care for a period of time, they carry the risk of financial losses if the cost of care exceeds the amount of premium dollars. Some managed care models create situations of shared risk between insurers and care providers. For example, primary care physicians may be told that a portion of the fees that are due to them (e.g., 15 percent) will be withheld until the end of the year. If expenditures on the medical care of their patients exceed certain targets, some portion or all of the withheld amount may be retained by the insurer. Withhold programs can target expenditures on particular services (e.g., pharmaceuticals, referrals to specialists, X-rays, and laboratory tests) or total medical costs (10). Physicians thus share some of the risk, up to the amount withheld, of costs exceeding premiums, and generally take on more of the responsibility for managing patients' care. Assuming that physicians will be more restrained in their recommendations for expensive treatment, managed care entities may be less aggressive about prospective and concurrent review and other means of direct control over resource utilization under this approach.

- Capitation. Insurers sometimes prefer to transfer *all* of the risk associated with a given population of patients by contracting capitation agreements with care providers. Under this model, groups of physicians or healthcare systems agree to accept a certain amount of money (usually quoted as a fixed sum "per patient per month") to provide all the treatment that a group of patients may require. If expenses can be held below the level of the capitation amount, the group or system will profit from the arrangement. But every dollar spent on patient care comes directly from the capitated entity's bottom line. Modifications of this approach that blur the boundaries between risk sharing and capitation can be seen, including capitation only of outpatient or primary care, and the establishment of "risk corridors," which set limits on both the potential profits and potential losses of the capitated entity (e.g., 20 percent of the capitated payments can be retained as profit, and the entity will not be expected to cover overages in excess of 20 percent of revenue). Physician groups and hospital systems are usually given the most leeway in managing care in a fully capitated model. The more risk that is shared, the greater the degree of control over utilization that is likely to be ceded by the insurer.

With managed care constantly evolving, it is probable that permutations will arise that represent hybrids of these models or that reflect entirely new approaches. But at its core, managed care—regardless of the precise approach taken—comprises a set of techniques for controlling costs of medical care that operates by constraining the discretion of both physicians and patients.

Physicians' leeway in recommending treatment options to their patients is limited by requirements for prospective and concurrent review of their choices, because the managed care company's refusal to authorize payment effectively precludes use of the recommended option for most patients. Referrals to specialists or non-medical health professionals (e.g., physical therapists, dietitians) may be restricted to a small group in the managed care entity's network, or may require preauthorization. Choices of medication are often limited by the formularies developed by managed care companies, which may exclude higher-priced medications in favor of generic drugs or other less expensive alternatives. As physicians move from modified fee-for-service to risk sharing and capitation models, internalized pressures come to bear on their decisions, as they face the reality that recommendations for more care, or simply more expensive care, will have a direct, negative impact on their financial status.

Patients, too, face constraints on their choices under managed care, above and beyond the limitations experienced by their physicians. Their selection of physicians and other caregivers is effectively limited to those who have contracted with their managed care entity. Some treatment options (e.g., long-term dynamic psychotherapy, experimental surgical techniques) may be precluded by the company's policies. And patients may no longer be able to control the dissemination of information from their medical records, as managed care companies request detailed data, or even copies of actual records, to make coverage decisions.

Managed care has ushered in a new world of medical care. To what extent do these innovations call for compensatory changes in the doctrine of informed consent?

"Economic" Informed Consent

As a consequence of the growth of managed care, physicians, medical organizations, ethicists, and legal experts have begun to suggest that the exclusion of economic factors from consent disclosure is no longer justifiable. A variety of arguments is presented in support of this position, including appeals to physicians' fiduciary duties and to the principle of patient autonomy that underlies the doctrine of informed consent. The bottom line, however, is the same: in the current structure of insurance coverage for medical care, it is fundamentally unfair to deprive patients of information concerning the financial pressures that may influence their physicians' treatment decisions.

The most straightforward argument in favor of offering patients information about the economic structure of care derives from the materiality standard of disclosure defined in the early informed consent cases. In the words of Haavi Morreim, a medical ethicist, "Although the concept of materiality can be vague, an incentive system strong enough to prompt significant alterations in care can reasonably be considered material [to a patient's decision]" (11). Patients who are unaware that financial factors may be shaping their physicians' recommendations are likely to assume that decisions are being made only on the basis of their medical interests. Once aware of the pecuniary interests that might be affecting their doctors' decisions, though, they may be more likely to ask questions, challenge conclusions, and seek alternative opinions.

Shea v. Esensten, a case decided by the federal Court of Appeals for the Eighth Circuit, posed this situation starkly (12). The patient in *Shea*, a man of only forty, repeatedly complained to his family physician of chest pain, shortness of breath, dizziness, and tingling in his arm—classic symptoms of ischemic heart disease. Despite the patient's extensive family history of cardiac problems, the physician advised him that he was too young to have heart disease and did not need to see a cardiologist. Even when the man offered to pay for his own referral to a heart specialist, the physician allegedly talked him out of it. Unbeknownst to the patient, however, his HMO offered financial incentives to its doctors to avoid referrals to specialists and imposed penalties if they exceeded their quota. A few months after the patient's death from heart disease, his widow sued the HMO under the federal Employee Retirement Income Security Act (ERISA), alleging that had her husband known about the physician's financial incentives, he would have sought an independent second opinion from a cardiologist at his own expense.

The facts in *Shea*, taken at face value, indicate how data about financial incentives can be as material to a patient's decision as a description of the risks of surgery or the side effects of medication. Patients who are deprived of such information may not be able to exercise appropriate caution in evaluating physicians' recommendations. Believing that no other options exist, they may fail to pursue viable alternatives. This condition hardly constitutes the informed decision making envisioned by the progenitors of the law of informed consent. Moreover, since the impact of an incentive scheme on physicians' decision making will increase with the strength of the incentive (13), the potency of the argument for disclosure grows in such cases as well. As physician organizations are beginning to recognize the centrality of economic information for patients' decision making, some are responding accordingly. One example is reflected in a resource document published by the Council on Psychiatry and Law of the American Psychiatric Association, which recommends that incentive arrangements be discussed openly by psychiatrists at the beginning of any treatment relationship (14).

An alternative to the materiality rationale for disclosure of financial incentives is based on the fiduciary duty that exists between doctor and patient. Fiduciaries are obligated to act in the best interests of persons who seek their assistance. The law imposes fiduciary duties on physicians to permit patients to rely with confidence on their doctors' superior information and expertise, secure in the knowledge that patients' best interests will be the primary goal of the relationship (15). Although there is not a great deal of case law addressing these issues, several courts have indicated sympathy with a duty to disclose economic information that is rooted in physicians' fiduciary obligations. The first opinion to move in this direction was *Moore v. Regents of the University of California*, where the issue in contention was whether physicians had a duty to reveal to a patient their financial interest in developing a potentially valuable cell line from his spleen, which they were about to remove (16). In its ruling for the patient, the California Supreme Court held that "1) a physician must disclose personal interests unrelated to the patient's health, whether research or economic, that may affect the physician's professional judgment; and 2) a physician's failure to disclose such interests may give rise to a cause of action for performing medical procedures without informed consent or breach of fiduciary duty" (16, p. 150).

Indeed, *Shea v. Esensten* itself was decided ultimately on fiduciary grounds. The Eighth Circuit held that ERISA's statutory recognition of a fiduciary duty for providers of care in employee benefit plans is sufficient to require disclosure of financial incentives, and permitted the case to go to trial: "When an HMO's financial incentives discourage a treating doctor from providing essential health care referrals for conditions covered under the plan benefit structure, the incentive must be disclosed and the failure to so do is a breach of ERISA's fiduciary duties" (12, p. 629). An intermediate level court in Illinois reached a similar conclusion on common law grounds in a case with nearly identical facts, *Neade v. Portes* (17).

To this point, the discussion has focused on disclosure of financial incentives, but either a materiality or a fiduciary approach might also require disclosure of other kinds of information related to managed care. Patients might find it helpful to know about the process by which utilization of services will be reviewed to determine if their care will be compensated; the standards to be applied in such review; their rights to appeal adverse determinations; and the limits on the privacy of their medical records as a consequence of these review procedures. Disclosure of other economically based limits on their care—for example, limited referral networks, restricted formularies—arguably might also be helpful in assisting them to make meaningful decisions about their treatment.

Supporters of "economic informed consent," however, are by no means unanimous about *who* should be required to make the necessary disclosures. Ordinarily, the obligations of disclosure and obtaining consent devolve upon the patient's physician. That is the model described throughout this book, and some commentators and even some professional organizations have argued that it

should apply here as well (11,14,15). Stronger and more numerous voices, however, have expressed concern about the difficulties associated with imposing this
burden on patients' treating physicians. Doctors today typically contract with
many insurers, and each company may have a somewhat different incentive structure and review procedures; indeed, these may differ across various plans managed by the same company. It may be next to impossible for physicians to remain
aware of all this information for each patient. More significantly, a number of
commentators have pointed to the likely adverse impact of physicians' disclosures on the doctor–patient relationship (18,19). In essence, the physician may be
called on to start the relationship by telling the patient about the potential conflicts of interest that the physician faces (e.g., "The more care I give you, the less
money I make"), an awkward beginning that is likely to undermine the trust on
which the treatment will rest.

This is not an argument for withholding this potentially pivotal information
from patients, but it may constitute one of several reasons to shift the burden
elsewhere. David Mechanic and Mark Schlesinger make the case that "[r]outine
disclosure by [insurance] plans is preferable to disclosure by physicians early in
patient relationships because it is less likely to undermine the initial development
of interpersonal trust crucial to patient–physician relationships" (18, p. 1696).
Managed care plans, too, can be construed as having a fiduciary obligation to reveal to their beneficiaries the nature of the determinants that will affect the provision of medical care (11). Placing the burden on the plans has the added advantage of requiring the most knowledgeable parties to make the disclosure, and may
provide patients with a basis for choosing among managed care plans (20). Perhaps not surprisingly, the American Medical Association supports requiring
HMOs and other insurers, rather than physicians, to disclose financial incentives
and other matters (13), and federal Medicare and Medicaid managed care programs have implemented regulations requiring disclosure of a limited amount of
such information in some circumstances (21). Several states have adopted more
extensive disclosure requirements (22). Disclosure by managed care plans, however, may not necessarily absolve physicians and facilities of all obligations.
Some scholars argue that physicians have a concomitant duty to reveal financial
influences on their decisions (11), while almost everyone agrees that doctors
must at least respond honestly to their patients' queries about these matters (23).

When should these disclosures of economic information take place? Susan
Wolf offers the most comprehensive approach, favoring provision of information
about economic incentives at multiple times including when a worker accepts a
job, since if an employer offers only a single health plan, accepting the position is
tantamount to making a decision about insurance coverage; when the beneficiary
selects a health insurance plan, so that if more than one plan is offered, genuine
choice is possible; and at the time of choosing a primary care physician, when information can be proffered regarding the physician's "rationing and disclosure

styles" (5). Although the last of these, as noted earlier, is the subject of controversy, at a minimum disclosure by managed care plans should occur prior to enrollment, with physicians disclosing additional information relevant to a particular patient's care when appropriate circumstances arise. Thus, patients might receive a comprehensive disclosure from their insurer before deciding to enroll and then be told in general terms of the process for utilization review before that occurs, or as discussed later under *Disclosure of Alternatives to "Authorized" Treatment*, of their options when benefits are denied.

One might reasonably ask whether placing responsibility for disclosure on health plans and insurers remains within the ambit of informed consent law. Informed consent has always been grounded in the doctor–patient relationship and the clinical decisionmaking context. Insurers may have certain obligations toward those persons who contract with them, but these seem more in the nature of duties based on fiduciary principles in contract law or administrative regulation than they are related to the negligence-driven process traditionally associated with informed consent. Perhaps it might be more fitting to think of placing disclosure duties at least partially on the managed care entities themselves as constituting an alternative to sole reliance on the informed consent doctrine to promote economic disclosure.

How likely is it that we will see movement toward the implementation of "economic informed consent"? As Mark Hall observed, "it is clear that virtually no existing source of law—federal or state, statutory or judicial—requires the disclosure of HMO physician incentive payments, and such disclosure is nearly unheard of in practice" (22, p. 520). A handful of decisions aside (24,25), the courts have never been eager to embrace broader concepts of informed consent and to mandate presentation of additional information that might be of great interest to patients and that could easily be construed as material to their decisions. Examples of information that need not be disclosed under current law, at least in the absence of a specific patient request, include the amount of experience that a physician has had with a particular illness, or the number of times that a surgeon has performed a proposed procedure. And the Georgia Supreme Court has decided that even a physician's drug use need not be revealed to patients (26).

It might also be maintained that informed consent law as we know it would be a poor tool to protect patients' rights in this area. Recovery of damages in an action alleging failure to obtain informed consent is predicated on the patient-plaintiff's demonstrating that "but for" the failure to disclose the information in question, the patient would have chosen differently and avoided the consequent harms. There are likely cases in which the plaintiff can successfully make this showing; *Shea v. Esensten*, discussed previously, may well be such a case. But often the plaintiff will be hard-pressed to persuade a jury that—having heard all of the risks and benefits of the proposed course of action, and having decided to proceed anyway—her course of action would have been different if only she had known the arcane details of her physician's financial compensation scheme (27).

There have, however, also been powerful indications that the general public believe that their physicians should be frank with them about the factors that influence their care. Early in their evolution, managed care companies typically included "gag rules" in their contracts with physicians that precluded physicians from speaking openly with patients about their treatment (28). Some of these clauses were extremely broad, like this one from an Ohio HMO: "Physician shall take no action nor make any communication which undermines the confidence of enrollees, potential enrollees, their employers, plan sponsors, or the public in Choice Care, or in the quality of care which Choice Care enrollees receive" (29, p. B13). Others were more focal, only restricting disclosures about treatments not covered by the plan (30). As knowledge of the gag rules spread, the public became incensed that their physicians had information potentially relevant to patients' care that they were unable to share. By late 1997, only two years after the first antigag rule statute was passed, thirty-six states had adopted statutes eliminating or constricting the reach of gag clauses in managed care contracts (31). The federal government acted similarly for Medicare managed care programs (28). Although antigag clause statutes have their limitations (32), they do seem to reflect a consensus against restrictions on physician disclosure.

Thus, in addition to whatever requirements may be imposed on HMOs and other managed care plans by means of regulation or interpretation of their fiduciary obligations, it seems likely that informed consent law will continue to evolve in the direction of encouraging greater disclosure of at least some "economic" information by physicians. How rapidly this movement will come and how far it will extend both remain to be seen. What physicians should do in the meantime, we consider in the final section of this chapter.

Disclosure of Alternatives to "Authorized" Treatment

Financial incentives and mechanisms of review may not be the only information of which patients in a managed care plan would want to be made aware that are unaddressed by the traditional rules of informed consent. Equally critical to their decision making is a reasoned consideration of the options for their care. But many managed care plans have attempted to prevent physicians from revealing all the medically appropriate options that patients may have, and some legal commentators have argued that patients might reasonably be asked to sign away their rights to such information when they enroll in a managed care plan. Given that the disclosure of alternative forms of treatment to that favored by the physician has been considered a mainstay of informed consent since the earliest cases, how has that principle come to be called into question?

As noted previously, the essential innovation of managed care is systematic limitation of the discretion of both physicians and patients in choosing treatment options. Denial of coverage for treatment recommended by physicians is a common occurrence in the world of managed care (33). Only by means of these limitations can managed care plans hope to restrain the growth of medical costs. Managed care companies recognized early in their development that if patients were fully aware of the restrictions, patients would demand access to additional options for their care where they thought them beneficial. This was, the companies knew, a "no win" situation for them. If they declined to provide the additional, more costly, options, they would end up with dissatisfied policyholders and a good deal of adverse publicity. Capitulating to patients' demands, however, would undercut their foundational cost-containment strategy.

In response to this dilemma, most companies initially attempted to use "gag clauses" to restrict physicians' disclosure of information about treatment options, other than those they had authorized. Beyond the restrictions discussed in the preceding section, these clauses often required physicians to wait until a proposed treatment was approved by the managed care company's prospective review procedures before informing patients of their recommendations for treatment. Mention of unauthorized treatment options was forbidden (34). Even when a gag clause failed to specify these restrictions, the general prohibition against impairing the confidence of the patient in the company could be interpreted as covering these issues.

Warren Holleman and colleagues reported a chilling example of such a clause in operation (30). The case involved a thirty-five-year-old man with schizophrenia, who was covered by a managed care plan through his wife's employer. After consulting with a psychiatrist, his family physician recommended an expensive new medication that required frequent laboratory monitoring. Upon inquiry of the managed care company, the physician was informed that the drug was not included in the plan's approved formulary. At that point, "the utilization reviewer at the insurance company reminds the physician that if she tells the patient about the new drug the insurance company will stop all payment for any treatment for this patient and might remove the physician from the plan. Angry and incredulous, the physician checks her contract and finds clauses to this effect in fine print" (30, p. 223).

The apparent demise of gag clauses due to the wave of legislation and federal regulation in the late 1990s means that such blatant efforts to restrict disclosure of treatment alternatives to patients are unlikely to be repeated today. However, physicians are by no means free from pressure by managed care entities to withhold information from patients (32). Consolidation of the managed care industry has led to fewer entities that now control access to larger numbers of patients (35). Physicians may therefore be dependent on the goodwill of a given company for their continued ability to treat 20, 30, or even 40 percent of their patients. Since in most instances the plans retain the right to terminate physicians from their panels at will (36) (judicial attempts to establish limits on this power have been rare and legislative efforts weak [32]), there is no small value to the physician in being seen as a "team player" or to use a term frequently heard in contemporary medical practice, "managed care friendly." Having too many of one's patients appeal to the managed care company for coverage of expensive treatment options, especially if it is clear that their information has come from the physician, may be a black mark against a doctor (37). Stories of physicians terminated from managed care plans on these grounds circulate through medical circles, though documentation of how frequently this occurs is hard to come by (28,38). Nonetheless, knowing this, physicians may impose some degree of self-restraint on the information they convey to their patients.

In the face of these pressures to withhold information about treatment alternatives from patients, there has been considerable adverse reaction from physicians and ethicists alike. The American Medical Association has held that physicians "should continue to promote full disclosure to patients enrolled in managed care organizations. The physician's obligation to disclose treatment alternatives to patients is not altered by any limitations in the coverage provided by the patient's managed care plan. Full disclosure includes informing patients of all of their treatment options, even those that may not be covered under the terms of the managed care plan" (13, p. 334). Although concern has been expressed that the courts have not been aggressive in supporting patients' rights to hear about the options for their care (39), the American Medical Association's approach reflects the consensus of legal commentators (5,15,31,40,41), as well as being consistent with the principles of disclosure in informed consent law as they have always been understood. Clinician-commentators have offered similarly strong support for disclosure (30,42–45).

But not everyone believes that this adherence to the principle of disclosure of treatment alternatives solves the problem. Hall, a lawyer by training, has been the most vociferous critic of requiring physicians to tell patients of unauthorized options (22,46). In his view, managed care's promise to restrain healthcare costs represents an important societal goal. That goal, however, is likely to be endangered, for reasons discussed earlier, if patients are made fully aware of the possible treatment options to which access is being denied. In his words, "in order for affordable insurance to exist, some degree of financial autonomy must be relinquished to physicians or others" (22, p. 514). Thus, he searches for and finds a mechanism that he thinks would justify depriving patients of this information.

Hall proposes that at the time of enrollment in a managed care plan, patients provide consent to the future withholding of information about treatment options that the plan elects not to cover. He argues that this agreement can be seen either as prior consent to the rationing decision that the plan will make, or as a waiver of the right to be informed of such information in the event that it becomes relevant to one's care. In essence, under either approach, "when an insurance subscriber knowingly enrolls in a constrained system of financing, he buys into an entire cost-constrained medical philosophy and set of practices" (22, p. 559). A managed care company looking to implement Hall's plan would disclose to prospective enrollees: the goal of "economical insurance," the identity of the person who makes medical spending decisions in the plan, the sources (but not the full content) of the rules that govern those decisions, "a fairly specific description of the financial incentives that influence physicians' decisions," and "an explanation of what patients can expect to be told when potentially beneficial treatment is not recommended due to its cost" (22, p.p. 583–584). In general, however, Hall anticipates that physicians "will not always point out where their professional judgment differs from those who practice under more expensive forms of insurance or who follow differing styles of medical practice" (22, p. 584).

Hall's proposal, along with similar arguments (47), is interesting in demonstrating what it would take to reconcile informed consent law with the managed care industry's preferred level of disclosure to patients: explicit waiver by patients (or its equivalent) of their right to be told of alternative options for their care. It has, as might be expected, attracted a great deal of critical attention (5,39,42), which has focused on two difficulties with the proposal, both related to the fundamental unfairness of withholding material information about treatment options from patients.

First, although Hall claims that persons can, on enrollment in a plan, freely and effectively waive their right to subsequent information, he recognizes that this would require enrollees to make knowledgeable choices among their insurance options. However, persons selecting a managed care plan who receive the disclosure that Hall suggests are unlikely to have any meaningful idea of the rights they are signing away or the potential effect of their action. They will know—if they read and understand the fine print, a dubious proposition in itself—that some officer of the plan will be making "medical spending decisions," but will have no basis for comprehending the unrevealed rules on which those decisions will be based. Even if prospective enrollees get the idea that some treatment options will not be covered by the plan, they will remain in the dark regarding the types of treatment involved and, of course, in the usual case, will not be able to anticipate whether those exclusions will affect them directly or will be irrelevant to their care. (Hall describes the unavailable treatment options as of "marginal benefit," a term that, if used in the disclosure for enrollees, will suggest—perhaps deceptively—little sacrifice on their part.) In the state of bewilderment attending most decisions regarding insurance coverage, it is difficult to imagine a knowledgeable consent or waiver taking place.

Perhaps even more significantly, it is not clear that a large proportion of persons will have any decision to make at all. Hall envisions potential subscribers choosing among insurance plans on the basis, in part, of the degree of information the competing plans will provide about treatment options, a benefit likely to involve some added cost. But a substantial percentage of employees (one survey estimated the number in excess of 40 percent, and it may now be greater [48]) are offered only one health insurance option, typically the least expensive one available to their employer. Even public Medicaid programs are more frequently turning the patients they cover over to the care of a single insurer (9). The continuing consolidation of health insurers suggests that the availability of options may decrease still further in the future (35). In the absence of a choice of plans with varying approaches, no real consent or waiver of disclosure is possible; at best, enrollees will merely accede to the inevitable. Hall himself, in a telling conclusion to his elaborate proposal, admits that his approach can only work when subscribers have valid options among plans. Given that this is frequently not the case today, he concedes that his proposal must be deferred until that condition obtains (22). Even then, however, the meaningfulness of the prospective consent involved in this approach will remain questionable.

In the end, it is difficult to avoid the conclusion that fairness to the patient and physicians' fiduciary duties demand disclosure of all reasonable treatment options, even those that an insurer may decline to reimburse. This course is required as well by our current understanding of the principles of informed consent. In the words of ethicist Ruth Faden, "with the resolution of this issue hangs in the balance the future and the meaning of informed consent. As the options available to patients, and the information about these options, decrease, so, too, does the meaningfulness of obligations to obtain a patient's informed consent" (49, p. 379).

The managed care system remains in a chronic state of flux, with case law and statutory rules that might affect consent procedures lagging behind the profound changes in the current economically oriented oversight of medical care. It is possible, nonetheless, to suggest some steps that physicians may want to take to meet their obligations to their patients. That is the task of the following section.

An Approach to Informed Consent in an Era of Managed Care

Three points of contact between physician and patient seem critical for the unfolding of a reasonable set of duties related to informed consent in the age of managed care: the initial meeting, the time when recommendations for treatment are being made, and the moment at which coverage of treatment has been rejected by the managed care company.

The first meeting between physician and patient—especially in primary care or other settings where an extended relationship is likely—is the optimal point for a general discussion of the framework within which the doctor–patient dyad will function. Almost invariably, in the current climate, that will include some mention of the impact that managed care is likely to have on the relationship. Physicians may want to call patients' attention to the reality that many treatment choices on which doctor and patient agree will need to be reviewed prospectively by the managed care entity responsible for the economic oversight of the patient's insurance coverage. Simply because the two parties most directly involved have jointly decided on what they consider to be the optimal course of action does not ensure that the crucial third party will agree to pay for it. As much as managed care has been discussed in the media and is the focus of public concern, there are still many patients who are unaware of the applicability of this principle to their own care. The risk that a prolonged course of treatment may be interrupted by a denial of further benefits at some point in the future may need to be mentioned as well. To the extent that the physician can identify treatment interventions that are likely to be relevant to the patient's condition, but will not be covered by the insurer (e.g., experimental procedures), this may also be a good time to point that out to the patient.

Should the physician use this occasion to reveal the financial incentives that may be operative in this case? We are inclined to agree with those commentators who have suggested that it would be best if someone other than the treating clinician carried this burden. Preferentially, the responsibility of disclosing the incentive structure of a particular insurance plan should fall on the insuring entity itself. [For one approach to disclosure, see the model information form for health plans devised by Morreim (11).] Given the understandable reluctance of managed care companies to reveal these details, legislation is likely to be required to accomplish this. In large medical systems, whether hospital- or clinic-based, it may be possible to have employees designated specifically to review insurance issues, including incentive schemes, with new patients (50). Of course, nothing should prevent physicians who feel strongly that they want to discuss these issues with patients from doing so, and at a minimum, patients' questions should be responded to frankly.

The second key point for discussion of managed care–related matters is when a diagnosis has been made and physician and patient are in the midst of selecting among treatment options. Here is where it falls to the physician—regardless of the preference of the patient's insurer—to disclose all medically reasonable options for care. This is also the point at which some description of the utilization review process can be offered, including how long the process is likely to take. (Note that where fully capitated models are in use, review may be conducted internally by the medical group or hospital system that holds the contract for delivering the patient's care.) Some patients, because of either their personal status and values or the nature of their condition or treatment, will have particular concerns about the privacy of their medical treatment; they may appreciate a description of the information that will need to be released for review purposes. In some cases, patients may elect to pay out of pocket or even to forgo treatment altogether to avoid further dissemination of their medical record information.

In the event that the mutually agreed upon treatment plan is rejected by the managed care company, the third and final critical point for disclosure and discussion arises. Here, patients need first to be told of their right to appeal the reviewer's decision, and of the physician's willingness to assist in that process (51). Most managed care companies have created mechanisms for internal appellate review, often involving several levels of personnel, culminating in a decision by the plan's medical director. Some states have mandated the creation of independent review systems, not controlled by the patient's insurer (52). Although the process can be time-consuming, costly (the independent review mechanisms often carry a fee), and difficult for patient and physician to negotiate, the decision on whether to proceed ought to rest in the patient's hands.

As they consider whether or not to undertake an appeal, patients will probably want to know what other options exist for their care. Physicians are sometimes leery of offering what in their view are "second best" choices in this situation, but their fears are misplaced. Treatments other than the one the physician would select are often chosen by patients, for example, when the doctor recommends surgical intervention, but the patient prefers a combination of medical management and ongoing monitoring. As long as the physician has been open about the risks and benefits of each approach, including the fact that these alternatives are not the ones that she recommends most highly, there ought not to be concern regarding potential liability on the grounds of having deviated from the standard of care. Rather, the physician is best understood as aiding the patient to make the optimal decision about treatment, given the very real constraints imposed by the absence of insurance coverage for the preferred option.

Patients may also want to consider the cost of paying for treatment on their own, either as the ultimate resort or while awaiting a decision on their appeal of a denial of coverage. This means that physicians will have to provide an estimate of the costs involved, information that may not be at their fingertips for hospital-based diagnostic procedures or interventions. Certain procedures are commonly funded in this way: long-term psychotherapy, for example. Others are within the reach of many patients; recall that the patient in *Shea v. Esensten* had considered paying out of pocket for a consultation with a cardiologist (12). Even patients without obvious means of paying for expensive treatment may be able to call on resources from relatives or their community. The example of a community fundraising drive to pay for experimental cancer treatment is probably familiar to most people. Thus, this possibility should always at least be raised by the physician.

In suggesting that physicians undertake this set of duties toward patients, we want to underscore that most of these issues have yet to be addressed in law, whether common or statutory. There is some case law to indicate, for example, that physicians may have a duty to appeal adverse utilization review decisions by managed care companies on their patient's behalf (53), but no consideration has yet been given by the courts to the information that should pass between doctor and patient in that situation. It is possible that the courts will define physicians' duties more narrowly or more broadly (e.g., requiring physician disclosure of information about financial incentives) than we have here.

Nevertheless, it is difficult to believe, in this circumstance of legal ambiguity, that physicians will go far wrong in looking for guidance to the principles underlying the doctrine of informed consent. Managed care has created new circumstances and constraints under which patients must make difficult choices about their care. Providing them with the information that most reasonable people would deem material to their decision making should fulfill physicians' ethical and potential legal obligations.

References

1. Iglehart, J.K. (1994) Physicians and the growth of managed care. *N Engl J Med*, 331:1167–1171.
2. Starr, P. (1982) *The Social Transformation of American Medicine*. New York: Basic Books.
3. Natanson v. Kline, 350 P.2d 1093 (Kan. 1960).
4. Canterbury v. Spence, 464 F.2d 772 (D.C. Cir. 1972).
5. Wolf, S.M. (1999) Toward a systemic theory of informed consent in managed care. *Houston Law Review*, 35:1631–1681.
6. Bodenheimer, T. and Sullivan, K. (1998) How large employers are shaping the health care marketplace. *N Engl J Med*, 338:1003–1007.
7. Jensen, G., Morrisey, M., Gaffney, S., and Listan, D. (1997) The new dominance of managed care: insurance trends in the 1990s. *Health Affairs*, 16(1):125–136.
8. Brown, R.S. and Gold, M.R. (1999) What drives Medicare managed care growth? *Health Affairs*, 18(6):140–149.
9. Health Care Finance Administration: National summary of Medicaid managed care programs and enrollment, June 30, 1999. *www.hcfa.gov/medicaid/trends99.htm* (accessed July 18, 2000).
10. Grumbach, K., Osmond, D., Vranizan, K., Jaffe, D., and Bindman, A.B. (1998) Primary care physicians' experience of financial incentives in managed-care systems. *N Engl J Med*, 339:1516–1521.
11. Morreim, E.H. (1997) To tell the truth: disclosing the incentives and limits of managed care. *Am J Managed Care*, 3:35–43.
12. Shea v. Esensten, 107 F.3d 625 (8th Cir. 1997).
13. Council on Ethical and Judicial Affairs, American Medical Association (1995) Ethics in managed care. *JAMA*, 273:330–335.
14. Council on Psychiatry and Law, American Psychiatric Association (1995) Resource document: the professional responsibilities of psychiatrists in evolving health care systems. APA State Update, October.
15. Mehlman, M.J. (1990) Fiduciary contracting limitations on bargaining between

patients and health care providers. *University of Pittsburgh Law Review*, 51:365–417.

16. Moore v. Regents of the University of California, 271 Cal. Rptr. 146 (Cal. 1990).
17. Neade v. Portes, 710 N.E.2d 418 (Ill. Ct. App. 1999).
18. Mechanic, D. and Schlesinger, M. (1996) The impact of managed care on patients' trust in medical care and their physicians. *JAMA*, 275:1693–1697.
19. Levinson, W., Gorawara-Bhat, R., Dueck, R., et al. (1999) Resolving disagreements in the patient-physician relationship: tools for improving communication in managed care. *JAMA*, 282:1477–1483.
20. Sorum, P.C. (1996) Ethical decision making in managed care. *Arch Intern Med*, 156:2041–2045.
21. Gallagher, T.H., Alpers, A., and Lo, B. (1998) Health Care Financing Administration's new regulations for financial incentives in Medicaid and Medicare managed care: one step forward? *Am J Med*, 105:409–415.
22. Hall, M.A. (1997) A theory of economic informed consent. *Georgia Law Review*, 31:511–586.
23. Hall, M.A. and Berenson, R.A. (1998) Ethical practice in managed care: a dose of realism. *Ann Intern Med*, 128:395–402.
24. Hiding v. Williams, 578 So.2d 1192 (La. Ct. App. 1991).
25. Estate of Behringer v. Medical Center at Princeton, 592 A.2d 1251 (N.J. Super. Ct. 1991).
26. Albany Urology Clinic v. Cleveland, 272 Ga. 296 (2000).
27. Perry, C.B. (1994) Conflicts of interest and the physician's duty to inform. *Am J Med*, 96:375–380.
28. Pear, R. (1996) U.S. bans limits on HMO advice in Medicare plan. *New York Times*, Dec. 7, 1996, p.1.
29. Pear, R. (1995) Doctors say HMOs limit what they can tell patients. *New York Times*, Dec. 21, 1995, p. A-1.
30. Holleman, W.L., Holleman, M.C., and Moy, J.C. (2000) Continuity of care, informed consent, and fiduciary responsibilities in for-profit managed care systems. *Arch Fam Med*, 9:21–25.
31. Miller, T.E. (1997) Managed care regulation in the laboratory of the states. *JAMA*, 278:1102–1109.
32. Krause, J.H. (1999) The brief life of the gag clause: why anti-gag clause legislation isn't enough. *Tennessee Law Review*, 67:1–44.
33. American Medical Association (1999) Kaiser/Harvard survey highlights need for strong patients' bill of rights. Press release, July 28, 1999.
34. Pear, R. (1996) Laws won't let HMOs tell doctors what to say. *New York Times*, Sept. 17, 1996, p. A-9.
35. Feldman, R.D., Wholey, D.R., and Christianson, J.B. (1999) HMO consolidations: how national mergers affect local markets. *Health Affairs*, 18(4):96–104.
36. Potvin v. Metropolitan Life Insurance Co., 997 P.2d 1153 (Cal. 2000).
37. Meyer, M. (1997) Bound and gagged: HMOs need to be reformed—but in the right way. *Newsweek*, March 17, 1997, p. 45.
38. Bass, A. (1995) Therapists say insurer gag order hurts patients. *Boston Globe*, Dec. 20, 1995, p.1.
39. Krause, J.H. (1995) Reconceptualizing informed consent in an era of health care cost containment. *Iowa Law Review*, 85:261–386.
40. Annas, G.J. (1998) A national bill of patients' rights. *N Engl J Med*, 338:695–699.

41. Miller, F.H. (1992) Denial of healthcare and informed consent in English and American law. *Am J Law Med*, 18:37–71.
42. Appelbaum, P.S. (1993) Must we forgo informed consent to control health care costs? *Milbank Q*, 71:669–676.
43. Bursztajn, H.J. and Brodsky, A. (1999) Captive patients, captive doctors: clinical dilemmas and interventions in caring for patients in managed health care. *Gen Hosp Psychiatry*, 21:239–248.
44. Miller, I.J. (1996) Ethical and liability issues concerning invisible rationing. *Prof Psychol Res Pract*, 27:583–587.
45. Strom-Gottfried, K. (1998) Informed consent meets managed care. *Health Soc Work*, 23:25–33.
46. Hall, M.A. (1993) Informed consent to rationing decisions. *Milbank Q*, 71:645–668.
47. Havighurst, C.C. (1992) Prospective self-denial: can consumers contract today to accept health care rationing tomorrow? *University of Pennsylvania Law Review*, 142: 1637–1712.
48. Blendon, R.J., Brodie, M., Benson, J.M., Altman, D.E., Levitt, L., Hoff, T., and Hugick, L. (1998) Understanding the managed care backlash. *Health Affairs*, 17(4): 80–110.
49. Faden, R. (1997) Managed care and informed consent. *Kennedy Institute of Ethics Journal*, 7:377–379.
50. Kuczewski, M.G. and Devita, M. (1998) Managed care and end-of-life decisions: learning to live ungagged. *Arch Intern Med*, 158:2424–2428.
51. Appelbaum, P.S. (1993) Legal liability and managed care. *Am Psychol*, 1993:251–257.
52. Frieden, J. (2000) More states implement external appeals laws. *Clinical Psychiatry News*, March 2000, p. 48.
53. Wickline v. State, 228 Cal. Rptr. 876 (Cal. App. 2d Dist. 1986).

11

Patients Who Refuse Treatment

From its inception, the law of informed consent has been based on two premises: first, that a patient has the right to receive sufficient information to make an informed choice about the treatment recommended; and second, that the patient may choose to accept or to decline the physician's recommendation. The legitimacy of this second premise should be underscored because it is too often belied by the everyday language of medical practice. *Getting a consent* is medical jargon that implies that patient agreement is the only acceptable outcome. Indeed, the term informed consent itself suggests that patients are expected to agree to be treated rather than to decline treatment. Unless patients are viewed as having the right to say no, as well as yes, and even yes with conditions, much of the rationale for informed consent evaporates.

Nonetheless, the medical profession's reaction to patients who refuse treatment often has been less than optimal. The right to refuse treatment is frequently ignored in practice because it is inconsistent with the history and ethos of medicine (1,2). Physicians are trained to treat illness and to prolong life; situations in which they cannot do either—not because of limitations of knowledge or technology, but because patients or third parties reject their recommendations for care—evoke profound feelings of frustration and even anger. It would not be too much to suggest that these confrontations challenge an essential element of the medical identity. Physicians' reactions to these situations are varied. Some will contend with patients over their refusal, while others, having assimilated a distorted version of patients' right to refuse treatment, may too quickly abandon their patients to the consequences of their choices, thereby depriving them of the guidance for which patients traditionally have turned to their physicians.

Regardless of the quality of care offered to patients or the degree of concern of those who treat them, some patients will have reasons of their own to decline treatment. Before considering how clinicians might respond to these situations, this chapter reviews the status of the law regarding treatment refusal, surveying a legal landscape that has seen dramatic changes in the last decade.

Legal Attitudes Toward Refusal of Treatment by Competent Patients

The right of a competent patient to refuse treatment is now universally recognized by the legal system. Indeed, in the words of one commentator, the "net effect" of court decisions on this issue "has been to bring the right to refuse treatment about as close to absolute as anything ever gets in law" (3, p. 241). The vast majority of decisions have come from state courts, and have been based on patients' common law right to give or withhold informed consent (4) or on state constitutional provisions (5). In its decision in *Cruzan v. Director, Missouri Department of Health* in 1990, the United States Supreme Court recognized a person's right to refuse treatment based on a liberty interest derived from the fourteenth Amendment to the United States Constitution. Using matter-of-fact language that was as telling as the conclusion it reached, the Court noted, "The principle that a competent person has a constitutionally protected liberty interest in refusing unwanted treatment may be inferred from our prior decisions" (6). Thus, the right to decline medical interventions has the strongest possible legal grounding.

As recently as the late 1980s, however, the status of competent patients' right to refuse treatment was much less clear. Although refusal has always been implicit in the doctrine of informed consent, the courts had carved out numerous exceptions for which they refused to enforce the rule. Patients who were pregnant (7), had minor children who were dependent on them (e.g., 8,9), were suffering from non-terminal illness (10), or sought to refuse nutrition or fluids (11) were often denied the right to reject proffered medical care. One by one, however, each of these barriers has fallen.

Pregnant women were often compelled to undergo procedures—most notably cesarean sections to deliver their babies—when physicians judged that their refusals endangered the lives of their fetuses (12). This practice came to a head in *In re A.C.,* an emotionally charged case from the District of Columbia (13). A.C., who was twenty-five weeks pregnant, was found to have had a recurrence of bone cancer, with one of her lungs nearly filled by an inoperable mass of tumor. Her doctors' judgment was that the fetus she carried had little chance of survival unless delivered immediately by cesarean section—an intervention, in her sedated and intubated condition, that she appeared to refuse. Complicating the situation was the equivocal probability (estimated at 50 percent–60 percent) that the prematurely delivered baby would survive even after a cesarean, and the substantial likelihood that the stress of an operative procedure would lead to the earlier demise of the patient herself. Nonetheless, after a hearing at the patient's bedside, a trial court ordered the procedure to be carried out, citing the state's interest in protecting the unborn child. Mother and child alike died soon after the surgery. The D.C. Court of Appeals, ruling nearly a year after the event, rejected the lower court's rationale, holding that the right of a competent woman to make decisions about her own medical care took precedence over whatever interest the state might have in preserving the life of the fetus. This approach has since become the norm; as a rule, courts will not overturn the medical treatment decisions of a pregnant woman to preserve the potential life of her fetus (14).

Closely related to the pregnancy cases are situations involving refusal of treatment by patients—usually women—with dependent minor children. These cases have arisen frequently with Jehovah's Witnesses, whose religiously based refusal of blood transfusions often provokes life-endangering situations. Many of the early decisions involving Jehovah's Witnesses overrode their refusals, despite the deference typically afforded by the courts to decisions based on religious motivations, out of concern for the fate of their minor children (8,9,15,16). In the 1990s, however, the tide in American courts swung decisively against compelling treatment on these grounds (14). The strength of these opinions varies; some courts speak in fairly absolute terms of the patient's common law, statutory, or constitutional right to decline transfusions (17,18), while others rest their holdings more narrowly on the presence of a supportive household or other family members who could ensure that the children were not abandoned (19, 20). But the outcome of all recent cases has been the same: the right of refusal has been upheld. In the words of one court, "The citizens of this state have long had the right to make their own medical care choices without regard to their physical condition or status as parents" (17).

The refusal of blood products cases exemplify another situation in which courts previously shied away from enforcing patients' refusal rights: patients with conditions that would be likely to respond to treatment, but whose lives would be endangered without it. The early landmark treatment refusal cases tended to involve situations in which patients were terminally ill, and their holdings often made reference to that fact (4,21). For a time, it was unclear whether the right to decline treatment would be extended to non-terminal patients. Even the Jehovah's Witnesses cases left this somewhat uncertain because of the greater deference that might be accorded to religiously based refusal. Indeed, it appeared that to promote the interests of minor children and to preserve the integrity of the medical profession, some courts would employ whatever rationale could be called upon, including finding patients incompetent, to deny patients' right to refuse treatment in non-terminal situations (10).

However, a line of cases in which treatment was declined by people with severe neurological impairments seems to have resolved this issue. Beginning with the celebrated case of Elizabeth Bouvia, who sought to end life-sustaining care required by her severe cerebral palsy (22), and continuing with other decisions involving patients with traumatic quadriplegia (23–25), the courts have made clear that patients who are not terminally ill in the usual sense of that term can decline treatment, even if the result would be their otherwise postponable deaths. (That a number of the people involved in these cases subsequently decided not to terminate their life-sustaining care raises important issues regarding psychological factors in treatment refusal, considered later under *Assessing Refusal of Treatment.*)

Despite the triumph in case after case of patients who are seeking to vindicate their refusal of treatment, the courts frequently assert that patients' right to refuse treatment is not absolute. Four countervailing state interests, derived from the ruling of the Massachusetts Supreme Judicial Court in *Superintendent of Belchertown State School v. Saikewicz* (26), are said to require weighing against the right of refusal in any particular case: (*1*) the preservation of life, (*2*) the protection of third parties, (*3*) the prevention of suicide, and (*4*) the protection of the ethical integrity of the medical profession. Though these may seem to be weighty factors, they play the role of strawmen in these decisions. The courts, beginning with the *Saikewicz* court itself, uniformly find that none of them are substantial enough to outweigh patients' rights of self-determination with respect to refusal of medical treatment. The right of medical patients to refuse unwanted treatment is now unquestioned.

An independent line of cases deals with the rights of involuntarily committed psychiatric patients to refuse treatment. Historically, in practice if not in theory, involuntary commitment was considered to represent an exception to the usual rules of informed consent (27). Even once the time had passed that all committed patients were considered ipso facto to be incompetent, it was assumed that whatever gave the state the power to confine these persons against their will provided authority to treat them as well. Indeed, it appears that so long as commitment was predicated on patients' presumed need for treatment (the somewhat vague, traditional standard for civil commitment in most jurisdictions), it did not occur to anyone to challenge the practice of treating them, once confined, over their objections. The change in commitment law in the 1960s and 1970s, which led to the substitution of criteria based on dangerousness to oneself or others for need-for-treatment criteria, however, led to challenges to the power of the states to treat competent, committed patients (27).

Almost all courts considering the issue have concluded that involuntarily committed psychiatric patients retain at least a qualified right to refuse unwanted treatment, even if that would delay their discharge from the hospital (28). The courts, interestingly, have differed somewhat in their analysis of the nature of this right. Two general lines of court decisions exist (29). In the first, the right of refusal has been rooted in the basic assumptions of the law of informed consent, and efforts to treat involuntarily have been made to turn on an adjudication of incompetence (e.g., 30). In the second, acknowledgment is made of the right of refusal, but involuntary commitment is seen as limiting that right, so that involuntary treatment can be instituted after a review of the appropriateness of the proposed regimen, irrespective of patient competence (e.g., 31). Here again the state is viewed as having an overriding interest in reducing the degree of dangerousness displayed by the patient and in restoring the patient to a level of functional ability such that he can be discharged from the hospital.

Jurisdictions also differ over whether review of competence and/or the appropriateness of treatment must be conducted by a court or a clinical/administrative review body, or whether it can be left to clinicians themselves. Several jurisdictions without court rulings on this issue simply retain the practice of treating patients over their objections, though some require a concurring opinion about the appropriateness of the selected treatment from a second clinician. The only clearcut United States Supreme Court decision on refusal by psychiatric patients came in the prison context (32). Treatment over the objections of prisoner-patients was permitted after a clinical/administrative panel in the prison reviewed the appropriateness of the proposed care and determined that the prisoner met the state's dangerousness-based commitment criteria. A finding that the prisoner was incompetent was not mandated. Whether the Court would rule similarly in a civil context is an open question.

Legal Attitudes Toward Refusal of Treatment on Behalf of Incompetent Patients

Among the earliest cases addressing patients' refusal of treatment were several in which the patient was entirely incapable of making a decision about treatment and someone else sought to decline further care on the patient's behalf. Karen Ann Quinlan, for example, lay in a New Jersey hospital, in a persistent vegetative state, apparently dependent on her respirator for life support (33). When her father, serving as guardian, sought a judicial order barring interference with his removing her from the respirator and granting him immunity from criminal prosecution, a lower court rejected his request. The New Jersey Supreme Court, however, recognized that Ms. Quinlan had a right to discontinue life-support measures, grounded in the constitutional right to privacy, and that her father could exercise that right on her behalf. His decision had to be made on the basis of the choice that she herself would make, were she capable to do so. (See the discussion of the additional requirement for ethics committee review imposed by the *Quinlan* court in Chapter 5.)

With *Quinlan* as the starting point, one court after another has acknowledged that incompetent patients retain their right to decline unwanted treatment, and that substitute decision makers can exercise that right on their behalf (34). As noted in Chapter 5, a rough consensus has evolved regarding how the decision should be made, based on a hierarchy of mechanisms. At the highest level of preference, when the patient has given explicit indications of what her choice would be—either in a formal advance directive or in less formal writing or conversations—that choice should be followed. In the absence of a definitive choice, the decision maker should rely on what evidence may exist regarding the patient's inclinations, and make a "substituted judgment" on that basis. Finally, many jurisdictions will permit a decision to be made on the basis of the patient's best interests—that is, whether the burdens of treatment outweigh the benefits—when no evidence is available as to how the patient would have made the decision.

Some variation exists among the states in these procedures. New York, Michigan, and Missouri, for example, demand clear and convincing evidence of the patient's desires while previously competent before life support can be discontinued (6,35,36). In these states, a person who was previously competent but failed to leave sufficient evidence of his or her wishes cannot have life-sustaining treatment terminated. The same may be true in some states for patients who have been incompetent for their entire lives (35). What counts as clear and convincing evidence appears to vary considerably, with the only certainty being that a written advance directive is likely to suffice. Other states, such as Massachusetts, insist paradoxically that a substituted judgment standard be used even for patients who have never been competent and thus for whom no evidence can be ascertained of their probable desires (26). This is clearly a fictional inquiry for never-competent patients and reduces in practice to application of a best interests standard (26). Most jurisdictions, however, follow the first schema outlined previously.

When the patient is incompetent, the question of who can decide on the patient's behalf is salient (37). The courts generally have held that judicial involvement is not required, though recourse still may be had to the courts when contention exists over whether the patient is incompetent or who should make the decision regarding treatment, or when certain extraordinary or controversial treatments or procedures are involved (e.g., abortion, sterilization, psychosurgery). When patients have identified substitute decision makers in advance directives, decisionmaking power should be lodged in their hands. Otherwise, physicians routinely look to family members to make decisions for their loved ones. A majority of states now have statutes indicating the order of priority in which family members should be approached. Conflict between family members at the same level of priority (e.g., between two adult children of an elderly patient) may require judicial intervention if informal attempts at mediation fail.

Children are one group of legally incompetent patients for whom the courts may be less willing to allow surrogates to make decisions to reject needed care. When parents refuse care for life-threatening conditions, even on religious grounds, the courts have usually, but not always, ordered treatment to be provided. Most courts have been of the view that parents do not have the right to deprive children of the opportunity to live to the age at which they can make their own decisions about how they want to order their lives. The cases in which courts have been more accepting of parental refusals have usually involved conditions that were not life threatening for the child (38,39), but this too is not always the case (40). As public tolerance for religiously based refusals has declined, criminal prosecution of parents whose children have died because of refusal of medical treatment has increased (41,42).

The Dilemma of Refusal of Treatment in the Clinical Setting

It should come as no surprise that the medical profession has been torn by the dilemma of patient refusal. Physicians are ordinarily deeply invested in promoting patients' health and convinced of the benefits of their interventions. There is an inherent frustration for physicians when patients reject treatment that physicians believe is needed (43). In fact, it is in just such situations that the conflict between autonomy and health appears most stark and unresolvable.

Respecting patients' refusals may involve a compromise of the interest in health, but this will not always be the case. Patients will often be choosing between no treatment and treatments of limited or uncertain efficacy, frequently on the basis of the side effects that must be endured. A patient who suffers nausea or constipation from medication designed to reduce chronic pain might well choose to forgo it, if the effects of the drug are more troubling than the condition itself. Similarly, patients choosing among breast cancer treatments that are more or less disfiguring can be understood, given continuing controversy over the relative benefits of each approach, if they choose one that preserves their body intact. Whether or not the trade-off between treatments—or between the choice of treatment and no treatment—is roughly equivalent in medical terms, our society has given competent patients the right to make that choice.

Moreover, patients will sometimes be right, even from a strictly medical perspective, to refuse offered treatment. They may be aware, for example, that the same or a similar approach has been tried previously without success. Patients may recollect an allergic reaction or other serious side effect to a particular medication in the past. Or patients may accurately perceive from the physician's discussion of treatment options that a given intervention is likely to be of marginal utility. Thus, the first reaction that should follow a patient's refusal of treatment is reconsideration by the physician of whether the treatment is truly indicated for this person.

Assessing Refusal of Treatment

Assuming that they have satisfied themselves regarding the appropriateness of their recommendation, physicians can fulfill their obligations to their patients by assuring that, as when patients choose to accept treatment, patients' refusals are informed and made in accord with their basic values. To accomplish this physicians must assess the bases for patients' refusals, and shape appropriate responses. This reaction to refusal can be viewed as an extension of the process model of informed consent. The mutual monitoring process need not end simply because the patient has turned down a recommendation for treatment.

As self-evident as the need to uncover the motivations for refusal may appear, studies of physicians' responses to patients' refusals suggest that tailored responses are the exception rather than the rule. Clinicians frequently react in the same fashion to patients' refusals. Appelbaum and Roth reported that physicians often attempted to persuade refusing patients to undergo the recommended treatments without first taking the time to ascertain the basis for the patients' refusals (44). This approach reduced physicians to general exhortations to their patients to accept treatment because of its importance to their care, or attempts to address the concerns the physicians thought were on patients' minds rather than those that were really at issue.

The reasons many physicians fail to pursue a more targeted approach to patient refusal are similar to those that generally inhibit physician–patient communication. Doctors are busy and may seek to resolve an unexpected difficulty in the decision process in what seems like the most expeditious way. They may also believe that patients are unlikely to understand detailed explanations and that, as a rule, exhortation is more appropriate than education. And refusal of a physician's recommendations is often taken by the physician as a personal affront (45). Refusal of treatment is seen by physicians as a rejection of the person making the offer, particularly when physicians have made extra efforts on a patient's behalf. As a result, physicians may feel angry, frustrated, and unwilling to explore the underlying basis of refusal.

Any effort to respond meaningfully to patients' refusals must overcome these tendencies and begin with a thorough exploration of the reasons for refusal (44,46,47). The sensitive mutual monitoring envisioned by the process model of informed consent can continue as the refusal provides a focus for the interaction.

Rather than emphasizing disclosure, the process now focuses on clarification of how the situation is seen by the patient. Patients are sometimes initially reluctant to reveal their reasons for refusal, because they feel embarrassed about having inconvenienced their physicians or fearful of some sort of retaliation if their reasons are not good enough. Sometimes patients may even lack a conscious awareness of all the reasons. Physicians need to take the lead in identifying the bases for refusal.

In doing so, physicians ideally should be guided by an understanding of the factors that tend to provoke patients' refusal of treatment. Of particular concern are those considerations that may interfere with the expression of a knowledgeable, autonomous choice. Put somewhat differently, the focus should be on issues that may lead to poorly informed choices or choices that fail to reflect patients' underlying values. The literature on refusal of treatment by medical patients, unfortunately, is heavily weighted with anecdotal papers (46–58). Systematic studies of the issue are rare (44,59). A large number of studies have addressed the problem of treatment refusal by psychiatric patients (reviewed in 27), but their conclusions are not completely transferable to the general medical context. Nonetheless, existing knowledge does offer a starting point for the exploration of patients' refusals.

Research suggests that when patients' refusals are poorly informed, a number of factors interact to that end. The primary cause of poorly informed decision making is the failure of physicians to inform patients about treatments or diagnostic procedures, much less to discuss their purpose, benefits, and risks (44,60). Other studies have shown that physicians consistently underestimate the amount of information patients would like to have before making medical decisions (61–64). Physicians often fail to elicit patients' underlying concerns, thereby making the physicians' failure to respond appropriately to them all but inevitable (65). Patients can also be supplied with too much or too complex information, so that their ability to assimilate it is overwhelmed. Language barriers may impede comprehension (66). Patients may receive conflicting information from one or several sources and end up bewildered about the facts surrounding their care (44,46,67). Physicians may have difficulty in conveying, and patients in understanding, the uncertainty inherent in medical procedures (2, pp. 165–206; 68). The empirical approach—involving trial-and-error efforts at selecting treatment—may be discomfiting for both physicians and patients to talk about.

Some of the difficulties in communication may derive from structural factors within the health-care system. The organization of care in a modern medical center, for example, may require patients to be involved with a large number of physicians and other healthcare workers. Confusion may arise over who really is the person with whom to talk about one's care, conflicting information may be provided, or no information may be offered, if everyone assumes that someone else is taking the responsibility (69). Economic pressures, often translated into productivity requirements, may limit the amount of time physicians feel they can spend in discussion with patients in either the hospital or the office (70).

Clearly, a multiplicity of factors can contribute to poorly informed patients. Not all of the responsibility can be laid at the door of the medical profession. Patients are often exceedingly reluctant to ask questions about information they desire or to seek clarification regarding issues about which they are confused (63,71). In a typical finding, the authors of one study concluded, "Results indicated that, even though patients expressed a strong desire for medical information, they showed little communication behavior designed to elicit this information" (71). Patients' reluctance to ask questions probably relates to deeply imbedded cultural notions of deference to physicians, as well as to reluctance to display ignorance—especially after what the physician appears to consider an adequate disclosure. Physicians' verbal and non-verbal responses to questions may also serve to discourage further inquiries. Nonetheless, some efforts to train patients to be more assertive in acquiring relevant medical information from caregivers have demonstrated success in changing patients' behavior (72,73).

Low levels of comprehension, of course, do not automatically translate into refusals of treatment. Most badly informed patients are more than willing to acquiesce to their physicians' recommendations for care. But poor understanding can lead patients to underestimate benefits of treatment, overemphasize risks, or even misinterpret the nature of their conditions and their likely natural course in the absence of intervention. Patients may be confused about the nature of the diagnostic procedure or treatment being recommended, after having heard it described only in technical terms (e.g., "We recommend performance of an angioplasty with insertion of an intraarterial stent") or in medical slang (e.g., "You'll be on bypass while we do the CABG").

How can physicians ensure that patients' refusals of treatment are not grounded in misunderstanding or misinformation? By monitoring patients' understanding, physicians can craft a redisclosure to focus on these areas of confusion. To pinpoint issues requiring attention, physicians might ask patients, for example, to explain the nature and purpose of the proposed treatment. The extent of patients' knowledge can be further clarified by questioning them about their views of the possible consequences of treatment and of its refusal. Besides uncovering simple misunderstandings, such questions may bring to the surface implicit beliefs about health, illness, and therapy that may lead patients to discount the information they are given (74,75). For example, a patient may believe that surgery on what the physician considers to be a potentially curable cancerous lesion is of no use because the diagnosis of cancer is equivalent to a death sentence that physicians are powerless to change.

Another concern about patient refusal is that it may fail to reflect patients' underlying values. Patients' emotional needs and styles of coping, the stresses of the treatment situation, and, in extreme cases, overt psychopathology can all result in decisions that are non-autonomous, in the sense that they do not reflect patients' value systems (76). Character traits such as rigidity, suspiciousness, ambivalence, or a need to be in control or to demonstrate independence (or conversely, passivity) can lead patients to refuse treatment even if, in the abstract, it is something they would desire (44). The maladaptiveness of these traits, which we all share to some degree, is heightened by the stress of hospitalization with its subtle depersonalization of patients and the threat to life and bodily integrity inherent in serious medical illness. The prospect of surgery, in particular, can produce severe anxiety, as patients confront fears of death, loss of control under anesthesia, and the prospect of unalterable change in their bodies (47).

Actual psychiatric illness, including psychosis, depression, and acute or chronic brain impairment, can exacerbate all of these reactions and lead to a decisionmaking process so compromised as to be considered incompetent. It should be emphasized, however, that refusal is only rarely a manifestation of psychiatric illness, and that psychiatric illness in itself is not sufficient to render patients incompetent (see Chapter 5).

The frequency with which these threats to autonomous decision making arise requires physicians to assess additional aspects of patient refusals. Physicians can inquire about the reasons why and the ways in which patients decided to reject the recommended care. Patients can be asked directly about the factors that entered into their decisions. To persuade patients to speak frankly about their decisionmaking processes, physicians must convey the belief that reasonable patients may actually make decisions that conflict with their physicians' recommendations. Physicians may find it useful to consult with other caregivers, especially nurses, and with family members to uncover limitations on autonomous choice that may not be immediately apparent. Questioning of family members, for example, may reveal that the patient has undergone subtle psychological changes or is unrealistically depressed about the prospect of being a burden to the family.

Responding to Refusal

With the information acquired by assessing patients' reasons for refusal and the influences on them, physicians are in a position to formulate appropriate responses. The initial response will often be simply to accept patients' decisions. If patients are well informed about the treatment options and have made choices that appear largely consistent with their underlying values, they clearly have the right to refuse treatment. Many physicians will have no difficulty accepting patients' decisions in such circumstances. Nonetheless, if the patients' values differ from the physicians' values, some physicians may feel uncomfortable merely acquiescing in the decision.

Patients' values, of course, deserve respect, but it would seem excessive to demand that physicians make no attempt to persuade patients simply because a matter of values is at stake. Indeed, such withdrawal from the dialogue with the patient may represent a failure of respect for the patient as someone who is worth the effort to attempt to convince of one's point of view (77). Physicians ought to be seen as advocates for the value of health, and their efforts to persuade patients of the importance of receiving treatment should be encouraged (see Chapter 8). Although some commonsense stopping point is required at which physicians acknowledge the disparity in underlying values and respect patients' choices, persuasion is a legitimate tool in the practice of medicine and should not be abandoned. If based on a desire to ensure the best possible outcome for the patient, this model of "enhanced autonomy" (77) is likely to be welcomed as a genuine expression of the physician's concern, even by a patient who continues to decline treatment.

Advocacy, however, must not be permitted to turn into coercion. Unfortunately, the line between persuasion and coercion is exceedingly fine, and physicians must be extremely sensitive to overstepping it. Threats to withhold all future care if the patient continues to refuse a recommended treatment are clearly inappropriate. Indeed, because of the prestige that inheres in the physician's position and the desire of patients to please them, physicians must be protective of patients' ultimate right to choose. Once the physician has laid out the basis for the recommendation for treatment, the final decision belongs to the patient.

The effort to persuade the patient is not a one-way process. Patients may be able to alter physicians' perceptions of the best course of treatment for them, and physicians need to remain open to this possibility. Best of all, the two participants may be able to reach a compromise that satisfies all interests. A medication the patient initially refuses, for example, may be started at a lower dose than the physician proposed, with incremental increases dependent on the absence of side effects.

Sometimes, in contrast to this situation, it will be clear that patients are making uninformed decisions. At this point, physicians must reinitiate the effort to educate the patient. A good assessment will have revealed the basis for the patient's lack of understanding and will suggest appropriate corrective measures. Additional information might be provided, the explanation simplified, or other people, such as family members, called in to aid the patient's understanding. All previous suggestions about offering information and monitoring patients' understanding are relevant here (see Chapter 8).

It will also be apparent sometimes that patients are well informed but their decisions do not reflect their own values. For example, to the extent that maladaptive character traits have led patients to become angry with their caregivers and thus reject attention, or that overt psychopathological factors are implicated, consultations with a psychiatrist may be of use. Evidence indicates that such consultations are underutilized in these circumstances, with psychiatrists being called in only when patients are clearly psychotic; their expertise in diagnosing and managing depression and problematic character traits tends to be ignored (44).

Once the problem has been identified, a response can be devised. Alteration of the environment may help. A patient in one study who described herself as a "night owl" consistently refused to have blood drawn when awakened early in the morning, which was the hospital's routine, but agreed to undergo the procedure when it was arranged for the technician to come later in the day (44). Family members may be enlisted to ease patients' anxieties, making it easier for them then to act according to their underlying values. A brief psychotherapeutic intervention may have the same effect. Indeed, for those patients for whom control over their lives is a major issue, a simple acknowledgment of their right to refuse treatment may be precisely what enables them to accept it. This may be what has occurred in several highly publicized cases involving persons with severe physical disabilities who fought prolonged battles to be allowed to die, only to decide in the end not to reject the intervention that was keeping them alive (58,78). The use of neuroleptic medication or the cessation of a medication that is clouding the patient's sensorium may restore decisionmaking capacity. The list of potential responses to impairments either in understanding or in autonomous action can be added to ad infinitum without encompassing all possibilities. The key lies in the individualization of response, which in turn depends on a careful assessment of patients' decision making.

What should physicians' responses be when all efforts at persuasion, education, and removal of obstacles to the expression of underlying values fail? If patients are believed to be incompetent, of course, a substitute decision can be sought either judicially or extrajudicially (see Chapter 5). Physicians should beware of too rapid a resort to the legal process. It can lessen the chance of resolving the situation short of an extended and expensive court proceeding, which can tear apart the fabric of the doctor–patient relationship, and is an unquestionable assault on patient autonomy. The law is a last resort to be reserved for otherwise intractable cases with potentially serious outcomes (e.g., when efforts to restore patient competence have failed and the patient's refusal risks serious disability).

Assuming that the patient is competent, the clinician is faced with two other options: continuing to treat in accord with the patient's wishes (or a negotiated compromise) without using the rejected treatment, or discharging the patient from further care. The latter option should be employed only when the physician is convinced that the refused treatment is absolutely crucial to the patient's care and that there are no alternatives the physician could ethically pursue. These occasions will be rare. When they occur, reasonable efforts must be made to find a physician willing to accept the stated limitations, so the patient will not be abandoned. In some situations, the courts have declined to allow facilities to transfer patients whose desire for care (expressed by patients or their surrogates) is in conflict with the institution's moral principles (79). Indeed, it has been argued that denying treatment to a non-compliant patient, insofar as the patient's behavior may be caused by an underlying psychological disorder, may violate the Americans with Disabilities Act (80). Careful self-scrutiny ought to take place before making a decision to terminate care, to be sure that the decision is based on the absence of other reasonable options and not on the physician's desire to strike back at a frustrating patient.

In some cases, of course, it will be the surrogate decision maker for an incompetent patient who refuses the proposed treatment. The physician's response here begins much as it does with a refusing patient: exploration of the basis for the decision and an attempt to clarify any misperceptions that may be identified. Surrogates who are themselves incompetent are not unheard of. If an incompetent surrogate is suspected, a court can be petitioned for the appointment of an alternate decision maker. Moreover, surrogates' decisions are supposed to be made in accordance with the governing standard in each jurisdiction, as discussed earlier. Should caregivers believe the surrogate is deciding otherwise—to the patient's detriment—recourse to the courts may be appropriate. But this is not a remedy to be pursued lightly, and certainly not simply because the physician or other caregivers disagree with the surrogate's choice.

Conclusion

Patients' refusals are among the most difficult situations physicians must handle. This is especially true if refusal is likely to lead to a patient's demise. Physicians must come to grips with the limits on their authority to order interventions and on their power single-handedly to combat disease and restore health. Even physicians who are generally supportive of the idea of informed consent may balk at its implications when patients refuse care that physicians believe will be highly beneficial. The reality, however, is that no human being is omnipotent. We all must face real limitations on our power to pursue our goals and advance our values. Having done what they can to ensure informed decision making by patients who are refusing treatment, as outlined previously, physicians can do no more. Their moral and legal obligations have been fulfilled. If in consequence patients are not treated precisely the way their physicians would have desired, that is the price we pay as a society for supporting individual freedom of choice.

Informed Consent and Refusal of Treatment

Patients' refusal of treatment is the nub of many physicians' opposition to the idea of informed consent (see Chapter 7). Not particularly resistant to sharing information with patients, these physicians are concerned that the emphasis on patients' choice inherent in the doctrine encourages refusals of treatment. Given physicians' orientation toward the value of health, this outcome seems to them undesirable. In medical terms, it could be considered a side effect of the idea of informed consent.

Theoretically it should be possible to study the effect of the idea of informed consent to treatment on the frequency of patient refusals, but it has not been done. Earlier in the history of informed consent, clinicians from time to time published anecdotal accounts of patients who had been led to refuse treatment, as a result of the information provided them, and the adverse outcomes that resulted (81–83). Such reports have become hard to find these days. Certainly, both the ethical and legal doctrines at the root of the legal requirement of informed consent anticipate that some patients will refuse treatment after receiving appropriate information; one might say that the opportunity to refuse is the point of the whole thing. It cannot be denied that some patients who otherwise would have accepted care might refuse apparently desirable treatment after participating in the process of informing and seeking consent.

On the other hand, and most noteworthy, the empirical and anecdotal studies of patients who refuse treatment almost never portray the process of obtaining informed consent as playing a causative role. The opposite appears to be true. Refusal of treatment and more subtle forms of non-compliance repeatedly have been linked to patients' being inadequately, not overly, informed. In other words, it is *failure* to live up to the idea of informed consent that has been shown to precipitate refusal of treatment (84). Physicians who neglect the careful discussion of treatment options, including their nature, purpose, risks, and benefits, seem much more likely to have patients overtly or covertly refuse their recommendations for care than their colleagues who adhere more closely to the idea of informed consent.

Of course, merely providing adequate information does not ensure that patients will accept treatment or that their decisions will be reasonable. As noted before, a refusal that is ill informed or in conflict with a patient's underlying values usually has complex antecedents. A patient's fear of surgery may combine with pressure from family members who distrust physicians to make it more likely that information that leaves the patient confused about the purpose of the procedure will result in refusal. Although each factor by itself might not have led to refusal, taken as a group they do. The prevention of poorly informed or non-autonomous refusal does not require that all the precipitating factors be dealt with. Removal of one may be sufficient to help the patient to make a better informed and more genuine choice. Of all the problems likely to be involved in these cases, the provision of information is the one most under physicians' control and thus easiest for them to remedy. If the dilemmas raised by ill-informed, non-autonomous refusal are to be addressed anywhere, the process must begin here.

Informed consent does indeed have a relation to refusal of treatment, but not the expected one. Rather than acting most commonly as a stimulus to refusing treatment, informed consent—particularly in the process model (see Chapter 8)—may actually serve a preventive function. Our present knowledge suggests that well-informed patients are less likely to refuse treatment than those who are poorly informed. Patients for whom the process of mutual monitoring has been successful—that is, whose physicians are aware of their beliefs, values, and attitudes toward treatment, and who in turn are cognizant of their physicians' beliefs, values, and attitudes—will rarely get to the point of using refusal as a weapon. If they do not wish to follow their physicians' recommendations and cannot negotiate an alternative, they may reject the treatment offered, but usually this will be done in the context of an ongoing physician–patient relationship. These facts should serve to reassure clinicians who may have tended to see informed consent as an alien construct imposed on them by the law and working to the detriment of patient care, rather than as a natural extension of the sensitive clinician's desire to build a working relationship with her patients.

References

1. Appelbaum, P.S. and Roth, L.H. (1984) Involuntary treatment in medicine and psychiatry. *Am J Psychiatry,* 141:202–205.
2. Katz, J. (1984) *The Silent World of Doctor and Patient.* New York: Free Press.
3. Meisel, A. (1998) *Legal aspects of end-of-life decision making.* In Steinberg, M.D., Youngner, S.J. (eds) *End-of-Life Decisions: A Psychosocial Perspective.* Washington, D.C.: American Psychiatric Press.
4. In re Conroy, 486 A.2d 1209 (N.J. 1985).
5. Norwood Hospital v. Munoz, 564 N.E.2d 1017 (Mass. 1991).
6. Cruzan v. Director, Missouri Department of Health, 497 U.S. 261 (1990).
7. Nelson, L.J. and Milliken, N. (1988) Compelled medical treatment of pregnant women: life, liberty, and law in conflict. *JAMA,* 259:1060–1066.
8. In re President & Directors of Georgetown College, Inc., 331 F.2d 1000 (D.C. Cir. 1964).
9. Raleigh Fitkin-Paul Morgan Memorial Hospital v. Anderson, 201 A.2d 537 (N.J. 1964).
10. Meisel, A. (1992) A retrospective on Cruzan. *Law Med Health Care,* 20:340–353.
11. In re Conroy, 464 A.2d 303 (App. Div. 1983).
12. Kolder, V.E.B., Gallagher, J., and Parson, M.T. (1987) Court-ordered obstetrical interventions. *N Engl J Med,* 316:1192–1196.
13. In re A.C., 573 A.2d 1235 (D.C. 1990).
14. Levy, J.K. (1999) Jehovah's Witnesses, pregnancy, and blood transfusions: a paradigm for the autonomy rights of all pregnant women. *J Law Med Ethics,* 27:171–189.
15. John F. Kennedy Memorial Hospital v. Heston, 279 A.2d 670 (N.J. 1971).
16. Application of Winthrop University Hospital, 490 N.Y.S.2d 996 (N.Y. Sup. Ct. 1985).
17. Fosmire v. Nicoleau, 551 N.E.2d 77 (N.Y. 1990).
18. Stamford Hospital v. Vega, 674 A.2d 821 (Conn. 1996).
19. In the Matter of Dubreil, 629 So.2d 819 (Fla. 1993).
20. Public Health Trust of Dade County v. Wons, 541 So.2d 96 (Fla. 1989).

21. Satz v. Perlmutter, 362 So.2d 160 (Fla. Dist. Ct. App. 1978).
22. Bouvia v. Superior Court, 225 Cal. Rptr. 297 (Ct. App. 1986).
23. State v. McAfee, 385 S.E.2d 651 (Ga. 1989).
24. McKay v. Bergstedt, 801 P.2d 617 (Nev. 1990).
25. Thor v. Superior Court, 855 P.2d 375 (Cal. 1993).
26. Superintendent of Belchertown State School v. Saikewicz, 370 N.E.2d 417 (Mass. 1977).
27. Appelbaum, P.S. (1994) *Almost a Revolution: Mental Health Law and the Limits of Change.* New York: Oxford University Press.
28. Winick, B. (1997) *The Right to Refuse Mental Health Treatment.* Washington, D.C.: American Psychological Association.
29. Appelbaum, P.S. (1988) The right to refuse treatment with antipsychotic medications: retrospect and prospect. *Am J Psychiatry,* 145:413–419.
30. Rogers v. Commissioner, Department of Mental Health, 458 N.E.2d 308 (Mass. 1983).
31. Rennie v. Klein, 462 F.Supp. 1131 (D.N.J. 1978).
32. Washington v. Harper, 110 S.Ct. 1028 (1990).
33. In re Quinlan, 355 A.2d 647 (N.J. 1976).
34. Meisel, A. (1995) *The Right to Die,* 2nd ed. New York: John Wiley & Sons.
35. In re Storar, 420 N.E.2d 64 (N.Y. 1981).
36. Martin v. Martin, 538 N.W.2d 399 (Mich. 1995).
37. Weir, R.F. and Gostin, L. (1990) Decisions to abate life-sustaining treatment for nonautonomous patients: ethical standards and legal liability after Cruzan. *JAMA,* 264:1846–1853.
38. In re Green, 292 A.2d 387 (Pa. 1972).
39. Matter of Seiferth, 127 N.E.2d 820 (N.Y. 1955).
40. Matter of Sampson, 317 N.Y.S.2d 641 (Family Ct. 1970).
41. Commonwealth v. Twitchell, 617 N.E.2d 609 (Mass. 1993).
42. May, L. (1995) Challenging medical authority: the refusal of treatment by Christian Scientists. *Hastings Cent Rep,* 25(1):15–21.
43. Levinson, W., Stiles, W.B., Inui, T.S., and Engle, R. (1993) Physician frustration in communicating with patients. *Med Care,* 31:285–295.
44. Appelbaum, P.S., and Roth, L.H. (1982) Treatment refusal in medical hospitals. In President's Commission for the Study of Ethical Problems in Medicine and Bio-medical and Behavioral Research, *Making Health Care Decisions: The Ethical and Legal Implications of Informed Consent in the Patient-Practitioner Relationship.* Volume 2, Appendices. Washington, D.C.: U.S. Government Printing Office; summarized in Appelbaum, P.S. and Roth, L.H. (1983) Patients who refuse treatment in medical hospitals. *JAMA,* 250:1296–1301.
45. Mester, R. (1972) Psychiatrists' reactions to their patients' refusal of drugs. *Isr Ann Psychiatry and Relat Disciplines,* 10:373–381.
46. Himmelhoch, J., Davis, N., Tucker, G., et al. (1970) Butting heads: patients who refuse necessary procedures. *Psychiatry Med,* 1:241–249.
47. Scully, J.H. (1982) *Psychiatric Problems in Primary Practice, No. 3: Psychiatric Problems in Surgery* (pamphlet). Manati, Puerto Rico: Roche Products Inc.
48. McCartney, J.R. (1979) Refusal of treatment: suicide or competent choice? *Gen Hosp Psychiatry,* 4:338–343.
49. Goldberg, R.J. (1983) Systematic understanding of cancer patients who refuse treatment. *Psychother Psychosom,* 39:180–189.

50. Lansky, S.B., Vats, T., and Cairns, N.V. (1979) Refusal of treatment: a new dilemma for oncologists. *Am J Psychiatr Hemat/Oncol,* 1:277–282.
51. Hershkowitz, M. (1984) To die at home: rejection of medical intervention by geriatric patients who had serious organic disease. *J Am Geriatr Soc,* 32:457–459.
52. Cohen, M.A.A. and Dronska, H. (1988) Treatment refusal in a rootless individual with medical problems. *Gen Hosp Psychiatry,* 10:61–66.
53. Diamond, D.B. (1988) Psychologic conflict underlying bioethical dilemmas in a chronic disease hospital: empathy, treatment refusal, and the role of the consulting psychiatrist. *Gen Hosp Psychiatry,* 10:250–254.
54. Schindler, B.A., Blum, D., and Malone, R. (1988) Noncompliance in the treatment of endocarditis: the medical staff as co-conspirators. *Gen Hosp Psychiatry,* 10:197–201.
55. Dresner, N., Raskin, V., and Goldman, L.S. (1990) Medical psychiatric grand rounds on an obstetrics-gynecology service: refusing to terminate a life-threatening pregnancy. *Gen Hosp Psychiatry,* 12:335–340.
56. Wear, A.N. and Brahams, D. (1991) To treat or not to treat: the legal, ethical and therapeutic implications of treatment refusal. *J Med Ethics,* 17:131–135.
57. Kleinman, I. (1991) The right to refuse treatment: ethical considerations for the competent patient. *Can Med Assoc J,* 144:1219–1222.
58. Herr, S.S., Bostrom, B.A., and Barton, R.S. (1992) No place to go: refusal of life-sustaining treatment by competent persons with physical disabilities. *Issues Law Med,* 8:3–36.
59. Barry, P.P., Crescenzi, C.A., Radovsky, L., Kern, D.C., and Steel, K. (1988) Why elderly patients refuse hospitalization. *J Am Geriatr Soc,* 36:419–424.
60. Lidz, C.W. and Meisel, A. (1982) Informed consent and the structure of medical care. In President's Commission for the Study of Ethical Problems in Medicine and Biomedical and Behavioral Research, *Making Health Care Decisions: The Ethical and Legal Implications of Informed Consent in the Patient-Practitioner Relationship.* Volume 2, Appendices. Washington, D.C.: U.S. Government Printing Office.
61. Harris, L., et al. (1982) Views of informed consent and decisionmaking: parallel surveys of physicians and the public. In President's Commission for the Study of Ethical Problems in Medicine and Biomedical and Behavioral Research, *Making Health Care Decisions: The Ethical and Legal Implications of Informed Consent in the Patient-Practitioner Relationship.* Volume 2, Appendices. Washington, D.C.: U.S. Government Printing Office.
62. Strull, W.M., Lo, B., and Charles, G. (1984) Do patients want to participate in medical decisionmaking? *JAMA,* 252:2990–2994.
63. Shapiro, M.C., Najman, J.M., Chang, A., Keeping, J.D., Morrison, J., and Western, J.S. (1983) Information control and the exercise of power in the obstetrical encounter. *Soc Sci Med,* 17:139–146.
64. Waitzkin, H. (1984) Doctor-patient communication: clinical implications of social scientific research. *JAMA,* 252:2441–2446.
65. Marvel, M.K., Epstein, R.M., Flowers, K., and Beckman, H.B. (1999) Soliciting the patient's agenda: have we improved? *JAMA,* 281:283–287.
66. Woloshin, S., Bickell, N.A., Schwartz, L.M., Gary, F., and Welch, H.G. (1995) Language barriers in medicine in the United States. *JAMA,* 273:724–728.
67. Kravitz, R.L., Callahan, E.J., Paterniti, D., Antonius, D., Dunham, M., and Lewis, C.E. (1996) Prevalence and sources of patients' unmet expectations for care. *Ann Intern Med,* 125:730–737.
68. Bursztajn, H., Feinbloom, R.I., Hamm, R.M., et al. (1981) *Medical Choices, Medical*

Chances: How Patients, Families, and Physicians Can Cope with Uncertainty. New York: Delacorte Press.

69. Lidz, C., Meisel, A., Zerubavel, E., et al. (1984) *Informed Consent: A Study of Decisionmaking in Psychiatry.* New York: Guilford.

70. Kaplan, S.H., Greenfield, S., Gandek, B., Rogers, W.H., and Ware, J.E. (1996) Characteristics of physicians with participatory decision-making styles. *Ann Intern Med,* 124:497–504.

71. Biesecker, A.E. and Biesecker, T.D. (1990) Patient information-seeking behaviors when communicating with doctors. *Med Care,* 28:19–28.

72. Roter, D.L. (1977) Patient participation in the patient-provider interaction. *Health Educ Monogr,* 5:281–315.

73. Greenfield, S., Kaplan, S., and Ware, J.E. (1985) Expanding patient involvement in care. *Ann Intern Med,* 102:520–528.

74. Stimson, G.V. (1974) Obeying doctor's orders: a view from the other side. *Soc Sci Med,* 8:97–104.

75. Becker, M.H. (ed) (1974) *The Health Belief Model and Personal Health Behavior.* Thorofare, N.J.: Charles B. Black.

76. Miller, B.L. (1981) Autonomy and the refusal of lifesaving treatment. *Hastings Cent Rep,* 11(4):22–28.

77. Quill, T.E. and Brody, H. (1996) Physician recommendations and patient autonomy: finding a balance between power and patient choice. *Ann Intern Med,* 125:763–769.

78. Applebome, P. (1990) An angry man fights to die, then tests life. *New York Times,* February 7, 1990, p. A-1.

79. Miles, S.H., Singer, P.A., and Siegler, M. (1989) Conflicts between patients' wishes to forgo treatment and the policies of healthcare facilities. *N Engl J Med,* 321:48–50.

80. Orentlicher, D (1991) Denying treatment to the noncompliant patient. *JAMA,* 265:1579–1582.

81. Katz, R.L. (1977) Informed consent—is it bad medicine? *West J Med,* 126:426–428.

82. Patten, B.M. and Stump, W. (1978) Death related to informed consent. *Tex Med,* 74:49–50.

83. Kaplan, S.R., Greenwald, R.A., and Rogers, A.J. (1977) Neglected aspects of informed consent. *N Engl J Med,* 296:1127.

84. Roter, D.L. and Hall, J.A. (1989) Studies of doctor-patient interaction. *Annu Rev Public Health,* 10:163–180.

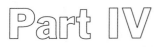

Part IV

Consent to Research

12

The Independent Evolution of Informed Consent to Research

Despite apparent similarities in the issues raised, informed consent in the research setting has evolved quite separately from informed consent to treatment. Consent to treatment is largely a creature of case law, with some subsequent statutory modification. Consent to research has been shaped by professional codes, statutes, and administrative regulations, with the courts playing a less important role.

Systematic medical research, of course, is a newer phenomenon than medical treatment. The eighteenth century saw some of the first efforts to demonstrate the etiology of diseases. One was Lind's controlled study of the effects of citrus juices in preventing scurvy (1). Pierre Louis's classic study, in the 1820s, of the efficacy of bloodletting as a treatment for pneumonia demonstrated the potential of clinical investigation, but his medical colleagues were slow to follow his lead (2). By the turn of the century, the pace of experimentation with human subjects was quickening. The etiologies of beriberi and pellagra, for example, were discovered using human volunteers.

In the early years of systematic medical investigation, only sporadic attention was paid to the circumstances under which research should be carried out, including the issue of consent. There are a few statements from leading physicians of the time, such as Paul Ehrlich and William Osler, endorsing the disclosure of information about the risks and benefits of experimental treatment. After a public scandal in Prussia in the 1890s, involving experimentation on unsuspecting patients who were inoculated with the spirochete that causes syphilis, the Prussian government required consent for any further research with human subjects (3). Shortly thereafter, Walter Reed, conducting his famous experiments in Cuba on yellow fever, developed a contract—very much like the modern consent form—for his volunteers to sign, which included a discussion of the risks they would be running (3). Public concern in Germany culminated in the 1931 promulgation of guidelines that required clear explanations of innovative or experimental treatments (4). Interestingly, this pre–war German code of ethics, which addressed human experimentation, was, in some ways, more extensive in its protections and principles than either the post–war Nuremberg Code or Helsinki Declaration (5). But the retrospective accounts of physician-investigators who were active at the time make clear that obtaining consent was simply not part of the everyday conduct of research in any part of the world (6).

Over the last fifty years, inspired by ethical concerns that human subjects not be abused, informed consent requirements have become fully applicable to biomedical research, including research performed in the context of clinical care where benefit to the individual patient may be forthcoming while new generalizable knowledge is generated. Almost "all contemporary debate on human experimentation is grounded in Nuremberg"(7, p. 3), and therefore the Nuremberg Code provides an appropriate starting point for evaluating the historical background of human experimentation in the United States. The code arose out of the prosecution of Nazi physicians during the Nuremberg War Crimes Trials of the 1940s—the so-called Doctors Trial. The physicians and scientists who took an active role in the Nazi racial extermination programs were charged with "murder, tortures and other atrocities committed in the name of medical science" (8, p. 67). Their "experiments" included the exposure of inmates to cold water or low air pressure to observe the events that would lead to their deaths, mass sterilization of inmates by irradiating their gonads, and injection of typhus and other pathogens in order to study the disease (9). The horrors that were perpetrated by, as one author notes, "men with white coats in SS boots," seemed somehow all the more horrific because of the involvement of physicians (10, p. 70). In fact, it was the legitimacy that this involvement lent to Adolf Hitler's "final solution" that prompted the Nuremberg tribunal to develop guidelines for biomedical research in order to prevent future abuses. The military judges at Nuremberg, outraged by the studies (which seemed to them to cross the line between experimentation and torture), asked the expert witnesses—most notably the American physicians Andrew Ivy and Leo Alexander—to articulate the universal standard of ethical research practices from which the Nazi experimenters had deviated.

Ivy obtained the endorsement of the American Medical Association for three basic principles of human experimentation: "1) The voluntary consent of the person on whom the experiment is to be performed must be obtained, 2) The danger of each experiment must have been investigated previously by means of animal experimentation, and 3) The experiment must be performed under proper medical protection and management" (11, p. 142). With considerable modification and elaboration by the judges of the Nuremberg tribunal, these standards were incorporated in the court's final judgment against the Nazi physicians in the case of *United States v. Karl Brandt* (12). The resulting document has come to be known as the Nuremberg Code.

Central to the Nuremberg Code is the concept of subject consent. Two of the ten sections of the code deal with informed consent; the remaining eight sections establish limits on the power of researchers to inflict harm on subjects in the name of science. The first section begins with the following assertion:

> The voluntary consent of the human subject is absolutely essential. This means that the person involved should have legal capacity to give consent; should be so situated as to be able to exercise free power of choice, without the intervention of any element of force, fraud, deceit, duress, overreaching, or other ulterior form of constraint or coercion; and should have sufficient knowledge and comprehension of the elements of the subject matter involved so as to enable him to make an understanding and enlightened decision. This latter element requires that before the acceptance of an affirmative decision by the experimental subject there should be made known to him the nature, duration, and purpose of the experiment; the method and means by which it is to be conducted; all inconveniences and hazards reasonably to be expected; and the effects upon his health or person which may possibly come from his participation in the experiment. (13)

Thus stated, the code not only requires subject consent but also maintains that the consent be voluntary, competent and informed. Moreover, the code mandates the provision of certain information, including a description of the nature, duration, and purpose of the experiment, and the risks of participation. In addition, it states that the subject has the right to terminate participation "if he has reached the physical or mental state where continuation of the experiment seems to him to be impossible." It is these fundamental requirements that form the basis of later regulation of biomedical research.

However, the code had a number of shortcomings. First, the language employed failed to allow for research with those subjects who lack legal capacity to consent. Thus, research involving incompetent persons (i.e., children or adults with cognitive impairments that affect their capacity to make decisions) appeared to be impermissible. The restriction may be inadvertent and due to the particular victims involved in the Nuremberg case. Since many of the concentration camp prisoners were competent adults, the tribunal was concerned primarily with ensuring voluntary consent (5). In fact, this focus on preventing coercion can be seen in the present Department of Health and Human Services (HHS) regulations regarding research conducted with prison populations (see later under *Prisoners*). Moreover, there is some evidence that the code was intended to address only the "pure" research context, not research that has the potential to provide a direct therapeutic benefit to the subject. If so, the apparent prohibition on proxy consent is more understandable (14).

A second and more important problem was that the code lacked enforceability. The Nuremberg tribunal, casting about for a principled basis on which to condemn intuitively repugnant behavior, mistook the aspirations of a few leaders of medicine with regard to disclosure and consent for the practices of the vast majority of researchers (1). Although they were endorsed by a number of members of the medical community, the code's precepts did not reflect the common practice of researchers at the time. Even viewed as a statement of an ideal, the Nuremberg Code had limited immediate impact on worldwide research practices. As a decision of a court whose jurisdiction (to prosecute war crimes, not to issue proclamations regarding medical experimentation) arose sui generis, the code was not enforceable under the law of individual nations.

As various nations struggled with the problem of regulating medical research, the World Medical Association took steps to issue guidelines that attempted to remedy some of the concerns about the Nuremberg Code. The 1964 Helsinki Declaration responded to the medical profession's objections to an unqualified consent requirement and allowed for proxy consent or even a complete waiver of consent if in the subject's best interest (15). By distinguishing between "nontherapeutic clinical research"—for which consent must be obtained—and "clinical research combined with patient care"—for which physicians should try to obtain consent but only if in the patient's best interest, the declaration left considerable room for researchers to decide that they need not obtain consent in a particular case. For non-therapeutic research, however, the declaration made it clear that the subject must be fully informed (i.e., the nature, purpose, and risks of the research must be explained) and competent (but guardians could function as proxy decision makers for incompetent patients), and that the consent must be freely given and in writing.

In some respects the Helsinki Declaration went too far in the opposite direction from the Nuremberg Code. Instead of a hard and fast rule that the subject's consent must be obtained in all cases, the Helsinki Declaration appeared to allow physicians discretion to forgo consent under a number of circumstances. A comparison of the Nuremberg and Helskinki documents illustrates the competing interests of protecting individual rights versus accommodating the need for scientific progress and experimentation. Courts, which are concerned primarily with remedying individual harms, tend to focus almost exclusively on the former. Medical organizations, without ignoring the need for individual protections, are understandably concerned with the latter. Neither, alone, is an appropriate forum in which to shape the requirements for informed consent.

The second through fourth revisions of the Declaration of Helsinki expanded upon the principles articulated in the first document, but maintained the distinction between clinical and non-clinical research, thereby allowing physicians to circumvent consent requirements in the clinical situation (16).[1] Paradoxically, by permitting consent to be forgone in "clinical research combined with patient care," the declaration endorsed a standard that fell below the historic common law standard for consent to treatment. This oddity highlights the distinct and often disparate development of the regulation of consent to research versus development of the law relating to consent to treatment.

Had cases of abuse in research made their way through the courts, the rules governing treatment and research would probably have been more similar. The pre-1964 case law is all but barren of suits involving actual research settings. The small number of cases from the nineteenth century involved unique treatment approaches formulated by the defendants and directed at improving a particular patient's situation, not at the systematic acquisition of generalizable knowledge for the benefit of others (17). The decisions in many of these cases discouraged the idea of innovation by holding physicians closely to prevailing standards of care, from which they deviated at their own risk. A New York court in 1871, for example, stated, "Any deviation from the established mode or practice shall be deemed sufficient to charge the surgeon with negligence, in the case of an injury arising to the patient" (18). Later cases were a bit more hospitable to innovation but required patient knowledge of and consent to the novel practice. "We recognize the fact that, if the general practice of medicine and surgery is to progress," wrote the Michigan Supreme Court in 1935, "there must be a certain amount of experimentation carried on; but such experiments must be done with the knowledge and consent of the patient or those responsible for him, and must not vary too radically from the accepted method of procedure" (19). Still, despite their language, this case and the cases that followed dealt with innovation (or what is sometimes termed "experimental treatment") and not with the conduct of systematic research.

By the early 1960s, non-binding codes were almost everywhere the sole means of regulating research. Their provisions concerning informed consent varied substantially. Although the codes themselves were often unenforceable, they set the stage for the extensive statutory and administrative regulation that was to ensue.

The United States took the lead in the development of administrative regulations. The antecedents date to the opening of the Clinical Center of the National Institutes of Health (NIH) in 1953, when loose guidelines were formulated for subject consent (20). (The independent evolution of rules, intermittently enforced, governing human subjects research in the United States military is well described by Moreno [3].) Since it was believed that experimental procedures used with patients should not be subject to regulation, lest the doctor–patient

---

[1]The fifth revision of the Declaration, adopted in October 2000, establishes basic principles for all medical research, and no longer distinguishes between different types of research with respect to informed consent requirements.

relationship be impaired, the application of the guidelines was limited to volunteers without physical illnesses. Even for this group, written consent was required only when there was a possibility of an unusual hazard (21). Research funded by NIH but conducted by researchers elsewhere in the country remained free of regulation; researchers were "to be guided by their own professional judgment and controlled by their own ethical standards as well as those of their institution" (22, p. 409).

The amount of extramural research funded by the NIH grew, and it awarded a contract in 1960 for a study of ad hoc procedures for the regulation of research in major medical centers around the country. Fifty-two departments of medicine responded to a questionnaire. Only nine had procedural documents to guide their investigators in the ethical design and implementation of research protocols. Five others said they were planning to develop guidelines or favored doing so. Only two of the existing documents covered all clinical research being performed in the institution. Twenty-two departments had committees that reviewed the protocols being implemented in their institutions, but none became involved in questions concerning the recruitment of subjects (22).

In 1962, the same year the survey was performed, a congressional committee was conducting hearings to review the regulatory procedures of the Food and Drug Administration (FDA), the agency responsible for monitoring the testing of new medications in the United States. The hearings were already under way when the news broke of a large number of congenital deformities caused in Europe by the drug thalidomide. In response to public concerns generated by the thalidomide tragedy, Congress enacted the Drug Amendments of 1962 (22). The new law tightened controls on the approval process for new medication in the United States. It also required, in clinical trials of new drugs, that subjects be informed of the investigative purpose for which the medications were being used, and that their consent be obtained (23). A large loophole was created by permitting researchers to dispense with consent "where they deem it not feasible or, in their professional judgment, contrary to the best interest of such human beings." Although an FDA official indicated that the agency intended to interpret the exceptions in the statute narrowly, the FDA itself did not tighten its regulations until 1966, when it elaborated on the consent requirement, drawing heavily on language in the Nuremberg Code and Helsinki Declaration (23,24).

Meanwhile, NIH had formed an internal study group to devise a uniform policy on the regulation of experimentation. In 1966 the Public Health Service, parent body of NIH, issued a brief statement of policy on both intramural and extramural research programs funded by NIH (20). Grant recipients were required to

> provide prior review of the judgment of the principal investigator or program director by a committee of his institutional associates. This review should assure an inde-

pendent determination: 1) of the rights and welfare of the individual or individuals involved, 2) of the appropriateness of the methods used to secure informed consent, and 3) of the risks and potential medical benefits of the investigation. (20, p. 52)

With this step, the federal government cast the mold for all subsequent regulation of the research process. From this point on, regulation provided for a decentralized, institution-based, prospective review of research, with informed consent explicitly required as part of the process of subject recruitment. The Public Health Service regulations, extended to encompass all research funded by the Department of Health, Education, and Welfare, were modified on several occasions, with required procedures growing steadily more complex.

Much of the pressure to expand the regulations came from continuing revelations about unethical research practices. In 1963 it was revealed that investigators at the Jewish Chronic Diseases Hospital in Brooklyn, New York, had injected live cancer cells into elderly patients without their knowledge or consent (25). The investigators had reasoned that the procedure involved little or no risk and that informing the subjects would likely frighten them. In a 1966 article Henry Beecher chronicled twenty-two human subject experiments that involved ethically unacceptable or questionable procedures, including the failure to obtain informed consent from the subjects (26). One case in particular raised a number of concerns. It involved the deliberate injection of viral hepatitis into developmentally disabled children at the Willowbrook State School in New York. Waiting lists for the school were long, and parents were promised admission in exchange for their consent to their children's participation in the experiment. In addition to the coercive aspects of the exchange, parents were not given a full disclosure of the risks involved and, in fact, were often misled as to the nature of the experiment. Following Beecher's documentation of unethical research, a number of other abuses in medical experimentation came to light. One of these was the 1971 discovery of the syphilis observation experiments at the Tuskeegee Institute in Alabama (27). Although the experiment began in the early 1930s, it continued into the 1970s, at least twenty years after penicillin became the accepted treatment for syphilis. Approximately 400 African-American men were studied during the time period, none of whom were told about the study, nor informed about possible treatments for the disease. In another revelation, the U.S. Army acknowledged in 1975 that they had given unwitting civilians hallucinogenic compounds in order to observe their psychological reactions. At least one of the subjects had died (28). Of particular concern was the use of vulnerable populations: developmentally disabled children, elderly persons, and members of disadvantaged minority groups. Even if these individuals had been asked to consent, there was concern that either inability to understand or coercive pressures would have rendered their consent invalid.

In 1978 the National Commission for the Protection of Human Subjects of

Biomedical and Behavioral Research published the Belmont Report. The commission identified three ethical principles that should govern human subject research—respect for persons, beneficence, and justice. Among other things, the commission addressed the issue of informed consent and noted the possibility of research involving "subjects that one might consider as incompetent" (29, p. 13).[2] Without specifying particular guidelines for proxy consent, the report stressed that each group should be evaluated separately, and that a subject's wishes should be taken into account to the greatest extent possible. In addition, a third party should be appointed to act on behalf of the subject and thus substitute his consent for that of the subject's. The report advocated the use of a reasonable person standard of information disclosure and reiterated the role of Institutional Review Boards (IRBs) in ensuring that "sufficient information will be disclosed" to the subjects (29, p. 11). Moreover, it stressed that investigators should avoid the use of vulnerable subjects when possible and that research involving unreasonable risks should not be conducted.

Current Regulation

In 1991 HHS issued revised regulations endorsed by almost all Federal Departments funding human subjects' research—the so-called Common Rule. Subjects (or their legally authorized representatives) must give "legally effective informed consent" (30). There are eight basic elements of information that must be provided to either the patient or the patient's legally authorized representative: (1) a statement that the study involves research, as well as a description of the research and its purposes; (2) a description of reasonably foreseeable risks; (3) a description of reasonably expected benefits; (4) disclosure of appropriate alternatives; (5) a statement about maintenance of confidentiality; (6) for research involving more than minimal risks, an explanation about possible compensation if injury occurs; (7) information about how the subject can have pertinent questions answered; and (8) a statement that participation is voluntary (i.e., that refusal to participate involves no penalties or loss of benefits). The regulations also state that appropriate subjects should be given information regarding: (1) unforeseeable risks; (2) circumstances under which the subject's participation will be terminated; (3) additional costs that the subject may incur; (4) the consequences of a subject's decision to withdraw; (5) the dissemination of findings developed during the study that relate to a subject's willingness to continue (31); and (6) the approximate number of total subjects (30). The consent must be documented in writing and must be signed by the subject or the subject's legally authorized representative (30, §50.27; 32). Institutional Review Boards (IRBs) are given pri-

[2]The list included "infants and young children, mentally disabled patients, the terminally ill and the comatose."

mary responsibility for assuring research oversight, including evaluation of the scientific merit of the research, whether the risks and benefits balance out in favor of enrolling human subjects, and whether legally effective informed consent could and would be obtained. A separate section of the Code of Federal Regulations addresses research that is subject to oversight by the Food and Drug Administration (FDA) (32). It sets forth the same general elements of informed consent as stated previously and applies to all research subject to regulation by the FDA, as well as "clinical investigations that support applications for research or marketing permits for products regulated by the FDA"(32, §50.1(a)).

The power of the FDA and HHS, as administrative agencies, to regulate biomedical research differs fundamentally from the power of a court (e.g., the Nuremberg tribunal) or the various medical associations that have developed ethical guidelines. Since HHS's authority derives from its oversight of the monies it controls, the regulations focus on institutions that receive funding, rather than on individual investigators. The Common Rule applies to "all research involving human subjects conducted, supported or otherwise subject to regulation by any federal department or agency" [30, § 46.101 (a)]. Likewise, the FDA regulations target companies whose investigational drugs or devices are subject to agency approval. In effect, all federally funded research, as well as all research involving the development of new pharmacologic agents and medical devices, is covered. The regulations also state that the institution engaged in research must provide "a statement of principles governing . . . the discharge of its responsibilities for protecting the rights and welfare of human subjects . . . regardless of whether the research is subject to federal regulations" [(30, §103(b)(1)]. Since most major research institutions obtain some general federal funding (and therefore must comply with the HHS regulations), the result of this requirement is that almost all research at those institutions, even research that is not directly funded by the federal government, is subject to some oversight. Many institutions not originally covered have voluntarily adopted the HHS regulations; moreover, some states have enacted regulations that are similar to the federal requirements, thus broadening the scope of their impact (33).

Still there are many venues in which biomedical research occurs that are not subject to the federal regulatory scheme. The shift of many clinical trials to private practice settings has undoubtedly magnified this problem. There are no data on the volume of such research, nor data on what measures, if any, such settings have adopted voluntarily for the protection of human subjects. In 1997 a bill was presented to Congress that would have made all publicly and privately funded research subject to federal regulation and make investigators who violated the bill subject to criminal penalties (34). The bill was not passed, and its constitutionality is unclear. Moreover, its passage would not necessarily have assured protection for research subjects, since even in institutions currently covered by the federal regulations, the possibility exists for covert research—research that the investigator does not submit for review by the IRB and that does not otherwise come to its attention.

The Regulatory Approach

The most important conceptual difference between the regulation of consent in research and treatment settings is that consent to research is reviewed prospectively, while consent to treatment is ordinarily subject only to retrospective review, if reviewed at all. These differing approaches are a reflection of the origins of regulation in these areas. The very fact that consent to treatment has been left to judicial control, while consent to research is regulated by administrative bodies, points to the fundamental distinctions between the treatment and research processes (35). In the treatment setting, physician, patient, and society share a consensus about the overall goal—promoting the patient's health—and conflicts that arise usually turn on the question of whether the goal was pursued in the most appropriate way. Patients may charge, for example, that physicians undertook the task of diagnosis and treatment negligently, or that in their therapeutic zeal they failed sufficiently to respect patient autonomy. By granting patients access to the courts for independent review of their care, society provides a means of compensating patients who have suffered harms resulting from negligent practices, and of deterring physicians from engaging in such practices. The general confluence of patients' and physicians' goals and the relative rarity of conflicts lend themselves to a system with minimal oversight and selective retrospective review.

In the research setting, things are somewhat different. Researcher and subject may share some goals—for example, the advancement of knowledge—but are likely to be in conflict with respect to others. Subjects of clinical research (in which treatment is provided) will naturally be concerned about receiving optimal care for their conditions. Their physicians must balance the desire to treat optimally with the need to maintain a valid experimental situation (36,37). Subjects of non-clinical research (in which no treatment is provided, or in which there is no potential for direct therapeutic benefit) will have a natural interest in avoiding harm. Although researchers will generally share that goal, they may be somewhat more inclined than subjects to take risks in order to generate desired data.

The conflicts between researchers' interests and those of their subjects have been firmly in the public mind since Nuremberg. Indeed, the horror stories of researchers' failing to resolve the conflicts to their subjects' benefit have given continued impetus to regulation. This perception of real conflicts of interest in the research setting has stimulated more rigorous review than is found in the treatment setting. Prospective oversight of all research evolved primarily to prevent exploitation of research subjects.

There are obvious advantages and disadvantages to the prospective approach.

As noted, prospective review can be effective in preventing harms, without excluding the possibility of compensation should harm occur. Such review also provides some control over researchers who might not alter undesirable practices merely because of the remote possibility of a lawsuit for damages. Furthermore, prospective review permits the rapid formulation of a body of coherent rules, while retrospective review is limited to consideration of the particular circumstances presented by the case at hand.

However, universal prospective review does have substantial costs, including the cost of the personnel required to carry out the review and the valuable time lost awaiting approval. Another possible cost is that the complacent assumption may be engendered that the goals, design, and methods of conducting the research and obtaining informed consent from prospective subjects—once approved—are unimpeachably in accord with ethical principles. For example, there is a growing body of literature suggesting that in the review process IRBs focus primarily on the content of consent forms and pay little attention to numerous other aspects of research that affect its overall conformance with ethical norms (38,39).

Institutional Review Boards

Although a regulatory approach allows much more precise specification of controls on consent than an approach that relies heavily on case law, the decentralized review system and the absence of an appellate body do not provide a formal mechanism to distribute information among review boards and to establish precedent in the resolution of difficult cases (40). There has been some informal effort to share information about problematic cases (see discussions in 41), but the lack of a formal mechanism has contributed to the perception that the responses obtained from IRBs vary from institution to institution, depending on the composition of the panel and other idiosyncratic factors (42,43). Although the present HHS and FDA regulations articulate specific guidelines for IRB membership, functions and operations, review of research, expedited review procedures, and the criteria for approval of research (30,32), there appears to be substantial variation in the care with which IRBs address issues of informed consent (44).

In a 1993 article Jay Katz argued that, in general, IRBs fail to protect adequately the rights of patient-subjects and that a national commission should be established "to administer and review the human experimentation process" (45, p. 12). Specifically Katz does not believe that "members of IRBs will hold investigators to a standard of disclosure and consent that would protect subjects of research if doing so would place impediments on the conduct of research" (45, p. 41). There is a consensus that IRBs to date have rarely exercised their available powers to require monitoring of the manner in which patients are approached as potential subjects, are provided with relevant information before making their decisions to participate, have their questions about participation answered both before and after deciding, or are permitted to exercise their right to discontinue participation.

In June of 1998 the Office of Inspector General of HHS issued a series of reports on IRBs. The reports conclude that "IRBs are reviewing too much, too quickly, with too little expertise; conducting minimal continuing review of approved research; facing conflicts that threaten their independence; and providing little training for clinical investigators and board members" (46). With respect to informed consent, the report notes that "IRBs have all too little information about how the informed consent process really works and about how well the interests of subjects are being protected during the course of research" (47). Although the reports call for reform of the IRB system, they do not recommend dissolution of the current review structure. In fact, they stress the need for FDA and NIH to take a greater role in overseeing IRBs and in strengthening the review process. An update, issued in April of 2000, is more pessimistic. Noting that few of the recommended reforms have been enacted, it points out that IRB review of the consent process continues to be minimal and that significant legislative reform might be necessary (47). Concerns about continuing abuses in human subjects research led HHS Secretary Donna Shalala to suggest considerable reforms, including enactment of civil monetary penalties that could be imposed both on investigators and institutions for violations of informed consent (48).

IRBs can and should take a more active role in the oversight of informed consent. A number of recent court decisions have held hospitals liable for the failure to obtain informed consent (49), and at least one implied that the federal regulations place a responsibility on a hospital, through its IRB, to assure protections for informed consent (50,51). Although consent forms should not be ignored, IRBs should make efforts to evaluate the actual consent interaction, rather than to focus all attention on the wording and content of a single document.

In addition, IRBs should make special efforts to safeguard consent in research involving vulnerable or cognitively impaired subjects especially in research that has substantial risks (see later under *Special Populations*). These efforts may include requiring that investigators take additional steps to ensure voluntary and competent consent, such as direct observation of the consent process by a third party (perhaps an IRB member or team). An IRB can function as an institutional resource and establish guidelines for subject capacity, use of capacity screening mechanisms, surrogate consent, or other protections (52). For example, an IRB might draft a basic document explaining what is meant by substituted judgment or best interests and give examples of how proxies should apply the standards in specific cases. Furthermore, it could specify the level of certainty a proxy must demonstrate that a decision is in accord with the subject's probable wishes before making a decision to enroll the subject, with less certainty needed for lower risk studies and more certainty required for higher risk studies (53). In cases where there is a concern that proxies will not understand the experiment because of the complicated nature of the research, and there are high risks involved, the IRB might require that the investigators take additional steps to ensure comprehension, such as employing a neutral third-party educator. Furthermore, IRBs should carefully scrutinize investigators' conflicts of interest in research settings (54) and ensure that this information is part of the informed consent disclosure. In some cases, relying solely on disclosure to mitigate the conflict will be insufficient and additional safeguards will be necessary (55). The extent of the protections required will depend on the case, but IRBs can clearly take a more active role in this context (53,56).

Exceptions

Certain types of research are exempt from compliance requirements, and thus exempt from IRB review, under the federal regulations. These include: (*1*) research conducted in established educational settings, involving normal education practices, (*2*) research involving educational tests, survey procedures, interview procedures, or observation of public behavior [30, §§101(b)(2)–(3)],[3] (*3*) research involving collection or study of existing data, if either the data are publicly available or there are no identifiers that can be used to trace the information back to the subjects (57–60),[4] (*4*) research conducted to evaluate public benefit or service programs, and (*5*) research involving taste and food quality evaluations as long as the food does not come under the purview of the FDA [30, §101(b)].[5]

In addition to exemptions, HHS regulations provide for expedited IRB review of other kinds of research projects. Such review may be conducted by the chairperson or another designated member of the committee without awaiting a scheduled IRB meeting or consideration by the full complement of the IRB membership. Categories of research eligible for expedited review include projects in

---

[3]This applies unless the information gathered can be linked to an identifiable individual and disclosure of the responses could place the subject at risk of criminal or civil liability, or damage the subject's financial standing, employability, or reputation. However, if the subject is a public official or candidate for public office, then all research involving educational tests, survey procedures, interview procedures, or observation of public behavior is exempt.

[4]This raises interesting questions for DNA databanks. Since DNA is itself an identifier, it is unclear whether DNA samples can be used for research other than that for which the sample was originally taken without an individual's informed consent even if all other identifying variables are removed.

[5]HHS has the authority both to require specific research activities that are otherwise exempt under this section to meet all or some of the requirements of the regulations [30, §101(d)] and to exempt research that is otherwise covered by the regulations [30, §101(i)].

which no more than minimal risk is likely to accrue to subjects and the procedures involve only the following:

1. Clinical studies of drugs and medical devices only when (*a*) an investigational new drug application is not required; or (*b*) an investigational device exemption application is not required, or the medical device is cleared/approved for marketing and the medical device is being used in accordance with its cleared/approved labeling.

2. Collection of blood samples by finger stick, heel stick, ear stick, or venipuncture with a certain amount of restrictions.

3. Prospective collection of biological specimens for research purposes by non-invasive means.

4. Collection of data through non-invasive procedures (not involving general anesthesia or sedation) routinely employed in clinical practice, excluding procedures involving X-rays or microwaves. Where medical devices are employed, they must be cleared/approved for marketing.

5. Research involving materials (data, documents, records, or specimens) that have been collected or will be collected solely for non-research purposes (such as medical treatment or diagnosis).

6. Collection of data from voice, video, digital, or image recordings made for research purposes.

7. Research on individual or group characteristics or behavior (including, but not limited to, research on perception, cognition, motivation, identity, language, communication, cultural beliefs or practices, and social behavior) or research employing survey, interview, oral history, focus group, program evaluation, human factors evaluation, or quality assurance methodologies.

8. Continuing review of research previously approved by the convened IRB as follows:

(*a*) Where (*i*) the research is permanently closed to the enrollment of new subjects; (*ii*) all subjects have completed all research-related interventions; and (*iii*) the research remains active only for long-term follow-up of subjects; or

(*b*) Where no subjects have been enrolled and no additional risks have been identified; or

(*c*) Where the remaining research activities are limited to data analysis.

9. Continuing review of research, not conducted under an investigational new drug application or investigational device exemption where categories 2 through 8 do not apply but the IRB has determined and documented at a convened meeting that the research involves no greater than minimal risk and no additional risks have been identified (61).

Expedited review does not relieve investigators of the responsibility of formulating appropriate methods for obtaining informed consent. There are, however, conditions in which the requirement of subject or surrogate consent, which generally functions as a baseline protection, may be waived by an IRB. There are three specific situations for which the regulations allow research to proceed in the absence of informed consent. The first, highlighted by the HHS regulations, involves minimal risk research. HHS regulations allow an IRB to waive some or all of the requirements of informed consent if the IRB documents that:

1. the research involves no more than minimal risk,
2. the waiver will not adversely affect the rights and welfare of the subjects,
3. the waiver is necessary to carry out the research, and
4. when appropriate, the subject will be informed after participation [30, §116(d)].

One example of the application of IRBs' discretion in this area is in so-called deception research, where subjects are not told they are going to be part of a research study or not told the exact purpose of the study, but are debriefed afterward (see Chapter 13). Data suggest that informed consent regulations have not inhibited the use of deception (62). The most famous example is the Milgram electric shock experiment in the 1970s in which subjects, believing that they were administering increasingly higher levels of electric shocks to other subjects, were willing to follow instructions from an authority figure despite indications of severe harm to the subjects receiving the shocks (both the authority figure and the "subjects" receiving "shocks" were part of the research team) (63). Another example is a 1992 study of the accuracy of self-reports regarding illicit drug use where subjects were told they were part of a study of sexually transmitted diseases (64).

The second situation in which informed consent requirements may be waived is exemplified by the FDA regulations that allow a waiver of informed consent for emergency use of a test article when the following requirements are met:

1. the subject has a life-threatening condition necessitating the use of the experimental article;
2. the subject does not have the capacity to consent;
3. there is no time to obtain surrogate consent;
4. there is no alternative treatment that provides an equal or greater likelihood of helping the subject; and
5. an uninvolved physician reviews and evaluates the use of the article (32, §23).

In fact, both HHS and FDA guidelines make it clear that the regulations are not intended to limit emergency treatment [30, §116(f); 32, §25(d)]. As noted in Chapter 4, consent for treatment is generally assumed in an emergency situation. The FDA regulations expand this concept and allow the use of experimental treatment when standard treatment is inadequate. Although the preceding section permits a single use of an experimental treatment, it does not allow controlled studies to occur, though they may be necessary to evaluate the safety and efficacy of experimental treatments.

On October 2, 1996, with an assurance of compliance by HHS, FDA issued new regulations, creating an exception from informed consent requirements when:

1. subjects are in a life-threatening situation, available treatments are un-proven or unsatisfactory, and a controlled investigation is necessary;
2. obtaining informed consent is not feasible;
3. the research offers the possibility of direct therapeutic benefit to the subjects;
4. the investigation could not practicably be carried out without the waiver; and
5. additional protections of the rights and welfare of the subjects will be provided (65).

The rationale for allowing a waiver of informed consent under these circumstances is twofold. First, there is need for research to establish better treatments for emergency conditions. Second, such research could not meet existing requirements because most emergency situations involve subjects who lack capacity to consent, and the investigational intervention must be applied before surrogate consent can be obtained. Although allowing a waiver of informed consent undermines one of the most significant protections of human subjects, the guidelines attempt to compensate for this by providing for additional precautions. These include requirements of community consultation and public disclosure, as well as establishment of an independent data and monitoring committee to oversee the investigation [32, §24(a)(7)].

To a certain extent it is still unclear how the HHS and FDA exceptions should be read in conjunction. Both have accepted the emergency research exception. Since HHS regulations are effective for all entities covered by FDA regulations, the exception for minimal risk research is not problematic. However, the exception for emergency use of a test article remains a source of confusion. The FDA regulations apparently allow both a waiver of consent and a waiver of prospective IRB review (retrospective review is required), whereas the HHS regulations do not allow waiver of IRB review under any circumstances.

Consent Forms

The HHS regulations focus both on what information must be given to subjects and the manner in which information is given. The latter issue has two aspects. The first involves the format for providing information. In most cases a written consent form, setting forth the information relevant to the proposed research, is required and must be signed by subjects if they are to participate [30, §117(a))] With IRB approval, oral disclosure and a short form may be used; the short form, signed by the subject, contains a statement that the required elements of disclosure have been made orally. In addition, if oral disclosure is relied upon, a witness must be present for the disclosure and must sign the short consent form. Presumably this option for oral consent is a response to the objections of some investigators that for many studies in clinical settings, or social research projects involving naturalistic observation, subjects are not capable of assimilating or not likely to attend to a lengthy written document. In specified circumstances even the short form can be dispensed with: when the study presents no more than minimal risk, or when the signed document would be the only record linking the subject to the project and the major risk to the subject is breach of confidentiality. Waiver of the requirement for a signed consent form is solely at the discretion of the IRB, not the individual investigator.

A major review of a random sample of consent forms showed that many were seriously deficient, especially in communicating risk information to potential subjects (66). Another study found that 96 percent of the forms studied had a reading level above the target level (eighth grade) (67). Consent forms may be unclear, or too long, hindering the subjects' understanding (68,69). Although consent forms may serve as evidence of subjects' consent, as in the clinical setting they should not serve as a proxy for interaction between the investigator and subject. In fact, IRBs should encourage alternative consent mechanisms rather than focus exclusively on consent forms. Forms may ensure that standard information is conveyed to subjects, but they cannot ensure or even evaluate subject understanding of the information.

Voluntariness, Understanding, and Competence

One other way that the regulations affect the manner in which consent is obtained involves the problem of voluntariness. The regulations require that consent be sought "only under circumstances that provide the prospective subject or the [subject's legally authorized] representative sufficient opportunity to consider whether or not to participate and that minimize the possibility of coercion or undue influence" (30, §116).

The regulations address the related problems of understanding and competence almost as cursorily as voluntariness. With respect to understanding, they merely require that information be provided in language that subjects are likely to understand. There is no requirement that either the investigator or the IRB undertake any effort to ascertain adequacy of understanding, nor guidance for action in the event that a subject's understanding is deficient.

The regulations are equally vague about competence. They direct that when patients are incompetent, their legally authorized representative may consent on their behalf to their participation as a research subject. Who is a legally authorized representative is a matter to be determined by reference to state rather than federal law. This determination may be extremely confusing in a number of states (see Chapter 5). The problem is further complicated by the question of whether even judicially appointed guardians have the authority to consent to their wards' participation in research, especially where procedures are not intended to benefit subjects (53). Finally the regulations are silent on the question of what constitutes incompetence in a research setting. There are few cases or statutes that speak to this issue in the treatment setting, and none that address competence to consent to research (53,70).

Special Populations

Concerns about voluntariness, understanding, and competence form the basis for the regulatory protections of what are termed "special populations." In response to the debates of the late 1970s and early 1980s, the present regulations alert IRBs and investigators to the possibility of providing additional safeguards for persons who are "likely to be vulnerable to coercion or undue influence, such as children, prisoners, pregnant women, mentally disabled persons, or economically or educationally disadvantaged persons" [30, §111(b)]. Under the regulations, IRBs have the authority to appoint consent auditors, that is, third parties to observe the consent process in research; however, this is not mandatory [30, §109(e)]. In the twenty years since the regulations have been promulgated, these additional safeguards have rarely been used. Even though the IRB Guidebook specifically states that "IRBs must be sure that additional safeguards are in place to protect the rights and welfare of . . . vulnerable subjects (such as the mentally disabled)," IRBs still focus almost exclusively, and not always meaningfully, on consent forms (71).

The vulnerability of the groups listed can be divided into two areas: vulnerability due to circumstances and vulnerability due to cognitive deficits. Prisoners, pregnant women, and economically disadvantaged persons fall into the former category, while children and mentally disadvantaged persons fall into the latter. But the categories may overlap. Children, for example, vary greatly in their cognitive abilities (see Chapter 5), and the issue may be more a concern about coercion. And another example of blurred categories is demonstrated by a 1999 case that involved psychiatric research on teenage prison inmates (72).

The regulations provide specific guidelines for three populations: fetuses[6] and pregnant women (30, subpart B),[7] prisoners (30, subpart C), and children (30, subpart D). But it is generally accepted that additional protections also should be instituted for some cognitively impaired populations. In addition, recently there has been more discussion regarding protection for socioeconomically disadvantaged populations.

Pregnant Women

The regulations focusing on pregnant women restrict research that has no potential for direct therapeutic benefit to studies that involve minimal risk to the fetus. Thus, only in research that is designed to meet the health needs of the mother may the fetus be placed at greater than minimal risk. Research designed only to gain generalizable knowledge may not involve greater than minimal risk to the fetus, and the knowledge sought cannot be obtainable by other means. Moreover, the regulations stress the need to separate research participation from decisions to terminate the pregnancy—under no circumstances may the investigator play a role in determining the viability of the fetus, or the "timing, method, and procedures used to terminate a pregnancy" [30, §206(a)(3)]. In emphasizing this point, the regulations note that "[n]o inducements, monetary or otherwise, may be offered to terminate pregnancy" [30, §206(b)]. Finally, the regulations allow for research with non-viable fetuses when the purpose is to gain biomedical knowledge that is unobtainable by other means, as long as there is no artificial maintenance of vital functions[8] or conduct of "experimental activities which of themselves would terminate the heartbeat or respiration of the fetus" [30, §209(b)(2)]. Exceptions to the preceding requirements may only be accomplished with approval by a special Ethical Advisory Board established by the secretary of Health and Human Services.

Prisoners

Prisoners raise concerns about both voluntariness and capacity. Their competence has been questioned on the grounds that "judgment about an acceptable degree of

---

[6]Until recently, research on fetuses was prohibited by executive order. For a number of reasons, women of childbearing age have also been excluded de facto from research protocols. The resulting dearth of information about both women's health issues and the effect of certain substances on pregnant women (e.g., new AIDS vaccines) has led many people to argue that research subject populations should reflect the diversity of the population afflicted with the disease.

[7]The regulations also restrict research involving in vitro fertilization

[8]Experimentation with dead fetuses or fetal material may be addressed by state or local law.

risk requires contact with the free world as opposed to the prison environment. What may be an acceptable risk for a person inside prison may be totally unacceptable for that same person outside" (73). One of the major legal cases in this area, *Kaimowitz,* involved the adequacy of a prisoner's consent to participate in a study of an experimental psychosurgical procedure (74). Despite his initial insistence that he consented because he felt this was the only means of helping his problem, immediately upon release from the prison facility he withdrew consent for the procedure. The court stated that because "[i]nstitutionalization tends to strip the individual of the support which permits him to maintain his sense of self-worth . . . [a prisoner] has diminished capacity for making a decision about irreversible experimental psychosurgery." Robert Burt has argued further that the message given a prisoner about his self-worth distorts the ability to weigh the risks and benefits of participation in research; and rewards such as money, escape from boredom, and the goodwill of one's jailers constitute coercive pressures (75).

Initially these concerns led HHS and FDA to propose severe restrictions on research with prison populations, but backlash against the regulations resulted in the reformulation of the guidelines. At present the guidelines require IRBs reviewing such protocols to include at least one prisoner, or prisoner representative. Since the concern with this population is that "prisoners may be under constraints because of their incarceration which could affect their ability to make a truly voluntary and uncoerced decision" (30, §302), IRBs need to ensure that:

1. participation in the protocol does not entail such an improvement in general living condition, medical care, quality of food, amenities, or opportunity of earnings that the prisoner's ability to weigh the risks of research against the advantages is compromised;
2. nonprisoner volunteers would find the risks involved in the protocol acceptable;
3. subject selection is fair and equitable and control subjects are randomized;
4. informed consent information is presented in understandable language;
5. parole boards will not consider an individual's participation in making release decisions; and
6. follow-up mechanisms will take into account individuals' varying lengths of stay [30, §§ 305(a)(2)–(7)].

Types of research for this population are restricted. Only research that is (*1*) designed to study incarceration or related issues and involves minimal risk and inconvenience to the subjects, or (*2*) on conditions particularly affecting prisoners as a class, or (*3*) that has a "reasonable probability of improving the health or well-being of the subject" is permissible [30, §§ 306(a)(2)(i)–(iv)].

These restrictions have not been without controversy. Prisoners' competence, it is argued, is not different in its dimensions from that of non-prisoners. A federal court, prior to the issuance of the regulations, rejected the argument that prisoners could not provide valid consent (76). In another case, inmates of the Jackson State Prison in Michigan, where much testing of new drugs had been performed, sued to prevent the implementation of the FDA's 1980 regulations designed to restrict privately funded drug testing in prison (77). They alleged that they should have the right to decide whether the risks of participation outweigh the rewards, including improved living conditions and spending money. In response, the FDA reformulated those regulations to permit some private research not related to study of prison conditions. However, neither the initial regulations nor the reformulated ones were ever put into effect. As a result, privately funded research involving prisoners remains a matter of state regulation.

Children

Research protocols involving children are also subject to special regulation. In all cases both the consent of the parents or guardian and the *assent*[9] of the child, when she is capable of assenting, must be obtained. Research involving minimal risk is permissible without any additional safeguards if both consent and assent (where appropriate) are obtained. Research involving greater than minimal risk and the possibility of direct therapeutic benefit to the child is allowed only when the risk–benefit ratio "is at least as favorable to the subjects as that presented by [the] alternative[s]" [30, §405(b)]. Research involving greater than minimal risk and no potential for direct therapeutic benefit may be conducted only if:

1. the risk represents a minor increase over minimal risk;
2. the intervention or procedure involves experiences that are reasonably commensurate with those ordinarily encountered by the subject; and
3. the protocol is likely to yield generalizable knowledge about the subject's condition which is of vital importance to the understanding or amelioration of the condition (30, §406).

For research that is otherwise not permissible under the guidelines, one may obtain a waiver from the secretary of HHS (30, §407). The research must "present a reasonable opportunity to further the understanding, prevention, or alleviation of a serious problem affecting the health or welfare of children"[(30, §407(a)], the secretary must consult with a panel of experts (to determine that certain guidelines explicated in the Common Rule are met), and there must be an opportunity for public review and comment.

---

[9]"Assent" in this context refers to the child's agreement to participate in the research, after being provided with information appropriate to her age and cognitive abilities. Authorization for participation, or "consent," is obtained from parents or guardians.

The primary concern for all three special populations is their vulnerability to coercive pressures and thus their inability to give truly voluntary consent. The regulations focus on additional duties of IRBs and on limitations of the type of research that may be performed. One group noticeably absent from the above populations are persons with mental disabilities. As will be discussed in the section on cognitively impaired subjects, this population is also vulnerable to coercive pressures, but perhaps more important, subjects with mental disabilities may also suffer some form of cognitive impairment that may affect their ability to give informed consent.

Cognitively Impaired Subjects

Concerns about capacity to give informed consent arise in particular in a number of subject populations including persons with mental illness; AIDS patients (78); elderly persons, especially those suffering from dementia such as Alzheimer disease; people with organic brain damage; and substance abusers. The National Institute of Mental Health's Epidemiologic Catchment Area study estimates that 2.7 percent of the adult population (or 4,293,000 people) suffer severe cognitive impairment during the course of any year (79). These disorders may render some proportion of potential subjects incompetent to give consent for research, thus requiring that they not be entered into studies (even if they appear to be agreeing to participate) or that alternative mechanisms for authorizing their participation be developed. In addition, some severe illnesses that primarily affect organ systems other than the brain and some treatments for those illnesses will affect cognition.

In 1978 the Department of Health, Education and Welfare proposed rules that would deal with "individuals institutionalized as mentally disabled" (80). The purpose of the proposed rules was to set guidelines that would protect incompetent subjects. The proposal was not accepted for a number of reasons, most importantly because of objections that it singled out institutionalized populations for unwarranted special treatment. First, it was argued, vulnerability to coercive pressures is shared by a number of groups, not limited to institutionalized persons. Second, although the guidelines were intended to cover various groups of people,[10] the use of the term "mentally disabled" seemed to target unfairly persons suffering from mental illness and to inhibit research on their disorders.

Although concerns about this population are understandable, across-the-board protections for the mentally ill beyond those afforded to other medical patients and to volunteers are probably not justified by the available database (52,81–83).

---

[10]"Mentally disabled" individuals included those who are mentally ill, mentally retarded, emotionally disturbed, psychotic or senile, regardless of their legal status or the reason for their being institutionalized (80).

Certain high-risk groups of cognitively impaired populations may warrant special efforts (such as capacity screening), but these should be implemented selectively, with a focus on higher-risk studies to ensure a reasonable cost–benefit ratio of the additional protections. Of course, this does not mean that there are no problems in securing adequate informed consent from both the medically ill and the mentally ill (84). Empirical studies indicate that research is structured in a way that therapeutic and research goals often become intermixed and confused (39); patients/subjects frequently are not clear about which aspects of their treatment constitute ordinary treatment versus which aspects are controlled by the demands of a protocol (i.e., patients have a so-called therapeutic misconception) (85). But before it is concluded that persons with mental illness cannot understand or decide about research participation, it is essential that investigators make sustained, careful, and thorough attempts to educate potential subjects. There are a number of possible methods of increasing subject understanding, including employing innovative methods of information delivery and neutral third-party educators (86–88). As noted previously, however, these mechanisms are used rarely (89).

The National Bioethics Advisory Commission (NBAC), created by President Clinton in 1996, was charged with developing specific guidelines for research involving cognitively impaired subjects (90). NBAC made a number of recommendations regarding guidelines that should be applied to research with decisionally impaired subjects, but noted that implementation could occur either through changes in the existing regulations or by adding a new subpart specifically addressing this population of subjects. The recommendations include suggestions for IRB membership and review, creation of a national panel, mechanisms for approval of studies, informed consent, surrogate decision making, and future research into decisional impairment, as well as more controversial recommendations regarding mandatory independent competence evaluations.

Socioeconomically or Educationally Disadvantaged Persons

Socioeconomically or educationally disadvantaged individuals really comprise two different groups, although there may be a great deal of overlap between these populations. Although educationally disadvantaged individuals may not suffer from cognitive impairments, they may need many of the same types of protections as do impaired populations. These safeguards may include ensuring that consent forms and other explanations are provided in easily understandable language and that investigators take additional time to facilitate understanding.

Although many socioeconomically disadvantaged individuals also may be educationally disadvantaged, the concerns regarding these two populations are not identical. The primary concern in the socioeconomic area is the amount of compensation for research participation. It is generally accepted that money may be offered to research subjects to compensate for the time and discomfort associated with participation. However, it is less clear whether there should be special protections in place to ensure that subjects are not consenting to participation in high-risk research protocols that have no potential for direct therapeutic benefit based only on the monetary compensation offered. The issue becomes more complicated in the present-day situation where a large percentage of the population lacks healthcare coverage. Participation in a research study may be sought for the indirect therapeutic benefits gained, which may include access to healthcare facilities, basic health care, better attendant care, and/or additional monitoring of health conditions (91).

Whatever degree of uneasiness exists about the role of these factors in subjects' decision making, restricting socioeconomically disadvantaged populations from participating in research studies does not appear to be the solution. Quite the contrary, these populations may claim a right to participate in research not only for access to potential therapies but precisely for access to the indirect benefits. The Belmont Report notes that principles of justice require that no population disproportionately bear the burden of research, nor disproportionately gain the benefits of research (29, p. 19). But without additional guidance, the extent of the protections that should be put into place for these populations is left largely to the discretion of IRBs.

Conclusion

In the last three decades an extensive system of prospective regulation of research with human subjects has been erected. Much of the effort has been devoted to defining the proper nature of informed consent to research. Yet, as was true with informed consent in the clinical setting, the legal requirements provide only a part of the picture with which practitioners must be concerned. The existing regulations lay out the types of information that must be communicated to potential subjects. They give no guidance about the specific information that should be conveyed, the emphasis different elements of disclosure should receive, or the method of accomplishing meaningful explanation. Selection of an approach depends on an understanding of the differences between consent to treatment and consent to research.

Recent revelations about radiation experiments conducted by the United States government have prompted new concern about human subject protections (66). One study looked at subjects' attitudes about clinical research and found that informed consent did not seem an adequate protection of subjects' autonomous decision making—in fact, many subjects reported that their decision to participate was made before disclosure of risks and benefits and was based upon their trust in their physician (92). This may be evidence of the continuing persistence of the therapeutic misconception. A study of cancer patients found that the majority of subjects who consented to participation in a phase I trial (which has a low to non-existent probability of direct therapeutic benefit) did so because they hoped to improve their condition (93; see also 94). Even more disturbing was evidence that the referring oncologists shared the mistaken belief in the potential for direct therapeutic benefit.

"Research" over the past decade has shifted in the public's mind from an enterprise in which subjects need protection to one to which subjects demand access. The proliferation of new and deadly diseases, including AIDS, has decreased some of the emphasis on subject protections and increased the push to make new treatments available—even those that may not have been proven effective. The therapeutic misconception continues to pervade research, and the distinctions between standard therapy, experimental treatment, and research continue to blur. It is particularly striking that in 2000 President Clinton argued for increased involvement of the elderly in clinical trials and directed the Medicare program to cover such activities (95). Although it is undeniable that continued research is necessary to develop new treatments for disease, it is unclear whether insurance programs (such as Medicare) should cover experimental interventions, especially those offered as part of a research protocol that may or may not afford subjects any potential for direct therapeutic benefit.

Moreover, as research trials move from academic settings into community settings, additional concerns arise about conflicts between the roles of physician and investigator and the roles of patients and subjects. Subjects, especially those involved in clinical trials, are likely to rely heavily on their physicians' advice. This includes advice regarding research participation. But if physicians also miscalculate risks and benefits or are unclear about the distinctions between research and treatment, then subjects' trust may be misplaced. Unlike the treatment context, in research the physician-investigator's primary goal is not to benefit the individual patient (although this may be one goal), and the constraints of a research protocol may interfere with doing what is in the subject's best interest. Moreover, as research has been touted as a way for physicians and facilities to recoup lost revenues from regular patient care, physicians' conflicts of interest in this area have begun to receive increased attention. Finally, concern in the 1990s focused on international research endeavors (96), often undertaken in third world countries with subject populations that lack any access to health care and for whom informed consent is a foreign and almost meaningless concept (97). If we have learned anything in the fifty years since Nuremberg, it is that "there are [still] serious deficiencies in the current system for the protection of the rights and interests of human subjects" (98, p. 8). Although this does not mean that informed consent is useless in protecting subjects' autonomy, it does mean that steps must be taken to ensure that both physicians and subjects are truly informed and understand risks and benefits of research participation.

References

1. Bassinouni, M., Baffes, T., and Evrard, J. (1981) An appraisal of human experimentation in international law and practice: the need for international regulation of human experimentation. *Journal of Criminal Law and Criminology*, 72:1597–1666.
2. Louis, P.C. (1836) *Researches on the Effects of Bloodletting in Some Inflammatory Diseases*. Boston: Hilliard Gray.
3. Moreno, J.D. (1999) *Undue Risk: Secret State Experiments on Humans*. New York: W.H. Freeman.
4. Howard-Jones, N. (1982) Human experimentation in historical and ethical perspectives. *Soc Sci Med*, 16:1429–1448.
5. Grodin, M. (1992) Historical origins of the Nuremberg Code. In Annas, G.J., Grodin, M.A. (eds) *The Nazi Doctors and the Nuremberg Code: Human Rights in Human Experimentation*. New York: Oxford University Press.
6. Parson, W. (1984) Uniformed consent in 1942. *N Engl J Med*, 310:1397.
7. Annas, G. and Grodin, M. (1992) Introduction. In Annas, G., Grodin, M. (eds) *The Nazi Doctors and the Nuremberg Code: Human Rights in Human Experimentation*. New York: Oxford University Press.
8. Taylor, T. (1992) Opening statement of the prosecution, December 9, 1946. In Annas, G., Grodin, M. (eds) *The Nazi Doctors and the Nuremberg Code: Human Rights in Human Experimentation*. New York: Oxford University Press.
9. Proctor, R.N. (1992) Nazi doctors, racial medicine, and human experimentation. In Annas, G., Grodin, M. (eds) *The Nazi Doctors and the Nuremberg Code: Human Rights in Human Experimentation*. New York: Oxford University Press.
10. Lifton, R.J. (1986) *The Nazi Doctors*. New York: Basic Books.
11. Judicial Council (1963) Requirements for experiments on human beings. In Ladimer, I., Newman, R. (eds) *Clinical Investigation in Medicine: Legal, Ethical and Moral Aspects*. Boston: Boston University Law-Medicine Research Institute.
12. U.S. Adjutant General's Department (1947) The medical case. In *Trials of War Criminals Under Control Council Law No. 10 (October 1946–April 1949)*, Volume 2. Washington D.C.: U.S. Goverment Printing Office.
13. (1947) *The Nuremberg Code*. http://www.ushmm.org/research/doctors/Nuremberg_Code.htm (accessed October 11, 2000).
14. Glantz, L.H. (1992) The influence of the Nuremberg Code on U.S. statutes and regulations. In Annas, G.J., Grodin, M.A. (eds) *The Nazi Doctors and the Nuremberg Code: Human Rights in Human Experimentation*. New York: Oxford University Press.
15. World Medical Association (1964) *Declaration of Helsinki* http://www.bioscience.org/guides/declhels.htm (accessed October 11, 2000).
16. World Medical Association (1992) Declarations of Helsinki II, III, IV. In Annas, G.J., Grodin, M.A. (eds) *The Nazi Doctors and the Nuremberg Code: Human Rights in Human Experimentation*. New York: Oxford University Press.
17. Ladimer, I. (1963) Ethical and legal aspects of medical research on human beings. In Ladimer, I., Newman, R. (eds) *Clinical Investigation in Medicine: Legal, Ethical and Moral Aspects*. Boston: Boston University Law-Medicine Research Institute.

18. Carpenter v. Blake, 60 Barb. 488 (N.Y. 1871).
19. Fortner v. Koch, 261 N.W. 762 (Mich. 1935).
20. Frankel, M. (1975) The development of policy guidelines governing human experimentation in the United States: a case study of public policy-making for science and technology. *Ethics Sci Med*, 2:43–59.
21. Sessoms, S. (1963) Guiding principles in medical research involving humans, National Institutes of Health. In Ladimer, I., Newman, R. (eds) *Clinical Investigation in Medicine: Legal, Ethical and Moral Aspects*. Boston: Boston University Law-Medicine Research Institute.
22. Curran, W. (1970) Government regulation of the use of human subjects in medical research: the approach of two federal agencies. In Freund, P.A. (ed) *Experimentation with Human Subjects*. New York: Braziller.
23. Kelsey, F. (1963) Patient consent provision of the Federal Food, Drug, and Cosmetic Act. In Ladimer, I., Newman, R. (eds) *Clinical Investigation in Medicine: Legal, Ethical and Moral Aspects*. Boston: Boston University Law-Medicine Research Institute.
24. Katz, J. (1972) *Experimentation with Human Beings*. New York: Russell Sage Foundation.
25. Hyman v. Jewish Chronic Disease Hospital, 206 N.E.2d 338 (1965).
26. Beecher, H.K. (1966) Ethics and clinical research. *N Engl J Med*, 274:1354.
27. Jones, J. (1981) *Bad Blood*. New York: Free Press.
28. Barrett v. Hoffman, 521 F. Supp. 307 (S.D.N.Y. 1981),
29. United States National Commission for Protection of Human Subjects of Biomedical and Behavioral Research (1978) *The Belmont Report: Ethical Principles and Guidelines for the Protection of Human Subjects in Research.*
30. 45 C.F.R. 46.
31. Snider, D. (1997) Patient consent for publication and the health of the public. *JAMA*, 278:624–626.
32. 21 C.F.R. 50.
33. Levine, C., Dubler, N.N., and Levine, R.J. (1991) Building a new consensus: ethical principles and policies for clincial research on HIV/AIDS. *IRB*, 13:1–17.
34. Human Subjects Research Protections Act of 1997 S. 193, 105th Cong.
35. Morin, K. (1998) The standard of disclosure in human subjects experimentation. *J Leg Med*, 19:157–221.
36. Fried, C. (1974) *Medical Experimentation: Personal Integrity and Social Policy*. New York: American Elsevier.
37. Appelbaum, P., Roth, L., Benson, P., and Winslade, W. (1987) False hopes and best data: consent to research and the therapeutic misconception. *Hastings Cent Rep*, 17:20–24.
38. Gray, B., Cooke, R., and Tannenbaum, A. (1978) Research involving human subjects. *Science*, 201:1094–1101.
39. Appelbaum, P.S. and Roth, L.H. (1983) The structure of informed consent in psychiatric research. *Behav Sci Law*, 1:9–19.
40. Calabresi, G. (1970) Reflections on medical experimentation in humans. In Freund, P. (ed) *Experimentation with Human Subjects*. New York: Braziller.
41. *IRB: A Review of Human Subjects Research.* published by the Hastings Center.
42. Matthews, D., Sorenson, J., and Swazey, J. (1979) We shall overcome: multi-institutional review of a genetic counseling study. *IRB*, 1:1–3.
43. Goldman, J. and Katz, M. (1982) Inconsistency and institutional review boards. *JAMA*, 248:197–202.

44. President's Commission for the Study of Ethical Problems in Medicine and Biomedical and Behavioral Research (1983) *Implementing Human Research Regulations: The Adequacy and Uniformity of Federal Rules and of their Implementation.* Washington, D.C.: U.S. Government Printing Office.

45. Katz, J. (1993) Human experimentation and human rights. *Saint Louis University Law Journal*, 38:7–54.

46. Brown, J. (1998) *OIG Final Reports on Institutional Review Boards.* Washington, D.C.: Department of Health and Human Services.

47. HHS Office of the Inspector General (2000) *Protecting Human Subjects Research: Status of Recommendations.* Washington, D.C.: Department of Health and Human Services.

48. HHS Press Release, *Secretary Shalala Bolsters Protections for Human Research Subjects.* May 23, 2000.

49. University Hospitals Consortium (1997) *Legal and Risk Management Issues Associated with Clinical Research.* Oak Brook: University Hospital Consortium.

50. Kus v. Sherman Hospital, 644 N.E. 2d 1214 (Il. App. 1995).

51. LeBlang, T. (1995) Medical battery and failure to obtain informed consent: Illinois court decision suggests potential for IRB liability. *IRB*, 17(3):10–11.

52. Berg, J.W. and Appelbaum, P.S. (1999) Subjects' capacity to consent to neurobiological research. In Pincus, H.A., Lieberman, J. (eds) *Ethics in Psychiatric Research: A Resource Manual for Human Subjects Protection.* Washington, D.C.: American Psychiatric Association.

53. Berg, J.W. (1996) Legal and ethical complexities of consent with cognitively impaired research subjects: proposed guidelines. *J Law Med Ethics*, 24:18–35.

54. Spece, R.G., Shimm, D., and Buchanan, A.E. (eds) (1996) *Conflicts of Interest in Clinical Practice and Research.* New York: Oxford University Press.

55. Katz, J. (1996) Informed consent to medical entrepreneurialism. In Speece, R.G., Shimm, D., Buchanan, A.E. (eds) *Conflicts of Interest in Clinical Practice and Research.* New York: Oxford University Press.

56. Keyserlingk, E., Glass, K., Kogan, S., et al. (1995) Proposed guidelines for the participation of persons with dementia as research subjects. *Perspect Biol Med*, 38: 319–362.

57. Weir, R. and Horton, J. (1995) DNA banking and informed consent—Part 2. *IRB*, 17:1–8.

58. Weir, R. and Horton, J. (1995) DNA banking and informed consent—Part 1. *IRB*, 17:1–4.

59. American Society of Human Genetics (1996) Statement on informed consent for genetic research. *Am J Hum Genet*, 59:471–474.

60. Hunter, D. and Caporaso, N. (1997) Informed consent in epidemiologic studies involving genetic markers. *Epidemiology*, 8:596–599.

61. 63 Fed. Reg. 60353 and 60364 (November 9, 1998).

62. Adair, J., Dushenko, T., and Lindsay, R. (1985) Ethical regulations and their impact on research practice. *Am Psychol*, 40:59–72.

63. Milgram, S. (1974) *Obedience to Authority: An experimental view.* New York: Harper & Row.

64. McNagny, S.E. and Parker, R.M. (1992) High prevalence of recent cocaine use and the unreliability of patient self-report in an inner-city walk-in clinic. *JAMA*, 267: 1106–1108.

65. 61 Fed. Reg. 51498, 51528 (October 2, 1996).
66. Advisory Committee on Human Radiation Experiments (1995) *Final Report.* Washington, D.C.: U.S. Government Printing Office.
67. Philipson, S., Doyle, M., Gabram, S., Nightingale, C., and Philipson, E. (1995) Informed consent for research: a study to evaluate readability and processability to effect change. *J Investig Med*, 43:459–467.
68. Silva, M. and Sorrell, J. (1988) Enhancing comprehension of information for informed consent: a review of empirical research. *IRB*, 10:1–5.
69. Grisso, T. and Appelbaum, P.S. (1995) The MacArthur treatment competence study III: abilities of patients to consent to psychiatric and medical treatments. *Law Hum Behav*, 19:149–174.
70. Berg, J.W., Appelbaum, P.S., and Grisso, T. (1996) Constructing competence: formulating standards of legal competence to make medical decisions. *Rutgers Law Review*, 48:345–396.
71. Office for the Protection from Research Risks (1993) *Institutional Review Board Guidebook: Protecting Human Subjects Research.* Washington, D.C.: United States Department of Health and Human Services.
72. Weber, T. (1999) Drug test on teenage inmates probed. *Los Angeles Times.* August 16.
73. Bach-y-Rita, G. (1974) The prisoner as an experimental subject. *JAMA*, 229: 45–46.
74. Kaimowitz v. Michigan Dep't of Mental Health, 1 Ment. Dis. Law Rprt. 147 (Cir. Ct. Wayne County Mich. 1976).
75. Burt, R. (1975) Why we should keep prisoners from the doctors. *Hastings Cent Rep*, 5:25–34.
76. Bailey v. Lally, 491 F. Supp. 203 (D. Md. 1979).
77. Sun, M. (1981) Inmates sue to keep research in prisons. *Science*, 212:650–651.
78. Marks, E., Derderian, S., and Wray, H. (1992) Guidelines for conducting HIV research with human subjects at a U.S. military medical center. *IRB*, 14:7–10.
79. Regier, D., Narrow, W., Rae, D., et al. (1993) The de facto US mental and addictive disorders service system: epidemiologic catchment area prospective 1-year prevalence rates of disorders and services. *Arch Gen Psychiatry*, 50:85–94.
80. 43 Fed. Reg. No. 223, at 53954 (November 17, 1978).
81. Kaminiski, R. (1994) The importance of maintaining patient's continued and informed consent. *J California Alliance for the Mentally Ill*, 5:57–58.
82. Roth, L.H. and Appelbaum, P.S. (1983) Obtaining informed consent for research with psychiatric patients. *Psychiatr Clin North Am*, 6:551–565.
83. Roth, L.H., Appelbaum, P.S., and Lidz, C.W. (1987) Informed consent in psychiatric research. *Rutgers Law Review*, 39:425–441.
84. Appelbaum, P.S. and Grisso, T. (1988) Assessing patients' capacities to consent to treatment. *N Engl J Med*, 319:1635–1638.
85. Appelbaum, P.S., Roth, L.H. and Lidz, C.W. (1982) The therapeutic misconception: informed consent in psychiatric research. *Int J Law Psychiatry*, 5:319–329.
86. Schachter, D., Kleinman, I., Prendergast, P., et al. (1994) The effect of psychopathology on the ability of schizophrenic patients to give informed consent. *J Nerv Ment Dis*, 182:360–362.
87. Benson, P., Roth, L.H., and Appelbaum, P.S. (1988) Information disclosure, subject understanding, and informed consent in psychiatric research. *Law Hum Behav*, 12:455–475.

88. Carpenter, W., Gold, J., Lahti, A., Queern, C., Conley, R., Bartko, J., Kovnick, J., and Appelbaum, P. (2000) Decisional capacity for informed consent in schizophrenia. *Arch Gen Psychiatry*, 57:533–538.

89. Benson, P., Roth, L.H., and Winslade, W.J. (1985) Informed consent in psychiatric research: preliminary findings from an ongoing investigation. *Soc Sci Med*, 20: 1331–1341.

90. National Bioethics Advisory Commission (1999) Guidelines for research involving cognitively impaired subjects. Washington, D.C.: NBAC.

91. American Medical Association Council on Ethical and Judicial Affairs (1998) Subject selection for clinical trials. *IRB*, 20:12–15.

92. Kass, N., Sugarman, J., Faden, R., et al. (1996) Trust: the fragile foundation of contemporary biomedical research. *Hastings Cent Rep*, 26:25–29.

93. Daugherty, C., Ratain, M., Grochowski, E., et al. (1995) Perceptions of cancer patients and their physicians involved in phase I trials. *J Clin Oncol*, 13:1062–1072.

94. Schaeffer, M., Krantz, D., Wichman, A., Masur, H. and Reed, E. (1996) Impact of disease severity on the informed consent process in clinical research. *Am J Med*, 100:261–268.

95. White House Press Release, President Clinton Takes New Action to Encourage Participation in Clinical Trials, June 7, 2000.

96. Brody, B.A. (1998) *The Ethics of Biomedical Research: An International Perspective.* New York: Oxford University Press.

97. Levine, R.J. (1991) Informed consent: some challenges to the universal validity of the western model. *Law Med Health Care*, 19:207–213.

98. Faden, R. (1996) The Advisory Committee on Human Radiation Experiments: reflections on a presidential commission. *Hastings Cent Rep*, 26:5–10.

13

Fulfilling the Underlying Purpose of Informed Consent to Research

To a great extent the underlying purposes of informed consent in research settings resemble those in the treatment situation. Informed consent promotes individuals' autonomy by allowing subjects to make meaningful decisions about participation in research projects. Informed consent is also a means of reducing inequalities of knowledge and power in the researcher–subject relationship and thus increases the cooperation and compliance of subjects. Increased knowledge also enhances patients' abilities to make decisions that will protect them from unwanted and undesirable intrusions on bodily integrity, perhaps of even greater importance here than in treatment settings, because of the sorry history of abuses inflicted on research subjects.

Subject and Researcher—A Divergence of Interests

As great as the similarities are between consent to treatment and consent to research, the differences are equally great. In treatment settings, as already noted, clinicians and patients are presumed to share the same goal: promoting patients' health. They may disagree over the means, but a general coincidence of interests is ordinarily the rule. Charles Fried calls this confluence of interests the principle of personal care. "The traditional concept of the physician's relation to his patient is one of unqualified fidelity to that patient's health. He may certainly not do anything that would impair the patient's health and he must do everything in his ability to further it" (1, pp. 50–51). The essence of this principle is that physicians will not allow any other considerations to impinge on their decisions as to what measures are in their patients' best interests.

Since the goal of scientific investigation is the production of generalizable knowledge, not primarily the promotion of individual health, the interests of subjects and researchers are not identical. Clinician-researchers who are providing treatment to subjects in their research studies may feel this clash of interests most acutely as steps taken to protect the generalizability of the data may conflict with the maximization of benefit to individual subjects (2). The need to take this conflict into account in the decisionmaking process is largely responsible for the differences between consent to research and consent to treatment.

Research and the Loss of Personal Care

Divergences of interest between investigators and subjects exist on a gradient, with the fewest conflicts in research with normal volunteers and more conflicts when patients are recruited as subjects. Healthy volunteers may be motivated by altruistic identification with the goals of the research or by more mundane considerations such as monetary compensation. Differences in perspective may occur regarding the degree of risk that is acceptable, with subjects being more risk averse. Although from an objective standpoint no doctor–patient relationship exists, and thus the principle of personal care may be thought not to apply, the subjects may not take this view. They may assume that physicians or scientists would never take measures that might endanger research subjects, and thus rely too much on the researchers to avoid risks. Researchers will be torn between the desire to live up to this expectation and the need to implement their protocol, which may involve the imposition of some degree of risk. However, when both sides are aware of these conflicts and able to negotiate about them openly, they often can be resolved.

A second category of research can be more problematic: studies involving subjects who are suffering from illnesses but who will not receive treatment as part of the research. Included here are many investigations of the pathophysiology of disorders (e.g., electrophysiologic studies of cardiac conduction defects; brain magnetic resonance imaging of persons with psychiatric disorders). These studies may improve investigators' understanding of a disorder and contribute in the future to therapeutic advances, but they clearly are not intended to benefit individual subjects. Nonetheless, subjects may be hoping for therapeutic benefit and, as will be discussed later under *Subjects and the Therapeutic Misconception*, may have a difficult time relinquishing this expectation. Indeed, their interest in receiving personalized treatment may be sufficiently strong that subjects feel "used" or "abused" when it becomes clear that such benefit is not forthcoming. These feelings may be exacerbated when studies involve the actual provocation of symptoms of their disorders (e.g., stimulation of psychotic symptoms in schizophrenia with psychotomimetic agents; provocation of angina pectoris by cardiac stress testing). Researchers may assume that subjects share both the researchers' understanding of these studies as "non-therapeutic research" and their goal of advancing knowledge in the field. Unfortunately, this often is not the case.

Far and away the most striking potential for researcher–subject conflict of interest occurs in research with patients that tests the relative efficacy of therapeutic interventions. A number of commentators have noted that modern research methods are often responsible for actualizing this potential for conflict (1–5). These include the use of randomized assignment to the study's groups, detailed standardized scientific protocols, placebos in place of active interventions, and double-blind procedures. We consider each of these in turn.

The clearest example of the problem involves randomized assignment to experimental groups. Ordinarily, treatments are determined by patients' physicians based on individualized considerations of what would be most likely to help a particular patient. This process is short-circuited in controlled clinical trials by randomization, an important tool for minimizing bias in group assignment. The use of randomization is usually justified on the basis that controlled studies are only undertaken when clinicians do not have strong evidence that one treatment is superior to another (with the other sometimes being no treatment at all)—a condition referred to as clinical equipoise (6). Thus, although clinician-researchers may be surrendering the ability to select a treatment for their patients, and patients may be surrendering the potential benefits of that selection, it is argued that the patient-subjects do not suffer in this regard, since they are going to be assigned to one of a number of what are believed to be equivalent treatments.

This argument fails to take into account that existing knowledge does sometimes provide a reason to favor one treatment over another. Investigators may be impressed, for example, by the potential of a new medication used in uncontrolled trials and thus be led to undertake a controlled comparison. An experienced clinician in such a situation might simply use the innovative drug, even though no scientifically adequate data exist to support it. Besides a general belief that one treatment might be superior, a clinician may have reason to believe a given treatment would be preferable for a particular patient. This belief may be based on a pattern of familial response to treatment, idiosyncratic elements of the patient's presentation, or the patient's own past experience with similar treatments. Subjects entering clinical trials lose the putative benefit of this informed speculation on their behalf, perhaps one of the most valued aspects of the doctor–patient relationship.

Subjects in randomized trials also lose the right to select among treatments that, even if their main effects are identical, may have significantly different side effects. Or they may lose the ability to trade off potential efficacy in main effect against the severity of side effects. Treatment for breast cancer is the most frequently offered example here (7–8). To avoid the disfigurement of a radical mastectomy, a woman may be willing to take a chance on a procedure that may be (but is not proven) less effective, and is certainly less mutilating. This opportunity to take chances is lost when neither physician nor subject plays a role in deciding on treatment. Such a situation may further enhance feelings of helplessness in a hospitalized or seriously ill patient.

The constraints of a scientific protocol—the document that sets down what therapeutic interventions are and are not permissible in the conduct of a particular study—may also compromise individual decision making. In ordinary practice physicians might decide to raise or lower the dose of a medication, discharge a patient from the hospital, or add or delete adjunctive treatments. The rigidities of a protocol may limit a physician's ability to take these steps, regardless of patients' desires—short of dropping patients from the study, which neither physician-researchers nor patients may want to do (2,4,5). Entering a patient-subject into a protocol may also tend to freeze that patient's diagnosis, inhibiting refinement of the physician's conclusions.

Use of placebos has become one of the most controversial aspects of research methodology (9,10). Indeed, even the definition of a placebo is a matter of considerable contention (11). Some commentators, looking to such documents as the Declaration of Helsinki, contend that placebos should never be used when even partially effective treatments exist for a disorder (9,12,13). Arguing that the real question is whether the new treatment is better than the existing standard treatment, they would maintain instead that comparisons should be made with active compounds, or with historical controls. Proponents of placebo use, on the other hand, point out that the interpretation of research findings is often unclear unless a placebo control group is included. Comparable levels of efficacy, for example, between new and old active treatments may indicate a lack of sensitivity in the procedures used for assessment or a high level of treatment resistance in the particular sample at hand that rendered both treatments being tested equally ineffective (14–17). Moreover, historical controls may not be appropriate unless their equivalence with the sample being studied can be established (14). When patient-subjects receive placebo— and it seems likely for a variety of reasons that placebos will continue to be used regularly in the future— they are denied one of the key elements of personal care: a treatment that their physician believes will be helpful to them.

Finally, double-blind procedures, in which both patient-subjects and clinicians are kept in the dark about which group patients have been assigned to and what treatment they are receiving, are often considered essential to preventing bias in treatment or evaluation. In these situations subjects are at risk when information is unavailable to help physicians monitor a clinical course or diagnose adverse reactions (4).

How can these deviations from the principle of personal care that governs the usual relationships between clinicians and patients be justified? Indeed, when research has no therapeutic intent at all, what makes it legitimate for researchers to put subjects at risk of discomfort or overt harm? In our society, persons generally have been granted the right to place themselves at risk, especially for socially useful purposes, as long as they do so knowledgeably and voluntarily. (There are, of course, limits to the degree of risk ordinarily considered justified, and it is a generally accepted requirement that risks be proportionate to the likely gains from a study.) The losses associated with clinical research are usually considered to be ethically acceptable when a prospective subject is adequately informed about the alternatives to participation, the relative risks and benefits within and outside of the experimental protocol, and the existence of randomized assignment and other constraints placed on patients and physicians by the research protocol, and when the person voluntarily agrees to be a subject under these conditions.

Divergence of Interests and Informed Consent to Research

Given the critical role of informed consent in justifying research and the special difficulties that arise when patients are asked to forgo the benefits of personal care, decision making about research must go one step beyond decision making about treatment. In addition to disclosure of the nature, purpose, risks, and benefits of an intervention, along with the alternatives, decision making about research should involve a clarification of the differences between treatment and research, particularly the compromises of the principle of personal care that may have to be made. A focus and emphasis different from that of the treatment setting is required.

Many commentators have felt an uneasiness about violations of personal care (though they may not have used that term) inherent in much research. They have been led to suggest an additional goal of informed consent in research. Echoing Kantian considerations, the philosopher Hans Jonas, for example, expressed distress at the possibility that research subjects may come to be seen as manipulable means to researchers' ends rather than persons whose interests represent ends in themselves (18). The only corrective he saw to this problem is "such authentic identification [by the subject] with the cause that it is the subject's as well as the researcher's cause." He further stressed that "the appeal for volunteers should seek this free and generous endorsement, the appropriation of the research purpose into the person's own scheme of ends." Paul Ramsey, a theologian and ethicist, reached a similar conclusion that it is only "men's capacity to become joint adventurers in a common cause [that] makes possible a consent to enter into the relation of patient to physician or of subject to investigator. This means that *part-nership* is a better word than contract in conceptualizing the relation between patient and physician or between subject and investigator" (19, pp. 5–6).

Jonas and Ramsey, whose thoughts have profoundly influenced contemporary discussions of the ethics of research, sought to heal the conflict of interests by having the subject and investigator, like the physician and patient, work together toward a common goal. The means they envisioned for achieving this commonality involves a sufficiently detailed explanation of the research that enables the subject willingly to identify with and share the researchers' motivations. Although the worthiness of this goal is widely accepted and it may represent a valid ideal for which to strive, it is probably unattainable in most circumstances. Besides, talking about common goals may obscure real conflicts of interests and thus complicate and confuse the decisionmaking process. For example, the subject cannot be as single-mindedly devoted to the acquisition of data as the researcher when the subject alone accepts the risk of discomfort, injury, or even death, and the researcher's career is being built on the data. Clarity may be enhanced by pointing to differences where they exist, rather than papering them over with talk of a complete commonality of concerns. The requirement of informed consent provides a means of assuring an opportunity for conversation between investigators and prospective subjects. This opportunity should be used to explore not only matters included under the usual categories (risks, benefits, alternatives) but other matters of interest to potential subjects in deciding whether or not to participate in research.

Problems in Obtaining Adequate Consent

Clarifying the research situation so that potential subjects can participate meaningfully in the decisionmaking process is a difficult task. Obstacles can arise with respect to four elements: the investigator, the subject, the structure of the decisionmaking process, and communication of the necessary information.

Investigators' Perspective

Investigators' behavior remains an important stumbling block to a meaningful decisionmaking process. To some extent, investigators' failure to implement the doctrine of informed consent stems from a failure to assimilate its basic rationales. Appelbaum and Roth found that of seventeen investigators who worked with human subjects roughly half believed in the importance of informed consent as an ethical or practical principle, and the others rejected it as unattainable or as an unwarranted intrusion on the conduct of research (20). Investigators in Great

Britain and some other countries tend to be more overt about their negative views of informed consent, but they may merely be voicing the silent beliefs of many American researchers as well (21–23). Indeed, a recent proposal in the *New England Journal of Medicine* argued that in some cases physicians should not have to inform patients that they are being enrolled in a randomized controlled study. The authors stressed the benefits of research and concluded "blind insistence on informed consent is . . . harmful" (24).

Some researchers who hold negative views of the idea of informed consent believe that so much influence is exercised by the investigator over subjects that any attempt by them to protect their own interests, independent of the investigator, is meaningless (25). The subject has no alternative but to trust in the beneficence of the physician-investigator and the medical profession in general. Other critics believe that neither patients in treatment nor subjects in research are really able to understand the information necessary to reach an informed decision (26–28). J. C. Garnham, for example, claimed on the basis of his experience with forty-one volunteers that no one without medical training was able to acquire sufficient understanding of the risks of the research he conducted (27). Franz Ingelfinger argued similarly that without medical background to place risks and benefits into perspective, the result is what he called "informed but uneducated consent" (26).

Researchers' resistance to informed consent can also result from a concern that the consent process (as they practice it, usually along the lines of the event model) inhibits and biases the recruitment of research subjects (29). Just as the application of informed consent in clinical situations often involves a delicate balance between autonomy and health values, so its application to research involves a potential conflict with the investigator's commitment to generating new knowledge. Investigators have obligations not only to their subjects but also to their disciplines and to those who commit funds and other resources to the research.

Whether informed consent genuinely hinders research is unclear.[1] One reported attempt to conduct a randomized trial of cancer chemotherapy was stymied by subjects' refusals to agree to randomization when they were informed that it would be employed (30). Randomization appears to be a consistent problem in recruitment for cancer clinical trials (31). Another large national chemotherapy trial accrued subjects so slowly when using a standard consent procedure that its completion was threatened. The study was completed only when a controversial technique was used that allowed pre-randomization without explicit consent for subjects assigned to the control group (32). Three groups have reported that patient-subjects who consented to psychiatric research were markedly differ-

---

[1]In fact, this objection contradicts the previous objection, which claimed that informed consent is meaningless because all subjects can be convinced to participate.

ent from the patient population as a whole (33–35). Herbert Spohn and Timothy Fitzpatrick have convincingly linked at least part of that variance to the consent process (34). Concerns have also been reported that informed consent may alter the nature of research results. One study has found that subjects who received information about drug side effects frequently were able to break the double-blind in a placebo-controlled study (36). Several psychological experiments have demonstrated differences in subject response based on whether or not disclosure had previously been made as part of the consent process (37).

Other studies have shown no difference in response rates to questionnaires or in willingness to participate in research because of the informed consent requirement (38–40) or when more detailed disclosures were provided (41). There is also substantial evidence that volunteer subjects are always somewhat different from the population from which they are drawn (42). Moreover, the genuine cooperation a researcher obtains only from a subject who truly feels committed to the research may well offset much of the subtle undercutting of research that is of such concern.

Whether or not subject recruitment is adversely affected, the refusal of potential subjects to participate in a research project, even to the point of the project having to be abandoned, is entirely consistent with the nature of a democratic society. The scheme adopted by the Department of Health and Human Services for the regulation of research is a two-step process. It requires, in effect, approval both by a panel of the investigators' peers and by potential research subjects. Peer approval (that is, by the Institutional Review Board [IRB]) is merely conditional. It allows the researcher to begin to approach potential subjects. Their subsequent approval is also required before the research may be undertaken. In other words, IRB approval permits the research to be undertaken on the condition that individual subjects agree to participate. Without IRB approval, individual subjects cannot even be approached for participation. On the other hand, there is nothing implicit in approval by the IRB (or a federal funding agency) that a research project must, or even should, be undertaken. Approval means only that it may be, assuming the willingness of individual subjects to participate. Whatever license researchers have to do research is a license to do research on *willing* subjects only. Investigators are no more entitled to undertake a research project on unwilling subjects than non-investigator physicians are to practice a proven therapy on unwilling patients.

Even investigators who acknowledge the desirability of informed consent, however, may find it difficult not to allow the boundary between research and therapeutic functions to be blurred (5,43). Investigators may experience discomfort with the necessary compromise of personal care in research settings. One study investigated physicians' reasons for not entering eligible patients in a randomized clinical trial of surgery for breast cancer (32). The trial had difficulty maintaining a steady rate of recruitment. Sixty-six of ninety-one surgeons who participated as coinvestigators failed to enroll all eligible patients in the research project. Among the reasons they gave for not seeking the consent of potential subjects were concern with the doctor–patient relationship in a randomized clinical trial (73 percent), trouble with informed consent (38 percent), conflict between physician as clinician and as scientist (18 percent), and feelings of personal responsibility if treatments were proved to be of unequal efficacy (8 percent).

In addition to having problems acknowledging conflicts between the roles of researcher and clinician, investigators often have difficulty discussing with a patient-subject their own uncertainty about the best treatment. Ironically, that very uncertainty is what motivates and legitimates a research study; there would be no need to conduct it if the best treatment were already known. Katz has argued that physicians are systematically trained to avoid discussing uncertainty with patients (8), despite demonstrations that uncertainty may be the single most important concept for both patients and physicians to grasp in all medical encounters, not just medical research (44). In the problematic breast cancer protocol previously mentioned, 23 percent of surgeons who failed to enroll all eligible patients offered "dislike of open discussions about uncertainty" as a reason for their behavior (32).

Investigators' discomfort about informed consent can substantially affect the way in which consent is obtained. Studies of researchers' actual practices are rare. Some observational studies have suggested that members of the research team can underplay, distort, or even conceal information that would ordinarily be considered important in disclosure prior to obtaining consent (3,45). Some investigators avoid the term research altogether and describe instead the aspects of the study that might benefit the individual subject (3). A study of investigators' submissions to an IRB regarding what they would tell subjects about their research studies showed similar results: oral disclosures usually focused on the purpose and procedures of a study and neglected discussion of risks and alternatives (46).

Food and Drug Administration audits of clinical trials provide an estimate of the frequency of such problems. From 1977 to 1996, the FDA is reported to have conducted 4154 audits (47). "Fifty-three percent of the investigators were cited for failing clearly to disclose the experimental nature of their work. In 46 trials involving at least 1000 men, women and children, drugs were tested without any written evidence that subjects had consented" (47, p. 249). IRB reviews by the FDA between 1990 and 1996 (n=942) found cases at 16 percent of IRBs of failure to inform subjects of the experimental nature of procedures, at 13 percent of failure to offer alternatives, and at 10 percent of failure to specify risks and discomforts (47). These findings may actually understate the gravity of the problem. The FDA focused its investigations on audits of consent forms. Situations in which subjects signed seemingly adequate forms but were not given adequate oral explanations or opportunities to ask questions and have them answered would have gone unnoticed.

Subjects and the Therapeutic Misconception

Subjects, too, are not always comfortable with the differences in the nature of research and treatment. For example, patient-subjects in four psychiatric research projects voiced strong convictions that investigators were committed to acting solely in their best interests. This belief of patient-subjects that even in a research setting the principle of personal care will still apply has been called the "therapeutic misconception" (2,48). When not given information about how treatment decisions would be made, subjects fabricated reasonable-sounding explanations that placed their therapeutic interests first. Even when information was offered about the procedures that would be employed (e.g., randomization, double-blind, placebos), many subjects failed to acknowledge what they had heard, to apply it to their own circumstances, or to admit that the procedures served any interests other than their personal care.

In one study of this phenomenon, 69 percent of subjects were unaware that their assignment to treatment conditions would be randomized; 40 percent said explicitly that they expected that assignment would be made on the basis of their therapeutic needs. Similarly, 44 percent of subjects failed to recognize that the use of placebos and non-treatment control groups meant that some subjects who desired the experimental intervention would not receive it. With regard to double-blind procedures, 39 percent of subjects did not understand that their physician would not know which medication they would receive, and an additional 24 percent had only a partial understanding. Finally, when explicitly asked, only 9 percent of subjects could name a single way in which joining a protocol would restrict their options for the treatment they would receive; 50 percent of the subjects in the two medication protocols, in which adjustment of dosage was tightly restricted, said explicitly that they thought their dosage would be adjusted according to their individual needs (48).

One subject, for example, volunteered the information that assignment to active medication or placebo would be on a random basis. When she was asked directly how her own medication would be selected, she said she had no idea. She then added, "I hope it isn't by chance," and suggested that each subject would probably receive the medication needed. Given the conflict between her earlier use of the word random and her current explanation, the issue was pursued. She was asked what her understanding of random was. Her definition was entirely appropriate: "By lottery, by chance, one patient who comes in gets one thing and the next patient gets the next thing." She then began to wonder out loud if this procedure was being used in the current study. Ultimately, she concluded that it was not. Subjects apparently had been so socialized by their previous experiences in medical care settings, in which their expectation of personal care was realistic, that they were unable to adapt to the different norms of the research setting.

This type of therapeutic orientation toward research has been demonstrated in a wide variety of circumstances. For example, when a group of fourteen psychiatric outpatients were told they would be given sugar pills rather than pills containing active medication, about half of them reported that they believed that the pills contained active medication, and only three patients reported no doubts that the pills were placebos (49). The researchers attributed this response to "the force of prior experiences, which at times induced patients to disregard or to disbelieve the doctor's assertion" that no active medication was being given (49). These subjects' therapeutic misconception appeared to be firmly grounded in their difficulty distinguishing previous treatment experiences from the current research setting.

Several of the relevant studies come from cancer trials, where issues related to recruitment have been studied actively (50,51,51a). Penman and colleagues, for example, interviewed 144 cancer patients enrolled in a variety of phase II and phase III clinical trials (52). They reported, "Despite the statements in most consent forms that benefit could not be assured, 43 percent of patients stated they had no doubts at all about benefits from the treatment." Even more remarkably, the study by Schaeffer and colleagues of 127 subjects from four chemotherapy protocols at NIH showed that, despite being provided with information to the contrary, 100 percent of subjects in phase I studies, which are designed only to assess the maximum tolerated dose, described their protocols as having both treatment and research aims (53).

As part of its investigation of federally sponsored radiation research, the Advisory Committee on Human Radiation Experiments analyzed data from brief surveys of 1882 outpatients recruited from cancer and cardiology clinics, and from 90 in-depth interviews of patients who had been in research projects (54). They indicated that former subjects generally viewed their participation in research as in their best medical interests, in large part because "they could not imagine [their physicians] offering something not in their best interests." The report also noted, "Patient-subjects frequently expressed the belief that an intervention would not even be offered if it did not carry some promise of benefit; many certainly assumed that the intervention would not be offered if it posed significant risks."

A survey of attitudes toward research in a combined sample of patients and the general public showed an interesting discrepancy in responses. When asked why people in general should participate in research, 69 percent of respondents cited benefit to society at large. Only 5 percent cited benefit to the subjects themselves. However, when asked why *they* might participate in a research project, 52 percent said they would do it to get the best medical care, and only 23 percent responded that they would do it to contribute to scientific knowledge (55). In another study, among patient-subjects on a psychiatric research ward, the largest group of patients expressed the idea that "research is therapy—a patient and his family often believe that a prestigious research center will be able to cure him when other therapies and hospitals have failed" (43,56). Similarly, subjects frequently interpreted the word research to mean "finding out more about me" or "researching how to treat me better," an entirely personalized and therapeutic understanding of the research endeavor (2). Indeed, subjects' widespread misunderstanding of terminology used to describe research studies may help to sustain their therapeutic misconceptions (57,58).

The Structure of the Decisionmaking Process

Structural problems may also play a role in impeding the process of obtaining informed consent. Investigators often delegate the responsibility for informing and obtaining consent from potential subjects to subordinates who may be unable to clarify subjects' concerns. In a sample of seventeen investigators, only eight were ever directly involved in the disclosure and consent process, and only four were routinely involved throughout the disclosure (20). [In contrast, a study at four Veterans Administration hospitals revealed that 70 percent of thirty-seven principal investigators said that they or a coinvestigator were responsible for obtaining consent (59)]. Delegation of responsibility for informed consent to a junior person on the research team may not only demonstrate the investigator's belief that obtaining consent is of little consequence but also may place the process in the hands of an individual with less understanding of the ethical issues involved. Further, a research assistant who is responsible for recruitment of subjects may feel pressure to obtain subjects' consent and thus be led to distort or omit significant information. One study has shown that investigators infrequently monitor the performance of their subordinates to whom they delegate this responsibility (20).

A second kind of structural problem relates to the inherent pressures on subjects as they decide whether or not to participate. Clearly it would be unethical to withhold an otherwise available treatment in an effort to coerce a patient into joining a research project. However, there are occasions when the treatment the patient desires is only available as part of the research (e.g., when the research involves an investigational drug or a highly specialized procedure). The character of a situation in which the desired treatment is only available as part of a protocol places constraints on the degree of freedom with which a choice can be made. To be sure, there simply is no way to avoid the existence of such situations, and the degree and quality of limitation on free choice here is no greater than those encountered in everyday life, in which hard decisions and trade-offs must be made. The real danger is that patients, in their eagerness to become subjects of the study in order to receive the restricted treatment, will fail to attend to other information that might alter their assessment of the value of participation.

The Communication of Necessary Information

Difficulties in the communication of information can also form a barrier to the goals of informed consent. Complex research projects often require lengthy explanations of elements that are relevant to a potential subject's risk–benefit analysis. When these are committed to writing, the resulting consent forms often run many pages. Federal regulations governing the material that must appear on consent forms, including such items as whether treatment or compensation will be available if injuries occur, also contribute to the length of the forms. Subjects' comprehension of consent forms, and consequent willingness to participate, may be an inverse function of the forms' length (60; see also Chapter 9). Although numerous studies document the positive effects on subjects' understanding of decreasing the complexity of consent forms, improving their readability, and simplifying their format (61,62), there is no evidence that investigators as a group have taken this lesson to heart. Indeed, studies continue to show that consent forms remain consistently complex, even after IRB review (63,64).

What is true for consent forms probably holds for oral explanations as well. There is a lack of research on adequacy of oral disclosure. It seems likely that researchers' (often unconscious) addiction to jargon makes oral disclosure problematic for subjects. At the same time, simplification would probably increase the length of the explanation and might reduce the amount that subjects are able to comprehend.

A Reasonable Approach: Dispelling the Therapeutic Misconception

Obtaining informed consent to research requires good faith and some effort on the part of investigators. Neither the requirements of the law and relevant ethical codes nor the obstacles that commonly arise in the decisionmaking process prevent researchers from fulfilling the duty to obtain informed consent in a reasonable way.

Content of Disclosure

To some extent the decision about what information should be provided is more easily determined in research than in the purely therapeutic setting. Federal regulations (as outlined in Chapter 12), along with additional state and institutional requirements, specify in some detail the material that must be disclosed. In essence, the federal rules require disclosure of: the fact that the nature and purpose of the procedures are experimental, the risks and benefits, the alternatives (in therapeutic situations), and ancillary information on such issues as confidentiality, compensation for injuries, and the right to withdraw from the study. Institutional requirements may supplement these items—for example, asking investigators to inform subjects of the source of funding of their research.

The specificity conveyed by the federal rules and their progeny, however, is to a large extent spurious. Experienced investigators are aware that, particularly in complex investigations in which only a fraction of the available information can actually be disclosed, a large amount of discretion resides in the hands of researchers (and IRBs) to decide what should and should not be revealed. Since IRBs generally focus on written consent forms, ignoring the oral communication that ought to occur as well, investigators have the further ability to shape the tone and substance of the oral disclosure either to underscore or undercut the material in the consent form (45).

Even when they are supportive of the goals of informed consent, researchers may be confused about what subjects need to know in order to make informed decisions. This confusion is accentuated by the fact that anyone intimately familiar with a topic has difficulty empathizing with the problems of understanding faced by a person unfamiliar with the field. Guidance in this regard has tended to take the form of admonitions to adhere to existing regulations, which as we have seen are of little assistance, or to engage the potential subject as a collaborator (per suggestions of Jonas and Ramsey). The latter approach may only further confuse the investigator about what amount and level of material need be revealed.

A more focused approach derives from an awareness of the ways treatment and research differ. Taking this distinction as the conceptual core of disclosure provides a touchstone for investigators. Specifically, in covering the nature, purpose, overall risks and benefits, alternatives, and other specified disclosures required by the ethical mandate of informed consent as well as the federal regulations and state statutes or common law, investigators can ask themselves whether their planned disclosure will help potential subjects comprehend the differences between what they would undergo in the research project and their treatment in the ordinary clinical context. This approach is relevant even for research unlikely to have therapeutic benefit, since even here subjects are likely to extrapolate from the clinical setting and assume that research procedures are intended to benefit them or at the least not to cause them harm. One subject in non-therapeutic research explained that he had joined a research project despite the possible consequences of severe liver damage, because, he said, "Doctor, we know you wouldn't hurt us, and anyway the hospital wouldn't let you" (14).

The discussion between investigator and potential subject, and the consent form, should emphasize the distinction between therapy and research. Where the research consists of a study of a therapy or therapies—such as comparison of an accepted therapy with an innovative therapy, or comparison of a therapy (accepted or innovative) and a placebo, or comparison of all three—the focus must be on the distinction between therapy and research on therapy. Where the potential subject could obtain a particular therapy either in the context of the study or outside the study, much of the information to be provided is the same as in the purely clinical setting. The distinctive features to be called to potential subjects' attention are the nature and purpose of the research, the risks and benefits of being a subject, and the available options for obtaining the same or different therapies outside of the research setting. In particular, potential subjects need to be told about those features of being a research subject that do not exist in ordinary therapy, such as the possible use of placebos or the selection of treatment by randomization.

Such an approach, for projects in which therapies are being employed, can proceed in the following way: after being told that they are being asked to participate in a research project, potential subjects can be informed that the procedures in the project differ from those of the clinical care they would ordinarily receive. "Because this is a research project," the investigator might say, "we will be doing some things differently from what we would do if we were simply treating you for your condition." The investigator can then describe what the research is designed to demonstrate and how it will be conducted, with special emphasis on the aspects that differ from ordinary clinical care.

Although many of the elements of research design that differ most significantly from ordinary treatment are based on sophisticated statistical and methodological principles, they can often be explained quite simply. Potential subjects could be told about randomization in this way: "You will receive one of the three treatments we discussed, but the one you receive will be selected by chance, not because we believe that one or the other will be better for you." About placebos: "Some subjects will be selected by chance to receive sugar pills that are not believed to help the condition you have; this is done so we can find out whether the medications other patients get are really effective, or if many people with your condition would get better even with no active medication at all." About the use of protocols: "Ordinarily doctors change the amount of medication according to how their patients are doing. Here, in order to test the usefulness of the medications we are trying out, we will have to leave your dosage at the same level for four weeks—unless you suffer a severe reaction to it."

Once potential subjects have the distinctions between the research project and ordinary treatment clearly in mind, they can be told about the other risks of participation, as well as the benefits to themselves and others that might derive from the research project. Care must also be taken to ensure that subjects are informed of the risks and benefits of the underlying therapy or therapies on which research is being conducted, and to distinguish between the risks and benefits that arise from treatment in general, and risks and benefits that will accrue only as a result of participation in the project. The alternative of treatment outside a research protocol, if available, should be clearly outlined here, and the subject's right to elect a usual form of treatment or to withdraw from the study at any time should be stressed. Finally, any additional information relevant to a particular project or required by regulations can be provided. The understanding of potential subjects should be assessed continually, and additional information provided to correct misperceptions or misunderstandings as they occur and are detected. Subjects should also be given an opportunity to ask questions about the material that has been presented. In some cases, assistance in deliberating about entry into the protocol may be helpful (65).

This outline would be somewhat different for research in which no therapeutic methods were being employed that might benefit even some of the subjects. Yet the basic idea that needs to be communicated is much the same and could be stated thus: "Our primary goal is to obtain information about the issue we are studying, not to benefit you in any way. This is true even though you may find participation interesting or educational." Purpose and procedures can then be described, again emphasizing the fact that the selection of various experimental conditions is being made for experimental reasons and not with beneficial intent. Risks can then also be reviewed.

What is important about the approach described here is the effort to underline in potential subjects' minds the differences between research and treatment, or in some cases the lack of overall therapeutic intent. The precise wording and even the order of the disclosure can vary considerably, depending on the nature of the research project, the preferences of the investigators, and the potential subjects' educational levels. In their efforts to convey these distinctions, physicians should not lose sight of the fact that they are also obligated to adhere to the usual rules for obtaining informed consent that would prevail in the absence of a research protocol. That is, potential subjects must also be adequately informed of the risks, benefits, nature, and purpose of the investigated therapies themselves.

An additional issue that sometimes arises in the consent process is the deliberate use of deception for research purposes. Deception in the process of recruiting research subjects is frequently used in social psychological experiments, in an attempt to control the mindset that subjects bring to the experimental situation (37). Outright deception, though permitted by current federal regulations and the ethical code of the American Psychological Association (66), has been the subject of considerable criticism. Leading opponents of the practice have charged that deception does not actually produce a naturalistic situation, and thus its putative advantages may be a sham (67). A hot debate rages over these contentions (68). It is also argued that, in the long-term, deception may have an adverse effect on the entire research enterprise because researchers will eventually be able to enlist only cynical, distrustful subjects and may even forfeit public support for their research (67).

The most telling argument against deception is that it is disrespectful of persons. It serves the acquisition of knowledge while demeaning human dignity and is therefore simply incompatible with the underlying premise of informed consent, the entitlement of subjects to make knowing decisions about participation in research. Even were it proven effective, and its aftereffects mitigated completely by debriefing, deception still represents a serious intrusion on individual autonomy. Of course, subjects should have the freedom to consent to deception—that is, to agree knowingly to the researcher's withholding of some unspecified information from them. But complete deception cannot be justified within the framework of informed consent.

Disclosure as a Process

There are numerous benefits for both patients and physicians in a model that views consent as a process rather than an event (see Chapter 8). The same is true for subjects and investigators. Thus, the dialogue between investigator and potential subject outlined previously need not proceed linearly or take place as a single event. Particularly when potential subjects are accessible for a period of time, as inpatients or students might be, discussions can take place on a number of occasions, and the intervening periods can allow subjects to integrate and reflect on the information provided, to formulate questions, and to focus concerns (69). A subject's agreement to participate in research, signified by signing a consent form, should not be seen as the end of the process. Questions will arise; information will be forgotten; new concerns may come to the fore. The subject's right to withdraw at any time is a reminder of the need to view informed consent as a continuing, interactive process, with consent in effect renewed each time an experimental procedure takes place.

A variety of devices can facilitate this process. Allowing potential subjects to review written material and ask questions about it at a later time, prior to obtaining formal consent, can be useful. Additional information can then be provided as needed. All written material should attempt to strike a reasonable balance between clarity and brevity. Testing the comprehension of a sample of persons with educational backgrounds similar to those in the subject pool may be of use. Consent forms, required in most research settings, can play a useful role in informing subjects but must not be allowed to dominate the process (70; see also Chapter 9).

Recent years have witnessed a good deal of innovation in the informed consent process for research, much of it salutary. Investigators have introduced techniques including: the routine use of questionnaires to assess subjects' understanding after disclosure, but prior to consent (71); disclosures augmented by videotape and computer-based presentations (72–74); use of discussion groups, including subjects who have completed the study, to inform prospective subjects; involvement of family members in the consent process; a "try out" period during which subjects could experience some of the research procedures prior to being asked to give informed consent (75); and distribution of supplementary materials written at a low level of complexity. All of these may be reasonable approaches, though not all will be called for in every study. This proliferation of efforts to inform patients suggests wider recognition of the informed consent process as an educational effort, with teaching techniques developed for use in the classroom being brought to bear in the research setting.

Greater attention to ensuring that subjects' consent is meaningful has meant increased focus on the decisionmaking competence of research participants (76). As in the treatment settings discussed in Chapter 5, adult subjects are presumed to be competent to provide consent to research, though clearly some fall short of this ideal. Data characterizing those populations likely to be at greatest risk for incompetence are limited, focusing as might be expected on persons with psychiatric and dementing disorders (77–79). It is already apparent that not all psychiatric disorders increase the risk of incompetence and that there is great variability even among persons and populations with the same disorder (80). Moreover, it seems likely that many patients with serious non-psychiatric illnesses whose underlying conditions or treatments affect mentation may also be at risk of impaired capacity to consent to research.

For some groups of potential subjects for whom there is a particular reason to suspect elevated rates of incompetence, especially those being recruited to studies that pose greater risks of harm, it may be desirable to screen for reduced decisional capacity to obtain informed consent. Structured instruments for this purpose have been developed (81). Although there has been considerable controversy over who should do this screening—with some believing that investigators are too self-interested to be trustworthy (75)—members of the research team will be the most reasonable choice for this task in almost all cases (82). Another approach to detecting decisional impairment is simply to assess all potential subjects' comprehension after disclosure, a practice that is becoming more widespread in any event.

The key to dealing with decisional incapacity on the part of potential subjects is to recognize it as something that exists on a spectrum. Some persons show marginal impairment, while others have a severe lack of capacity. Detection of some degree of impairment, even a considerable degree, does not necessarily mean that subjects cannot provide a meaningful consent to research. Rather, it implies that these subjects will have a harder time learning, remembering, and manipulating the relevant information, and thus may require special efforts at education (83). These may include repetition of disclosures over a period of time, aided by devices such as computer-based learning programs and printed instructional materials. There are data to suggest that at least one category of subjects— patients with schizophrenia—respond well to such efforts (77).

Our discussion has proceeded as if the principal investigator were the only person directly involved in obtaining informed consent. In many projects this involvement is impossible. For example, in large-scale epidemiologic surveys, subjects may be recruited over a wide geographic area, and in projects with heavy subject flows, several subjects may be recruited simultaneously. It may simply be impossible for the investigators themselves to make time to obtain informed consent from all subjects. Thus, delegation of the responsibility inevitably occurs in many studies. This delegation is not necessarily bad, as long as investigators clearly communicate the importance of the process to the staff members responsible and assign the task only to persons who understand the ethical concerns underlying informed consent and who know enough about the projects to answer the questions likely to arise. Furthermore, staff should not be placed under such unreasonable pressures to meet subject enrollment quotas that they might be tempted to distort the disclosure process to attain that goal. The supervising investigators should obtain informed consent themselves at least a few times early in the course of a study, so as to become familiar with problems that may arise and better instruct their subordinates about them. Periodic checks on how informed consent is being obtained may be of use, too. This procedure would address the reported problems of investigators whose ideas about what kind of subject might be incompetent to consent to their study have never been communicated to the staff who must obtain consent, and who do not know how the staff handles the competence issue in practice (20).

As desirable as investigator involvement is, in some cases it may be optimal for someone else to be involved in addition or instead. Particularly in research on therapeutic procedures where the investigator also acts as the subject's physician, there may be a strong tendency on the part of subjects to merge in their minds the goals of research and treatment. The investigators themselves may be unwilling or unable to help subjects identify the non-therapeutic aspects of the proposed research or the additional risks it might entail. When those risks are particularly great, there is ample justification for IRBs to require that investigators' explanations be supplemented by information from an uninvolved party. This person, while not interfering with the communication of information that the investigator wishes to stress, can pay particular attention to the distinctions between treatment and research.

Balancing the Costs and Benefits

The approach to informed consent suggested here has costs and benefits. It seems reasonable to believe that the more clearly potential subjects understand the difference between research and treatment (and thus the additional risks they may incur from research participation), the more likely they may be to decline to participate in research. This phenomenon may slow down recruitment in some studies, bias samples, and perhaps prevent certain research altogether. No data are available to tell us how likely these consequences are, and some arguments exist against the underlying assumption. Some claim that subjects may be so impressed by the honesty and openness of investigators who reveal information that cuts against investigators' interests in recruiting subjects that they may decide to enroll in the study anyway on the grounds that the investigator is a person who can be trusted.

We are probably safe in assuming that some negative impact on subject recruitment is likely. But it may not be as great as is usually assumed. In particular, it may be mitigated by alternatives to randomized clinical trials (the most problematic type of research project where consent is concerned) and the techniques for correcting for resulting biases statistically (7). On the other hand, efforts to avoid the problem by obtaining consent only after randomization has occurred (83), or otherwise restricting the number of options disclosed to potential subjects (84, 85) are not good solutions because they impair subjects' power to make informed choices. What happens when means of mitigation are not available? Marcia Angell's response is to the point: "What can be done when nonrandomized designs are considered inadequate but randomization would be difficult because of patients' preferences for one treatment or the other? Not all problems have solutions. It simply may not be ethically possible to conduct a valid randomized clinical trial under these circumstances" (7). If our efforts to promote individual autonomy by allowing subjects to make informed decisions about participation may succeed only at the cost of slowing some scientific endeavors, that cost may have to be tolerated.

It would be wrong not to consider the potential benefits of an approach that emphasizes dispelling the therapeutic misconception. Well-informed patient-subjects may be more cooperative with research procedures and more willing to participate in later extensions of research projects. As Lee Park and colleagues noted, "Informing patients might be especially helpful in long term studies and follow-up studies in which patient cooperation would be facilitated by the patient's awareness of the significance of this participation not only for himself but for patients in the future. This kind of doctor-patient collaborative atmosphere would be conducive to the acceptance of arrangements in which patients could be called back or visited at home at predefined intervals" (86). For some types of research, subject cooperation may be a crucial determinant of success.

The advantages of having well-informed subjects are also clear when one considers what might happen if and when subjects discover that they have misunderstood the purposes of the study procedures and the degree of benefit to themselves. Subjects coming to such a realization during a study might drop out and thereby disrupt the conduct of the protocol. Subjects whose realization occurs only after the conclusion of a study may be left with anger and resentment against the researchers who they feel deceived them, even if their own desire to see research through therapeutic lenses contributed mightily to the deception. Such subjects will be unlikely ever again to consider research participation. As they tell their stories to sympathetic relatives and friends, they may contribute to a general perception that researchers treat patients as guinea pigs. The failure to distinguish between researchers and clinicians may contribute to a general perception that all physicians (or psychologists, sociologists, or scientists in general) cannot be trusted. Since most research is heavily dependent on public support—both for funding and for participation as subjects—the spread of such perceptions may constitute a threat to the research enterprise as a whole more serious than the inability to perform a few studies because of a scarcity of available subjects.

Well-informed subjects, while recognizing the potential conflict between their interests and those of investigators, nonetheless realize to some extent the goal of shared objectives advocated by Jonas and Ramsey. Such subjects are likely to prove strong allies in the future. They may benefit from learning more about the conduct of research, and in special cases their knowing participation may even have beneficial effects on their behavior in other areas (87). Disclosure of the type suggested in this chapter may make it easier for some investigators as well. The guilt that has been observed among researchers, which derives from their recognition that they are acting in ways that may be contrary to subjects' best interests, can be mitigated by limiting involvement to subjects who are truly aware of the risks they are running (5,86). A focus on informing patients and dispelling the therapeutic misconception will lead to greater respect for subjects' autonomy, and ultimately, perhaps, more cooperative subjects as well.

References

1. Fried, C. (1974) *Medical Experimentation: Personal Integrity and Social Policy.* New York: American Elsevier.
2. Appelbaum, P.S., Roth, L.H., and Lidz, C.W. (1982) The therapeutic misconception: informed consent in psychiatric research. *Int J Law Psychiatry,* 5:319–329.
3. Benson, P.R., Roth, L.H., and Winslade, W.J. (1985) Informed consent in psychiatric research: preliminary findings from an ongoing investigation. *Soc Sci Med,* 20:1331–1341.
4. Howard, J. and Friedman, L. (1981) Protecting the scientific integrity of a clinical trial: some ethical dilemmas. *Clin Pharmacol Ther,* 29:561–569.
5. Epstein, R.S. and Janowsky, D.S. (1969) Research on the psychiatric ward: the effects on conflicting priorities. *Arch Gen Psychiatry,* 21:455–463.
6. Levine, R.J. (1984) *Ethics and Regulation of Clinical Research.* Baltimore: Urban and Schwarzenberg, pp. 126–129.
7. Angell, M. (1984) Patients' preferences in randomized clinical trials. *N Engl J Med,* 310:1385–1387.
8. Katz, J. (1984) *The Silent World of Doctor and Patient.* New York: Free Press.
9. Rothman, K.J. and Michels, K.B. (1994) The continuing unethical use of placebo controls. *N Engl J Med,* 331:394–398.
10. Schechter, C., et al. (1995) The use of placebo controls (ltrs.). *N Engl J Med,* 332:60–62.

11. Kaptchuk, T.J. (1998) Powerful placebo: the dark side of the randomized controlled trial. *Lancet*, 351:1722–1735.

12. Aspinall, R.L. and Goodman, N.W. (1995) Denial of effective treatment and poor quality of clinical information in placebo controlled trials of ondansetron for postoperative nausea and vomiting: a review of published trials. *Br Med J*, 311:844–846.

13. Lapierre, Y.D. (1998) Ethics and placebo. *J Psychiatry Neurosci*, 23:9–11.

14. Makuch, R.W. and Johnson, M.T. (1989) Dilemmas in the use of active control groups in clinical research. *IRB: A Review of Human Subjects Research*, 11(1):1–5.

15. Streiner, D.L. (1995) The ethics of placebo-controlled trials. *Can J Psychiatry*, 40: 165–166.

16. Malone, R.P. and Simpson, G.M. (1998) Use of placebo in clinical trials involving children and adolescents. *Psychiatr Serv*, 49:1413–1414.

17. Kane, J. and Borester, M. (1997) The use of placebo controls in psychiatric research. In Shamoo, A. (ed) *Ethics in Neurobiological Research with Human Subjects: The Baltimore Conference on Ethics.* Amsterdam: Gordon and Breach Publishers.

18. Jonas, H. (1970) Philosophical reflections on experimenting with human subjects. In Freund, P.A. (ed) *Experimentation with Human Subjects.* New York: Braziller.

19. Ramsey, P. (1977) *The Patient as Person.* New Haven: Yale University Press.

20. Appelbaum, P.S. and Roth, L.H. (1983) The structure of informed consent in psychiatric research. *Behav Sci Law*, 1:9–19.

21. Little, P. and Williamson, L. (1997) Ethics committees and the *BMJ* should continue to consider the overall benefit to patients (ltr). *Br Med J*, 314:1478.

22. Baum, M. (1997) The whole population must be mobilized in the war against cancer (ltr.). *Br Med J*, 314:1482.

23. Madler, H., Myles, P., McRae, R., et al. (1998) Ethics review and clinical trials (ltrs.). *Lancet*, 351:1065–1066.

24. Truog, R.D., Robinson, W., Randolph, A., and Morris, A. (1999) Is informed consent always necessary for randomized, controlled trials? *N Engl J Med*, 340:804–807.

25. Beecher, H.K. (1966) Consent in clinical experimentation: myth and reality. *JAMA*, 195:124–125.

26. Ingelfinger, F.J. (1972) Informed (but uneducated) consent. *N Engl J Med*, 287:465–466.

27. Garnham, J.C. (1975) Some observations on informed consent in non-therapeutic research. *J Med Ethics*, 1: 138–145.

28. Farndon, J.R. (1998) Patients' understanding of clinical trials. *Lancet*, 351:1663.

29. Dennis, M., O'Rourke, S., Slattery, J., et al. (1997) Evaluation of a stroke family care-worker: results of a randomized controlled trial [with commentaries by McLean, S. and Dennis, M.] *Br Med J*, 314:1071–1077.

30. Lacher, M.J. (1978) Physicians and patients as obstacles to a randomized trial. *Clin Res*, 26:375–379.

31. Llewellyn-Thomas, H.A., McGreal, M.J., Thiel, E.C., et al. (1991) Patients' willingness to enter clinical trials: measuring the association with perceived benefits for decision participation. *Soc Sci Med*, 32:35–42.

32. Taylor, K.M., Margolese, R.G., and Soskolne, C.L. (1984) Physicians' reasons for not entering eligible patients in a randomized clinical trial for breast cancer. *N Engl J Med*, 310:1363–1367.

33. Schubert, D.S.P., Patterson, M.B., Miller, F.T., et al. (1984) Informed consent as a source of bias in clinical research. *Psychiatr Res*, 12:313–320.

34. Spohn, H.E. and Fitzpatrick, T. (1980) Informed consent and bias in samples of schizophrenia subjects at risk for drug withdrawal. *J Abnormal Psychol,* 89:79–92.
35. Edlund, M.J., Craig, T.J., and Richardson, M.A. (1985) Informed consent as a form of volunteer bias. *Am J Psychiatry,* 142:624–627.
36. Brownell, K.D. and Stunkard, A.J. (1982) The double-blind in danger: untoward consequences of informed consent. *Am J Psychiatry,* 139:1487–1489.
37. Adair, J.G., Dushenko, T.W., and Lindsay, R.C.L. (1985) Ethical regulations and their impact on research practice. *Am Psychol,* 40:59–72.
38. Singer, E. (1978) Informed consent: consequences for response rate and response quality in social surveys. *American Sociological Review,* 43:144–162.
39. McLean, P.D. (1980) The effect of informed consent on the acceptance of random treatment assignment in a clinical population. *Behav Ther,* 11:129–133.
40. Kokes, R.F., Fremouw, W., and Strauss, J.S. (1977) Lost subjects: source of bias in clinical research. *Arch Gen Psychiatry,* 34:1363–1365.
41. Simes, R.J., Tattersall, M.H.N., Coates, A.S., et al. (1986) Randomized comparison of procedures for obtaining informed consent in clinical trials of treatment for cancer. *Br Med J,* 293:1065–1068.
42. Rosenthal, R. and Rosnow, R.L. (1975) *The Volunteer Subject.* New York: Wiley.
43. Jacobs, L. and Kotin, J. (1972) Fantasies of psychiatric research. *Am J Psychiatry,* 128:1071–1080.
44. Bursztajn, H., Feinbloom, R.I., Hamm, R.M., et al. (1981) *Medical Choices, Medical Chances: How Patients, Families, and Physicians Can Cope with Uncertainty.* New York: Delacorte.
45. Lidz, C., Meisel, A., Zerubavel, E., et al. (1984) *Informed Consent: A Study of Decisionmaking in Psychiatry.* New York: Guilford.
46. Titus, S.L. and Keane, M.A. (1996) Do you understand? An ethical assessment of researchers' description of the consenting process. *J Clin Ethics,* 7:60–68.
47. Epstein, K. and Sloate, B. (1997) Informed consent is not always obtained in the United States. *Br Med J,* 3(15):249.
48. Appelbaum, P.S., Roth, L.H., Lidz, C.W., Benson, P., and Winslade, W. (1987) False hopes and best data: consent to research and the therapeutic misconception. *Hastings Cent Rep,* 17(2):20–24.
49. Park, L.C. and Covi, L. (1965) Nonblind placebo trial: an exploration of neurotic patients' responses to placebo when its inert content is disclosed. *Arch Gen Psychiatry,* 12:336–345.
50. Gotay, C.C. (1991) Accrual to cancer clinical trials: directions from the research literature. *Soc Sci Med,* 26:569–577.
51. Verheggen, F.W.S.M. and van Wijman, F.C.T.B. (1996) Informed consent in clinical trials. *Health Policy,* 36:131–153.
51a. Levi R., Marsick R., Drotar D., Kodish E. (2000) Disclosure and informed consent: learning from parents of children with cancer. *J Peds Hematol Oncol,* 222: 3–12.
52. Penman, D.T., Holland, J.C., Bahna, G.F., et al. (1984) Informed consent for investigational chemotherapy: patients' and physicians' perceptions. *J Clin Oncol,* 2:849–855.
53. Schaeffer, M.H., Krantz, D.S., Wichman, A., et al. (1996) The impact of disease severity on the informed consent process in research. *Am J Med,* 100:261–268.
54. Advisory Committee on Human Radiation Experiments (ACHRE) (1995) *Final Report.* Washington, D.C.: U.S. Government Printing Office.

55. Cassileth, B.R., Lusk, E.J., Miller, D.S., et al. (1982) Attitudes toward clinical trials among patients and the public. *JAMA,* 248:968–970.
56. Leigh, V. (1975) Attitudes and fantasy themes of patients on a psychiatric research unit. *Arch Gen Psychiatry,* 32:598–601.
57. Sugarman, J., Kass, N.E., Goodman, S.N., et al. (1998) What patients say about medical research. *IRB: A Review of Human Subjects Research,* 20(4):1–6.
58. Waggoner, W.C. and Mayo, D.M. (1995) Who understands? A survey of 25 words or phrases commonly used in proposed clinical research consent forms. *IRB: A Review of Human Subjects Research,* 17(1):6–9.
59. Riecken, H.W. and Ravich, R. (1982) Informed consent to biomedical research in Veterans' Administration hospitals. *JAMA,* 248:344–348.
60. Epstein, L.C. and Lasagna, L. (1969) Obtaining informed consent—form or substance. *Arch Intern Med,* 123:682–688.
61. Sugarman, J., McCrory, D.C., Powell, D., et al. (1999) Empirical research on informed consent. *Hastings Cent Rep,* (suppl.):S1–S42.
62. Bjorn, E., Rossel, P., and Holm, S. (1999) Can the written information to research subjects be improved?—an empirical study. *J Med Ethics,* 25:263–267.
63. Hammerschmidt, D.E. and Keane, M.A. (1992) Institutional review board (IRB) review lacks impact on readability of consent forms for research. *Am J Med Sci,* 304:348–351.
64. Goldstein, A.O., Fraiser, P., Curtis, P., Reid, A., and Kreher, N. (1996) Consent form readability in university-sponsored research. *J Fam Pract,* 42:606–611.
65. Widdershoven, G.A.M. and Verheggen, F.W.S.M. (1999) Improving informed consent by implementing shared decision making in health care. *IRB,* 21(4):1–5.
66. American Psychological Association (1982) *Ethical Principles in the Conduct of Research with Human Participants.* Washington, D.C.: APA.
67. Baumrind, D. (1985) Research using intentional deception: ethical issues revisited. *Am Psychol,* 40:165–174.
68. Baron, R.A. (1981) The "Costs of Deception" revisited: an openly optimistic rejoinder. *IRB: A Review of Human Subjects' Research,* 3(1):8–10.
69. Carpenter, W.T. (1974) A new setting for informed consent. *Lancet,* 1:500–501.
70. Lidz, C.W. and Roth, L.H. (1981) The signed form—informed consent? In Boruch, R.F., Ross, J., and Cecil, J.S. (eds) *Solutions to Legal and Ethical Problems in Applied Social Research.* New York: Academic Press.
71. Wirsching, D.A., Wirsching, W.C., Marder, S.R., et al. (1998) Informed consent: assessment of comprehension. *Am J Psychiatry,* 155:1508–1511.
72. Fureman, I., Meyers, K., McLellan, A.T., et al. (1997) Evaluation of a video-supplement to informed consent: injection drug users and preventive HIV vaccine efficacy trials. *AIDS Educ Prev,* 9:330–341.
73. Weston, J., Hannah, M., and Downes, J. (1997) Evaluating the benefits of a patient information video during the informed consent process. *Patient Education and Counseling,* 30:239–245.
74. Murphy, P.W., Chesson, A.L., Walker, L., Arnold, C.L., and Chesson, L.M. (2000) Comparing the effectiveness of video and written materials for improving knowledge among sleep disorders clinic patients with limited literacy skills. *South Med J,* 93:297–304.
75. Rikkert, M.G.M.O., van der Bercken, J.H.L., ten Have, A.M.J., et al. (1997) Experienced consent in geriatrics research: a new method to optimize the capacity to consent in frail elderly subjects. *J Med Ethics,* 23:271–276.

Fulfilling the Aim of Informed Consent to Research 303

76. National Bioethics Advisory Commission (1998) Research Involving Persons with Mental Disorders That May Affect Decisionmaking Capacity. Volume 1, Report and Recommendations. Rockville, Maryland: NBAC.
77. Appelbaum, P.S., Grisso, T., Frank, E., O'Donnell, S., and Kupfer, D. (1999) Competence of depressed patients for consent to research. Am J Psychiatry, 156:1380–1384.
78. Carpenter, W.T., Gold, J.M., Lahti, A.C., et al.(2000) Decisional capacity for informed consent in schizophrenia research. Arch Gen Psychiatry, 57:533–538.
79. Stanley, B., Stanley, M., Guido, J., et al. (1988) The functional competency of elderly at risk. Gerontologist, 28:53–58.
80. Berg, J. and Appelbaum, P.S. (1999) Subjects' capacity to consent to neurobiological research. In Pincus, H., Lieberman, J.A., and Ferris, S. (eds) Ethics in Psychiatric Research: A Resource Manual for Human Subjects Protection. Washington, D.C.: American Psychiatric Press.
81. Appelbaum, P.S. and Grisso, T. (2001) MacArthur Competence Assessment Tool—Clinical Research (MacCAT-CR). Sarasota, Fl.: Professional Resource Press.
82. Appelbaum, P.S. (1999) Competence and consent to research: a critique of the recommendations of the National Bioethics Advisory Commission. In: Shamoo, A. (ed) Research and Decisional Capacity—Response to the National Bioethics Advisory Commission's (NBAC) Report. Conference Proceedings. Amsterdam: Gordon and Breach Publishers.
83. Appelbaum, P.S. (1998) Missing the boat: competence and consent in psychiatric research (editorial). Am J Psychiatry, 155:1486–1488.
84. Zelen, M. (1990): Randomised consent designs for clinical trials: an update. Stat Med, 9:645–656.
85. Gallo, C., Perrone, F., DePlacido, S., and Giusti, C. (1995) Informed versus randomised consent to clinical trials. Lancet, 346:1060–1064.
86. Park, L.C., Covi, L., and Uhlenhuth, E.H. (1967) Effects of informed consent on research patients and study results. J Nerv Ment Dis, 145:349–357.
87. Siris, S.G., Docherty, J.P., and McGlashan, T.H. (1979) Intrapsychic structural effects of psychiatric research. Am J Psychiatry, 136:1567–1571.

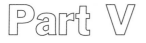

Part V

Advancing Informed Consent

14

The Limits of Informed Consent

It will come as no surprise to anyone who has read this far to know that we are enthusiastic supporters of informed consent. We believe that entitlement to adequate information and the right to make choices about one's medical treatment are fundamental ethical rights that are every bit as important in the healthcare arena as, for example, free speech and due process of law are in the wider society. Moreover, informed consent does not merely have deontological value. We have argued that, if done correctly, informed consent can often lead to better doctor–patient relationships, better patient adherence to treatment plans, and a fuller understanding of the disease process on the part of the healthcare provider.

Yet it is also important to understand the limits of informed consent so we do not try to make it do what it cannot do. For example, although informed consent may help in managing treatment, by itself it does not cure illness. The claims that have been made for informed consent, however, are sometimes almost that extravagant. Informed consent has been suggested as the means to protect patients from poor care (1–3), including involuntary care (4), and as a means to improve the outcomes of care (5, 6). It has been proposed as the solution to the problems of nursing homes (7) and as a device for compensating patients who are harmed by poor medical treatment (8). None of these are entirely specious ideas. Several of them, indeed, may be correct in part, but it is important for us to understand what informed consent cannot do as well as what it can. Just as free speech does not guarantee good government and due process of law does not guarantee justice, so too informed consent cannot solve all of the problems of the healthcare system.

In this chapter we explore some of the limitations of informed consent. Specifically, we want to suggest four propositions. First, informed consent is a mechanism for improving communication and decision making among healthcare providers and patients. However, it cannot create opportunities for autonomous choice when such choices are, in reality, lacking. Substantial constraints on patients are not necessarily obliterated simply because patients are given a formal opportunity to choose among various treatment options. Second, informed consent is a mode of decision making that has developed in a specific cultural context. It should not be assumed to function in the same way either in other societies or with individuals from different cultures. Third, informed consent may lose its impact when the parties to it lack a common interpretative framework, for example, if they approach the decisionmaking context with different conceptions of illness and its treatment. Finally, it is important to remember that, although in general an effort to get genuine informed consent will improve communication between doctors and patients, there are aspects of interpersonal communication that are not necessarily improved by disclosing all the facts in the situation. Interacting with patients who have substantially different expectations about the relationship may create a situation in which open communication will not necessarily produce the best result, at least in the short run.

Informed Consent in the Absence of Choice

Informed consent is supposed to enhance autonomy. A critical part of this process involves expanding individual choice. However, if because of the realities of a situation choice is not available, no informed consent procedure can create it. There are several circumstances in which this may be true. First, options may exist but the resources may not be available to make use of them. For example, a cardiologist may offer a patient with congestive heart failure a choice between conservative medical management and a heart transplant, but if the patient has no insurance, there is no real choice. A second, equally important way in which a real choice may not be available concerns situations in which the very structure of the setting impinges on autonomy. We offer a case study to demonstrate this type of limitation on the use of informed consent to augment autonomy.

Informed Consent and Autonomy in Nursing Homes

It has been widely recognized among providers of long-term care for the elderly that nursing homes severely constrain the autonomy of residents (9, 10). This has led to a wide variety of proposals about how informed consent and informed-consentlike procedures (including, for example, contracts signed by residents before entering the facility) could significantly enhance autonomy (11). Although there is some evidence that marginal gains may be made by such procedures, the autonomy problems in nursing homes and other "total institutions" are not easily amenable to change simply by presenting the subject with a formal choice.

The sociologist Erving Goffman points out some of the difficulties of attempting to make such changes in his classic study of what he calls "total institutions"—organizations in which individuals are watched over in a round-the-clock living and working situation that is largely cut off from the outside world. In particular, Goffman notes that:

> A basic social arrangement in modern society is that the individual tends to sleep, play, and work in different places with different co-participants, under different authorities, and without an overall rational plan. The central features of total institutions can be described as a breakdown of the barriers ordinarily separating these three spheres of life. (12)

Goffman suggests that total institutions substantially undermine personal autonomy.

> Total institutions disrupt or defile precisely those actions that in civil society have the role of attesting to the actor and those in his presence that he has some command over his world— that he is a person with "adult" self-determination, autonomy and freedom of action. (12)

Nursing homes that provide long-term care are good examples of total institutions. For our purposes, the issue is not whether they undermine autonomy, but the ways in which they do so. To the degree that this involves lack of information, deception, and failure to disclose risks and benefits, an informed-consentlike intervention might remedy the problem. Indeed, the first thing that an observer who is interested in autonomy and informed consent will note when visiting such an institution is the lack of decisions for residents to make. Although some facilities may work with residents and their families to make plans about forgoing life support, rarely are there discussions of day-to-day living issues. In fact, daily living is tightly structured by medically focused rules and by routines that apply (at least in theory) to all residents. They are designed, among other things, to allow the staff to complete their work as efficiently as possible. Requiring residents to live under uniform, highly restrictive rules clearly does not promote autonomy.

If informed consent is the solution, the resident should be offered choices, and have the risks and benefits and alternatives of each explained. It is easy to imagine an informed-consentlike rule that would specify that such organizations must provide clients with the maximum number of practical choices in directing their day-to-day living. But the lack of options is only a small part of the autonomy-limiting features of total institutions like nursing homes.

Although no single aspect of such organizations is necessarily ethically problematic when considered alone, the cumulative effect of living in a nursing home adversely affects a patient's ability to live a self-directed life. Concerns include:

- the absence of privacy—Residents' doors are always open so that residents can be monitored by staff.
- residents' social identities—Residents are reduced from people with long and complex personal histories to patients who are largely known by the "medicalized" stories (rich in medical detail, but containing little about the person) recorded in their charts.
- residents' rooms—All rooms are furnished identically with hospital stock furniture. Residents may not be permitted to bring with them such identity tokens as their furniture, family photographs, or other valued personal possessions.
- daily routines—Awakenings, mealtimes, and bedtimes are highly scheduled by staff and inflexible to the requests of residents.

An illustration of the last point can be seen in the way in which residents of a nursing home that we observed were awakened every morning. Each nursing assistant had a series of residents whom she had to assist in getting up and getting dressed. To accomplish these tasks efficiently, the nurses had adopted a policy in which they first woke up resident A, followed by resident B, resident C, etc. Then they went back to the beginning of the line and put resident A on the toilet, followed by B, etc. Then they returned to resident A and performed the next function, etc. This, of course, is more like an assembly line than an autonomous life.

Of course, these problems are present not only in nursing homes. Indeed, acute care hospitals also resemble Goffman's image of the total institution. Consider, for example, the characteristics of an Intensive Care Unit (ICU). Here, too, many of the same social structural features of a nursing home are present:

- the absence of privacy—Patients' cubicles do not even have doors. Temporary and minimal privacy is provided by a curtain.
- patients' social identities—Patients are reduced from people with long and complex personal histories to bodies who are largely known by the results of their medical tests.
- patients' rooms—These are furnished identically with hospital stock furniture.
- patients' schedule—Visitors are restricted to certain hours, and interactions with family or friends are at risk of being interrupted by medical or nursing personnel, who may insist that the visitors leave so as to allow some medical procedure to be performed.

The point is not that hospitals, or nursing homes for that matter, are poorly organized (although they may be). Nor is it that medical or nursing personnel in these settings are unkind to the people for whom they care. What is important is that these social structures substantially undermine autonomy. Simply increasing disclosure of information cannot solve these features of social structure.

The Cultural Context of Informed Consent

Although we often are tempted in the United States to think of informed consent as a universal human right, it exists in a cultural context. It is not an accident that the concept of informed consent in medical care developed here. The United States has a long tradition of commitment to individuality that crystallized in the founding documents of its political system, the Declaration of Independence and the Constitution. Drawing on the predominantly Protestant religious grounding of the new nation, these documents asserted the rights of all to follow the dictates of one's conscience independent of tradition and political coercion. Although these rights initially were accorded only to free white males who owned property, over the next two hundred years they have been expanded to include, to some degree, all members of society.

The concept of human rights is certainly not American in origin (13). Indeed, the French Enlightenment can probably be credited as the modern source of the concept of human rights, and the broader concepts of individualism have deep roots in Judeo-Christian religious beliefs. However, the differences in the European and the American concepts of such rights show that individual independence and autonomy are much more prominent in the American conception, while economic rights are more important in the Continental one.

This distinction could not be clearer than it is in health care. While the rest of the developed world has achieved universal access to health care (albeit with fairly strict governmental control on expenditures), the United States has developed the doctrine of informed consent and embedded it in a system of health insurance that allows very generous expenditures (albeit with increasing control on expenditures) for technically complex and expensive procedures, but provides no insurance for 45 million citizens. Although informed consent, as both a legal and an ethical doctrine, has been adopted by a number of countries—particularly in England and Scandinavia—it remains in many ways an American construct.

The point is not that the advocacy of informed consent by Americans is parochial or that those who seek to promote informed consent in other cultures are doomed to failure. Rather, it is important to appreciate that many cultures do not consider informed consent a universal human right of patients (14). The value of informed consent is not intuitively obvious to either patients or healthcare professionals in some cultural settings. To take an obvious example, the implications of a written consent form may depend, in part, on a patient's cultural background. In many peasant societies, written documents are suspect as something that lawyers develop for the rich landlords to take away peasants' traditional land rights. More fundamentally, individual autonomy is accorded less value than preservation of particular relationships or the authority of community norms.

Thus, there are problems not just with the technical requirements of informed consent, but with its theoretical underpinnings. Consider the notion that all competent adults have a right to control their medical care. In some societies, disagreement of a junior member of a family with the elders about the junior member's health care would be quite inappropriate. For example, in many African cultures, "[y]ounger members of traditional African families cannot make certain decisions, particularly in the area of health care, without referring to authority figures in the family. In the case of sickness, it may be the grandfather or grandmother who is the authority figure. A wife cannot give consent for any treatment, whether scientific or traditional, without the knowledge of her husband, even in an emergency" (15, p. 105). Similarly, Ahmed Okasha writes of Arab culture that "the collectivity of the community is valued rather than the individuality of its members. Decisions are made not at an individual level but at a familial, tribal or communal level, in the perceived collective interest." And he asks: "How can we adhere to our [international] ethical guidelines and at the same time not disregard the local values and norms of our target population?" (16, p. 18).

A somewhat different example of cultural difference related to informed consent concerns the second largest minority in America, the Latino population. There is ample evidence of a "familial" focus in the Latino community that crosses such different ethnicities as Mexican-American, Central-American, and Cuban-American groups in the United States (17). How can a culture that is deeply committed to family respond to the individualistic focus of informed consent? Consider the decision about treatment of terminal cancer. In a study of reported preferences of different ethnic groups in Los Angeles County, Leslie Blackhall and colleagues (18) found that 88 percent of African Americans and 87 percent of European Americans thought that patients should be told of a diagnosis of metastatic cancer, but only 47 percent of Korean Americans and 65 percent of Mexican Americans thought so. Similarly, Korean Americans and Mexican Americans were substantially more likely to believe that decisions about the use of life-support technology should be made by the family. Most informed consent theorists would assume that this decision is the patient's to make. Whether or not to consult the family is the patient's choice (of course, if they attend to the issue at all, most physicians would probably encourage their patients to discuss pending operations with their families). Contrast this with the situation in many non-Western cultures in which the expectation from all concerned is that the family needs to be the primary decision maker.

Another cultural difference concerns "truth telling." Joseph Carrese and Lorna Rhodes, in an ethnographic study of Navajos living on their reservation, report that Navajo culture strongly supports positive thinking and speaking and avoids negative discussions (19). This makes the sort of open and direct end-of-life discussions that bioethicists generally favor negatively valued in Navajo culture. Similarly, Mei-che Pang, although condemning the practice, notes that Chinese medical professionals have strong cultural support for their practice of not telling bad news to patients (20).

The cultural specificity of informed consent has two important implications. First, the effort to apply the doctrine in different societies other than those immediately derivative of American, and perhaps some European cultures, may well generate unsatisfactory or even counterproductive results. Second, even in the European and American contexts, healthcare professionals often find themselves treating patients whose cultural orientation comes from Asian, Middle Eastern, or Latin American societies for whom the concept of informed consent may be somewhat bewildering. Although encouraging such patients' participation in the decisionmaking process is part of their socialization into American culture, full patient participation will be difficult to achieve. Moreover, fully respecting the autonomy of these individuals dictates respecting their cultural values.

Divergent Frameworks of Significance

This book we have emphasizes that informed consent is a means of promoting autonomy. However, it is not necessarily the case that any time individuals are given the right to make a choice and the information with which to do it, their autonomy is enhanced. If the patient's and physician's ways of looking at and understanding the situation are not roughly congruent, the disclosure process may undermine rather than enhance the individual's sense and exercise of autonomy. We consider two situations below.

Gail Geller and colleagues recently reported on focus groups they conducted with women about genetic testing for breast cancer susceptibility (21). The discussions concerned whether or not the women would like such genetic information and what roles they would like their physicians to play in their decisions. The study found several different ways in which the women's background beliefs and understandings differed substantially from those that are usually taken for granted by medical professionals.

First, subjects had idiosyncratic beliefs about causation of breast cancer even before they talked with their physicians. In particular, "[s]ome women thought that 'breast cancer was caused by wearing saggy bras.' Others thought it was caused by being 'hit in the breast.' Rather than understanding growths in the body as expressions of the cancer, the understanding is that to have any sort of lump in the body, including welts from a violent assault, is to have cancer" (22, pp. 28–29).

Second, patients reported fatalistic or superstitious beliefs about cancer. Fatalists "believe that the diseases that befall them, and the timing of their death, are foreordained. Therefore, the individual has no control over whether . . . she will develop cancer. By contrast, some people believe that their thoughts and behaviors directly influence what happens to them: talking about bad things such as cancer might precipitate their onset. If they 'go looking for trouble,' God might punish them by giving them cancer" (21, p. 29).

Patients also often focus on personal experiences, stories of friends and acquaintances rather than statistical or other scientific evidence (21). For example, Geller and colleagues had a subject who reported, "It is my mother's side of the family that has breast cancer and I take after my father's side, I don't need to worry." Another subject whose mother died from breast cancer was convinced that she too would get it and was planning to get a prophylactic mastectomy whether or not her genetic tests showed increased susceptibility (21).

The point is not that the women in these examples are stupid or incapable of understanding what is going on. Nor is it that we cannot improve their understanding. The critical issue is that simply presenting a standardized body of information that is deemed "material" and giving them a choice will not lead to what most healthcare professionals would deem to be a decision based on rational reasons.

There are, however, other problems concerning divergent senses of meaning. Consider the case of alternative medicine and whether physicians and other conventional healthcare professionals ought to provide patients with information about alternative medical treatments. A large and growing portion of the public makes use of some form of "alternative health care"; thus, many people presumably believe that such care should be among the choices they can make. Whatever conventional healthcare professionals may think of chiropractic treatments or St. John's Wort, many competent people regularly choose to avail themselves of these therapies. However, if one believes that the essence of informed consent is an open honest dialogue, it is difficult to suggest to medical professionals that they need to present "all" of the alternatives, including those they believe to be ineffective or possibly harmful.

On the surface, it might appear that there is a simple answer to this problem. Physicians should be required to provide information about alternative treatments for which there is substantial empirical evidence of their effectiveness for the condition from which the patient suffers. Unfortunately, this requires a much higher standard for disclosure with respect to alternative medicine treatments than is required of conventional medicine, since physicians often recommend treatments that have no clear scientific evidence of effectiveness. Moreover, many practitioners of alternative medicines would argue, with some justification, that the research practices for assessing effectiveness are structured in such a way as to assure their failure even when their treatments work in everyday situations, since blinded trials remove the mental element that is so important in many alternate therapies. On the other hand, should physicians trained in scientific medicine really be required to describe neutrally alternatives that involve, in their terms, quackery? For example, should scientifically trained physicians be required to present, as a serious alternative, treatments that seek to adjust the balance of *chi* in the body?

Without trying to resolve the ethical question here, we would like to note that medicine, like other sciences, is based on theoretical assumptions and does not consist of simple bodies of evidence. A largely consistent theoretical framework underlies the modern practice of medicine. Thomas Kuhn (23) and other historians and philosophers of science have found repeatedly that science does not consist simply of accumulations of evidence. One way of viewing the current growth of alternative medicine is that it presents a variety of challenges to the dominant medical paradigm. It seems difficult to expect that physicians, who typically have made a major intellectual and emotional commitment to the medical paradigm, should engage in informed consent, as an aspect of medical practice, independently of the paradigm that the rest of medicine is based on. From the point of view of the average physician, to treat homeopathy as an appropriate alternative to penicillin is not simply an issue of what works; it would involve lying to the patient.

What these two examples (beliefs about breast cancer and alternative medicine) share, although they differ in many ways, is an absence of a common framework of meaning. Although in the first case patients were presented with options that made no real sense to them, and in the second case physicians find themselves caught in an intellectual, emotional, and moral bind if they disclose particular alternatives, the basic problem is the same. In both cases, disjunctive interpretative frameworks make the informed consent process stressful to one of the participants.

Emotional and Cognitive Preconceptions

One of the most widely accepted goals for informed consent is to promote more informed healthcare decisions in accordance with patients' values. This is the primary reason why information disclosure is required. We expect that the information will facilitate a rational decisionmaking process. Certainly the general proposition is true. One is more likely to make a rational decision the more accurate and complete the information that one has (24).

The provision of information is, for at least two reasons, hardly a universal guarantee of a rational decisionmaking process. First, information is absorbed

into already established structures of cognitive knowledge. We all have precon-
ceptions about situations that help us to understand what we learn from our environment. Indeed, as the work of the great developmental psychologist Jean
Piaget has shown, this is even true of newborn infants who process information
about their environment by assimilating it to inborn instinctual responses such as
sucking. As humans grow, their basic schemas for organizing new information
become increasingly rich and complex. Although such cognitive structures are
essential, they are far from infallible. Indeed, this is one of the main difficulties
that we have in understanding the information that others convey to us.

Perhaps the best example of this is the "therapeutic misconception" about research that we discussed in Chapter 13. Research subjects go into their physicians' offices expecting that they are going to get medical care. They assume that
the physician is primarily concerned with providing them the best possible treatment. Physicians who, regardless of their commitment to research, are inclined to
see caring for their patients as their first priority, often do not make the distinction
between research and treatment with their patients. The result is that patient-
subjects assimilate the information that they receive during disclosure into their
expectations as patients. Thus, we find subjects with end stage cancer going into
phase I protocols—whose goal is to assess the maximum level of a particular
anticancer drug that can be safely tolerated—believing that this is primarily a
therapeutic intervention. This misconception is demonstrated by the following interaction involving such a subject:

> SUBJECT: I had a bilateral mastectomy and I'm going through this. In my eyes it is
> preventative and I am going to live to be ninety-five. . . .
>
> INTERVIEWER: What does the project involve?
>
> SUBJECT: A stem cell transplant receiving high doses of chemo. And taking out my
> stem cells and then putting them back in once I have received the chemo which will
> destroy any teenie-weenie little minute chance of there being cancer.

A second problem is the fact that information disclosure is not only a cognitive
transaction but also a socioemotional one. We have already discussed this as a
positive aspect of the relationship. Providing information in a helpful manner can
become one way in which trust and confidence between healthcare provider and
patient can be increased. However, rational decisions by the patient do not always
result from this interaction.

Loren Roth, one of the early advocates for informed consent within psychiatry,
is fond of telling about his efforts to use informed consent when doing forensic
evaluations of prisoners concerning their competence to stand trial and their
criminal responsibility. As a representative of the court, he was obliged to report
on what he was told by the individuals whom he was evaluating. This often left

him in a position of acting against the best interests of these prisoners (since the information could be used in the criminal trial). As a way of minimizing this conflict (and in keeping with the ethics of forensic psychiatry) he decided to discuss in great detail with the prisoners whom he was evaluating his role as a representative of the court and their need to be extremely careful about what information they divulged to him.

The result was exactly the opposite of what he expected. The prisoners apparently assumed that anyone who would be so open and honest must be a very trustworthy doctor. The indirect result was that they told him much more than they might have otherwise and he had to discontinue the practice. In this case, and perhaps others, the socioemotional effects of full disclosure are not necessarily positive. They did not lead the patient to pursue rationally his own interests but, on the contrary, put him at risk in a way that he would not have been precisely because of the disclosure.

Conclusion

Anyone who has ever had a bacterial infection knows that antibiotics are appropriately called "wonder drugs." However, as we have learned repeatedly, they do no good and, eventually, do much harm when given for viral infections. So, too, is the situation with informed consent. Although it may be overstating the case to call informed consent a wonder drug for the physician–patient relationship, it has great potential for improvement of many aspects of health care. Like antibiotics, however, informed consent is not the best approach to solving all of the problems of health care. In this chapter we have tried to outline some of the situations in which informed consent may not live up to the expectations we have for it. Informed consent is no different from anything else in having limits. Recognizing these limits does not suggest any lessening of the general value of informed consent.

References

1. Glass, E. (1970) Note: Restructuring informed consent: legal therapy for the doctor-patient relationship. *Yale Law Journal,* 79:1572–1576.
2. Brennan, T. (1991) *Just Doctoring: Medical Ethics in the Liberal State.* Berkeley: University of California Press.
3. Fisher, S. (1986) *In the Patient's Best Interest: Women and the Politics of Medical Decisions.* New Brunswick, NJ: Rutgers University Press.
4. Szasz, T. (1963) *Law, Liberty and Psychiatry.* New York: MacMillan.
5. Kaplan, R. M. (1991) Health-related quality of life in patient decision making. *J Social Issues,* 47:69–70.

6. Greenfield, S., Kaplan, S., and Ware, J. (1985) Expanding patient involvement in care: effects on patient outcomes. *Ann Intern Med,* 120:520–524.

7. Collopy, B. (1988) Autonomy in long term care: some crucial distinctions. *Gerontologist,* 28 (supplement):10–17.

8. Meisel, A. (1977) The expansion of liability for medical accidents: from negligence to strict liability by way of informed consent. *Nebraska Law Review,* 56: 51–152.

9. Hofland, B. (1988) Autonomy in long term care: background issues and a programmatic response. *Gerontologist,* 28 (supplement):3–9.

10. Gamroth, L., Semradek, J., and Tornquist, E. (eds) (1995) *Enhancing Autonomy in Long Term Care: Concepts and Strategies.* New York: Springer.

11. Ambrogi, D. and Leonard, F. (1988) The impact of nursing home admission agreements on resident autonomy. *Gerontologist,* 28 (supplement):82–89.

12. Goffman, E. (1961) *Asylums: Essays on the Social Situation of Mental Patients and Other Inmates.* Garden City, NJ: Anchor Books.

13. Macklin, R. (1999) *Against Relativism: Cultural Diversity and the Search for Ethical Universals in Medicine.* New York: Oxford University Press.

14. Gostin, L.O. (1995) Informed consent, cultural sensitivity, and respect for persons. *JAMA,* 254:844–845.

15. Olatawura, M. (2000) Ethics in sub-Saharan Africa. In: Osasha, A. M., Arboleda-Florez, J., and Sartorius, N. (eds) *Ethics, Culture and Society.* Washington, D.C.: American Psychiatric Press, 103–108.

16. Okasha, A. (2000) Impact of Arab culture on psychiatric ethics. In: Osasha, A. M., Arboleda-Florez, J., and Sartorius, N. (eds) *Ethics, Culture and Society.* Washington, D.C.: American Psychiatric Press, 15–28.

17. Sabogal, F., Marín, G., Otero-Sabogal, R., VanOss Marín, B., and Perez-Stable, E.J. (1987) Hispanic familism and acculturation: what changes and what doesn't. *Hispanic J Behav Sci,* 9:397–412.

18. Blackhall, L.J., Murphy, S.T., Frank, G., Michel, V., and Azen, S. (1995) Ethnicity and attitudes toward patient autonomy. *JAMA,* 274:820–826.

19. Carrese, J. and Rhodes, L.A. (1995) Western bioethics on the Navajo reservation: benefit or harm. *JAMA,* 274:826–829.

20. Pang, M.S. (1999) Protective truthfulness: the Chinese way of safeguarding patients in informed treatment decisions. *J Med Ethics,* 25:247–253.

21. Geller, G., Strauss, M., Bernhardt, B.A., and Holtzman, N. (1997) "Decoding" Informed consent: insights regarding breast cancer susceptibility testing. *Hastings Cent Rep,* 27:28–33.

22. Kahneman, D., Slovic, P., and Tversky, A. (eds) (1982) *Judgment Under Uncertainty: Heuristics and Biases.* New York: Cambridge University Press.

23. Kuhn, T. (1970) *The Structure of Scientific Revolution.* Chicago: University of Chicago Press.

24. Janis, I. and Mann, L. (1977) *Decision Making: A Psychosocial Analysis of Conflict, Choice and Commitment.* New York: Free Press.

15

An Agenda for the Future

The cornerstone of our approach to informed consent is the belief that the right of patients to authorize their own medical treatment, usually called the right to autonomy in decision making, is a moral value worth promoting. When medical care is required, patients should be met by physicians' openness and willingness to present and discuss a variety of options, with the clear understanding that patients can play a role, if they desire, in shaping the ultimate decision. Our instinctive assumption that most patients would endorse this approach was confirmed by a large-scale study sponsored by the President's Commission (1). Patients do want to know about and have the option of influencing the nature of their medical care, even if they may not always exercise that option (2). Our society's deep-seated traditions of respect for the integrity of the individual reinforce the importance of protecting patients' interests in the medical decisionmaking process.

Legal initiatives by themselves are insufficient to accomplish these results (see Chapter 7). Endless proposals to refine the legal mechanisms by which the doctrine of informed consent is enforced are not likely to achieve their goals. The legal rules governing informed consent operate at a level of generality that makes it difficult for physicians to take them into account in dealing with patients. Some surveys have found that physicians are completely ignorant of the operative standard for disclosure in their state (1), and others have found that even when physicians are aware of the standard, they do not apply it properly (3).

More significantly, however, the medical setting seems relatively impervious to regulation in this area. Physicians and administrators have control over the structure of medical care and over the content of physician–patient interactions. Regardless of the law of informed consent, if the structure of hospital and office practice provides negligible opportunities for doctor–patient communication, little disclosure or shared decision making will occur. If physicians are resistant to the moral imperatives of informed consent, tinkering with standards of disclosure is unlikely to affect their behavior. Physicians, other healthcare personnel, and their attorneys are sufficiently imaginative and in control of the situation to devise means of defeating the intent of most legal regulation, perhaps even masking their response as mechanical compliance with its mandates. For example, although Congress enacted the Patient Self-Determination Act in order to ensure that all patients receive information about their rights to make medical decisions under state law, it has failed to result in significant differences in the number of patients who complete advance care documents (4).

For more than four decades legal stratagems have been employed to compel physicians, and now other healthcare professionals, to respect their patients as persons with the right to know about and help shape their medical care. Although some changes have occurred in doctor–patient interactions, we believe that in the long run attempts to force people to respect others are doomed to failure. One can create a framework in which respect can develop. One can even compel behavior similar to what would occur were respect to exist. But respect is so personal a characteristic that it either flows from a genuine source, or not at all. In essence, this is the paradox in which the law of informed consent has been caught. The legal requirements have gone as far as they can. The framework for respect has been created, and codes of behavior have been prescribed. And that has not been enough.

We do not believe that the legal requirements for informed consent should be dismantled, nor that they should be materially revised. Such action could not but be interpreted by physicians and other caregivers as a signal that informed consent is no longer to be taken seriously. But for further progress we must look elsewhere. Even granting the unlikely assumption that elements of physicians' overt behavior could be controlled by law, it is clear that attitudinal change must be accomplished by different means. Physicians must come to endorse the values underlying informed consent before they will behave accordingly.

A change in attitudes can only be brought about by systematic efforts to educate physicians. A two-pronged approach will be required. First, physicians should be exposed to the ethical principles behind the idea of informed consent, so they can come to understand and, most important, internalize them. Second, physicians must be persuaded that a model for the implementation of informed consent exists that does not compromise, but actually enhances, the physician–patient relationship and the delivery of medical care. Physicians must come to believe that the interests of autonomy and health can be reconciled in a manner that does not do unacceptable damage to the latter. This book conceptualizes and delineates such a model, which we term the process model of informed consent. The question remains how both the values and the model can be communicated to physicians.

As a first step, students in medical and other health professional schools must be taught to recognize that each party brings unique attributes and capacities to bear on medical decision making. Patients' contributions to the process are not inferior to those of physicians, but merely different in kind, and of irreplaceable importance, insofar as they best embody patients' systems of values, knowledge of their life situations, and experience of their illness. Students must learn about the ethical foundation of (patient) autonomy. Their anxiety about performing as clinicians, along with their nascent sense of professional identity, may make it difficult for them to accept the need to share information and decision making with patients. Students should be encouraged to place themselves in the position of patients, a role that is still more familiar to them than that of clinicians. They will also need to review the legal foundations of the patient–physician relationship, along with the clinical principles—now taught in many medical schools—on which effective physician–patient interaction rests.

Others before us have emphasized the importance, in achieving the goals of informed consent, of such education (5,6). Recommendations for model curricula in medical ethics and law have embraced these approaches (7,8), and they have begun to be implemented (9,10). But there is a great deal of work toward this end still to be done.

Discussions of informed consent issues in the preclinical or classroom years are of use but must be supplemented by hands-on training in the process model during clinical rotations. Students should be taught how to communicate information, facilitate patient participation, and handle questions of impaired competence and voluntariness. They should receive feedback on their performance in this area, just as in other aspects of delivering medical care. A number of medical schools are using simulated patient encounters for this purpose.

Many medical and other health professional schools have begun to revise their curricula in keeping with these ideas. Some have not. But it would be an enormous error to believe that efforts restricted to the years of formal schooling will be sufficient to change the attitudes of health professionals. Instruction at this level merely sets the stage for more crucial intervention later on. The initial years of functioning with responsibility in a clinical setting—for physicians, the years of residency—have the most powerful influence on enduring patterns of professional behavior. It is during these years that physicians really learn how to interact with patients. They model their behavior on that of their seniors and supervisors, and they experiment with a variety of approaches on their own. The benefits of years of excellent medical school instruction can be lost in a few months if residents' early steps in the right direction are not properly reinforced. Yet residency programs actually give less emphasis to ethical issues in health care than medical schools (11).

Currently, physicians in residency training too frequently learn from what they see around them that informed consent is a nuisance, an alien imposition of the legal system that must be tolerated because of possible legal consequences, but that can be dealt with in relatively mechanical ways, such as making sure patients sign consent forms before major procedures. They learn that patients must be listened to early in the evaluation process because they may be an important source of valuable diagnostic information, but that once the physician has made a diagnosis and decided on a plan of action, the patient's role goes no further than pro forma ratification of the physician's choice. They are taught by example that a system of medical care that minimizes doctor–patient interaction is acceptable, and that given economic pressures (e.g., demands for increased productivity as a result of reductions in payment by managed care organizations and the government), such minimization may even be desirable.

There is no hope for informed consent as an ethical doctrine or even as a meaningful set of legal rules unless this situation changes. Formal requirements for teaching about informed consent, which we now incorporate into residency accreditation guidelines in many specialties, are only a starting point. During residency training (and equivalent periods for non-physician health-care personnel), physicians must be taught that patients have a legitimate and important role to play in shaping decisions about their care, and that this role can be fulfilled in a reasonable manner. This teaching can only be accomplished by a combination of direct instruction and indirect modeling both of the importance of these attitudes and of the behavior that facilitates patients' playing this role. Innovative models of this sort are beginning to be developed (12,13). Since relatively few physicians today incorporate such an approach in their own practices, a small cadre of teachers will have to train a larger group of instructors for this purpose. At first, time for teaching this approach will need to be set aside, despite the already heavy time pressures on residents. As graduates of the initial years of teaching themselves assume supervisory roles, greater reliance could be placed on having residents model their supervisors' behavior, with formal didactic sessions taking a subordinate role.

One should not, of course, write off the physicians in practice today, who will be determining the shape of our medical care for many years to come. Remedial programs (though physicians might understandably resist such a designation) for physicians who have never been exposed to the idea of a collaborative approach to the doctor–patient relationship should be organized. It is likely, as well, that when older physicians are exposed to the new ideas and practices their juniors have learned (assuming the success of the other levels of training), their behavior will begin to change. Nonetheless, the difficulty of altering established patterns of interaction should not be underestimated. The primary emphasis must be on ensuring that another generation of physicians and other health-care personnel does not perpetuate the current unsatisfactory situation.

What are we likely to gain from an effort to improve the training of clinicians in regard to informed consent, considering the time, money (14), and energy it will cost? To be realistic, our expectations must be somewhat circumscribed. We consider utopian the idea that all patients could fully understand the risks, benefits, and alternatives recommended by their physicians. It is clear that not all patients, or even a substantial majority, will want to make their decisions about their medical care single-handedly—even if they could do so (2). Many patients may not want to participate in the decision-making process at all. How many decisions will be made differently is admittedly unclear.

None of these conclusions negate, in our eyes, the value of encouraging physicians to conform to the model of doctor–patient interactions and the process of medical decision making described in this book. The value is less that it will alter the outcome of the decisionmaking process than that it will change the nature of the process itself. Patients will be treated with the respect they deserve as autonomous individuals. To the extent that they make the effort to comprehend the information provided (and, of course, reasonable attempts should be made to ensure that the information is inherently comprehensible) and wish to participate, they will have the opportunity to do so. Even if they do not make the effort to grasp all of the data and their implications, or if they willingly cede decisionmaking authority to their physicians, they will still be treated as if the right to do otherwise is theirs, which in fact it is.

Not only do we believe that there are good reasons for promoting patients' rights in this area, but the realities of medical care in the electronic age provide further impetus for change. Patients have greater access to medical information than ever before—through the Internet, as well as through direct-to-consumer advertising of pharmaceuticals. It is becoming more common for a patient to enter a physician's office seeking a particular treatment, armed with a variety of information (including misinformation), rather than simply seeking a diagnosis. Moreover, new electronic communication media, such as e-mail, provide cost-effective and efficient ways to interact with physicians. Sometimes dubbed "the information age," the current era of medical care will challenge physician–patient interactions and subsequently change the face of informed consent (15).

The effects of widespread use of a process model of medical decision making, as described in this book, are unpredictable, but let us speculate on just how far-reaching they could become. When people are treated differently, they begin to respond differently. Patients who are treated as respected partners in medical care may begin to behave with a new level of responsibility. They may take more initiative to maintain their own health, comply with agreed-on regimens, and provide important information to their physicians. As active decision makers rather than passive recipients of care, they may acknowledge that they deserve partial credit for good results, but also partial blame for results that turn out poorly. A lessening of the tendency to blame physicians for adverse outcomes may reduce the desire to seek legal remedies through the malpractice system. A greater recognition of the degree of uncertainty in medical treatment, which can be expected to flow from a discussion of alternative courses of treatment, may also have the same effect.

The positive side effects of the model we have presented are, of course, largely speculative. Yet they may serve as a counterweight to the speculative disadvantages commonly given credence in medical circles: increased numbers of refusals of needed treatment, heightened anxiety among patients, and, above all, wasteful use of precious medical time. Even if the putative advantages were not to materialize, however, we would still urge adoption of our model. Informed consent—and by that we refer both to the idea of informed consent and the resulting legal requirements—is important because it ratifies and protects the autonomy of the individual patient. For us, and by now we hope for the reader of this book, that is justification enough.

References

1. Harris, L., et al. (1982) Views of informed consent and decisionmaking: parallel surveys of physicians and the public. In President's Commission for the Study of Ethical Problems in Medicine and Biomedical and Behavioral Research, *Making Health Care Decision: The Ethical and Legal Implications of Informed Consent in the Patient-Practitioner Relationship*. Volume 2, Appendices. Washington, D.C.: U.S. Government Printing Office.
2. Schneider, C.E. (1998) *The Practice of Autonomy: Patients, Doctors, and Medical Decisions*. New York: Oxford University Press.
3. Markson, L., Kern, D., Annas, G., and Glantz, L.H. (1994) Physician assessment of patient competence. *J Am Geriatr Soc*, 42:1074–1080.
4. Larson, E.J. and Eaton, T.A. (1997) The limits of advance directives: a history and assessment of the Patient Self-Determination Act. *Wake Forest Law Review*, 32:249–293.
5. President's Commission for the Study of Ethical Problems in Medicine and Biomedical and Behavioral Research (1982) *Making Health Care Decisions: The Ethical and Legal Implications of the Patient-Practitioner Relationship*. Volume 1, Report. Washington, D.C.: U.S. Government Printing Office.
6. Katz, J. (1984) *The Silent World of Doctor and Patient*. New York: Free Press.
7. Culver, C.M., Clouser, K.D., Gert, B., et al. (1985) Basic curricula goals in medical ethics. *N Engl J Med*, 312:253–256.
8. Gillon, R. (1996) Thinking about a medical school core curriculum for medical ethics and law. *J Med Ethics*, 22:323–324.

9. Walker, R.M., Lane, L.W., and Siegler, M. (1989) Development of a teaching program in clinical medical ethics at the University of Chicago. *Acad Med*, 64:723–729.

10. Carter, B.S., Roberts, A., Martin, R., and Fincher, R.M. (1999) A longitudinal ethics curriculum for medical students and generalist residents at the Medical College of Georgia. *Acad Med*, 74(Suppl):5102–5103.

11. Osborn, E.H., Lancaster, C., Bellack, J.P., O'Neil, E., and Graber, D.R. (1999) Differences in curriculum emphasis in U.S. undergraduate and generalist residency education programmes. *Med Educ*, 33:921–925.

12. Silverman, H.J. (1999) Description of an ethics curriculum for a medicine residency program. *West J Med*, 170:218–231.

13. Diekema, D.S. and Shugerman, R.P. (1997) An ethics curriculum for the pediatric residency program: confronting barriers to implementation. *Arch Pediatr Adolesc Med*, 151:609–614.

14. Teno, J.M. (2000) Advance directives for nursing home residents: achieving compassionate, competent, cost-effective care. *JAMA*, 283:1481–1482.

15. Miller, F. (1998) Health care information technology and informed consent: computers and the doctor-patient relationship. *Indiana Law Review*, 31:1019–1042.

Index